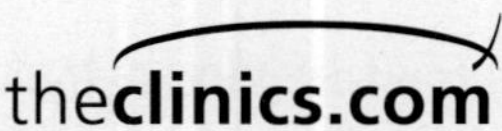

NEUROSURGERY CLINICS OF NORTH AMERICA

Intraoperative MRI Developments

GUEST EDITORS
Christopher Nimsky, MD
Rudolf Fahlbusch, MD

CONSULTING EDITORS
Andrew T. Parsa, MD, PhD
Paul C. McCormick, MD, MPH

January 2005 • Volume 16 • Number 1

SAUNDERS
An Imprint of Elsevier, Inc.
PHILADELPHIA LONDON TORONTO MONTREAL SYDNEY TOKYO

W.B. SAUNDERS COMPANY
A Division of Elsevier Inc.

The Curtis Center • Independence Square West • Philadelphia, Pennsylvania 19106

http://www.theclinics.com

NEUROSURGERY CLINICS OF NORTH AMERICA **Volume 16, Number 1**
January 2005 **ISSN 1042-3680**
Editor: Molly Jay

Neurosurgery Clinics of North America (ISSN 1042-3680) is published quarterly by Elsevier Inc. Corporate and editorial offices: 170 S Independence Mall W 300 E, Philadelphia, PA 19106-3399. Accounting and circulation offices: 6277 Sea Harbor Drive, Orlando, FL 32887-4800. Periodicals postage paid at Orlando, FL 32862, and additional mailing offices. Subscription prices are $205.00 per year (US individuals), $315.00 per year (US institutions), $225.00 per year (Canadian individuals), $380.00 per year (Canadian institutions), $265.00 per year (international individuals), $380.00 per year (international institutions), $133.00 per year (US students), and $133.00 per year (international students). International air speed delivery is included in all *Clinics* subscription prices. All prices are subject to change without notice. POSTMASTER: Send address changes to *Neurosurgery Clinics of North America*, W.B. Saunders Company, Periodicals Fulfillment, Orlando, FL 32887-4800. **Customer Service: 1-800-654-2452 (US). From outside of the US, call 1-407-345-4000.** E-mail: hhspcs@harcourt.com.

Neurosurgery Clinics of North America is covered in *Index Medicus*, *EMBASE/Excerpta Medica*, and *Current Contents/Clinical Medicine (CC/CM)*.

Printed in the United States of America.

CONSULTING EDITORS

PAUL C. MCCORMICK, MD, MPH, Professor, Department of Clinical Neurosurgery, Columbia University College of Physicians and Surgeons, New York, New York

ANDREW T. PARSA, MD, PhD, Assistant Professor, Department of Neurological Surgery, Neurospinal Research Center and The Brain Tumor Research Center, University of California San Francisco, San Francisco, California

GUEST EDITORS

RUDOLF FAHLBUSCH, MD, Department of Neurosurgery, University Erlangen-Nuremberg, Erlangen, Germany

CHRISTOPHER NIMSKY, MD, Department of Neurosurgery, University Erlangen-Nuremberg, Erlangen, Germany

CONTRIBUTORS

HERMANN ACKERMANN, MD, MA, Department of Neurology, University of Tübingen, Tüebingen, Germany

PETER M. BLACK, MD, PhD, Neurosurgeon-in-Chief, Department of Neurosurgery, Brigham and Women's Hospital, Harvard Medical School, Boston, Massachusetts

ROBERT J. BOHINSKI, MD, PhD, Assistant Professor, Department of Neurosurgery, University of Cincinnati College of Medicine, Cincinnati, Ohio

PETER W. CARMEL, MD, DMSc, Professor and Chairman, Department of Neurological Surgery, New Jersey Medical School, Newark, New Jersey

JEFFREY CATRAMBONE, MD, Assistant Professor, Department of Neurological Surgery, New Jersey Medical School, Newark, New Jersey

L. CELSO HYGINO CRUZ, Jr, MD, Clínica de Diagnóstico por Imagem, Multi-ImagemRessonância Magnética, Rio de Janeiro, Brazil

BORIMIR J. DARAKCHIEV, MD, Department of Neurosurgery, University of Cincinnati College of Medicine, Cincinnati, Ohio

RUDOLF FAHLBUSCH, MD, Department of Neurosurgery, University Erlangen-Nuremberg, Erlangen, Germany

OLIVER GANSLANDT, MD, Department of Neurosurgery, University Erlangen-Nuremberg, Erlangen, Germany

BRIGITTE GATTERBAUER, MD, Department of Neurosurgery, Medical University of Vienna, Vienna, Austria

WENDELL A. GIBBY, MD, Director, Riverwoods Imaging Center, Provo, Utah

WOLFGANG GRODD, MD, Professor, Section on Experimental Magnetic Resonance of Central Nervous System, Department of Neuroradiology, University of Tübingen, Tüebingen, Germany

STEPHEN GRUBER, PhD, Magnetic Resonance Centre of Excellence, and Department of Medical Physics, Medical University of Vienna, Vienna, Austria

WALTER J. HADER, MD, Assistant Professor, Division of Neurosurgery, Department of Clinical Neurosciences, University of Calgary, Calgary, Alberta, Canada

WALTER A. HALL, MD, Professor, Departments of Neurosurgery, Radiation Oncology, and Radiology, University of Minnesota Medical School, Minneapolis, Minnesota

ERNST HÜLSMANN, MD, Section on Experimental Magnetic Resonance of Central Nervous System, Department of Neuroradiology, University of Tübingen, Tüebingen, Germany

FERENC A. JOLESZ, MD, B. Leonard Holman Professor of Radiology, Vice Chairman for Research, Director, Division of MRI and Image Guided Therapy Program, Department of Radiology, Brigham and Women's Hospital, Harvard Medical School, Boston Massachusetts

JOHN J. KELLY, MD, Senior Neurosurgical Resident, Division of Neurosurgery, Department of Clinical Neurosciences, University of Calgary, Calgary, Alberta, Canada

FRITHJOF KRUGGEL, MD, Max-Planck-Institute for Human Cognitive and Brain Sciences, Leipzig, Germany

HEIKO LIPPMANN, PD, Max-Planck-Institute for Human Cognitive and Brain Sciences, Leipzig, Germany

VLADIMIR MLYNARIK, PhD, Magnetic Resonance Centre of Excellence, Medical University of Vienna, Vienna, Austria

EWALD MOSER, PhD, Scientific Director, Magnetic Resonance Centre of Excellence; Professor, Department of Medical Physics, and Department of Radiodiagnostics, Medical University of Vienna, Vienna, Austria

S. TERRY MYLES, MD, Professor, Division of Neurosurgery, Department of Clinical Neurosciences, University of Calgary, Calgary, Alberta, Canada

CHRISTOPHER NIMSKY, MD, Department of Neurosurgery, University Erlangen-Nuremberg, Erlangen, Germany

DENNIS S. OH, MD, Clinical Scientist and Fellow, Department of Neurosurgical Oncology, Brigham and Women's Hospital, Harvard Medical School, Boston, Massachusetts

KARL ROESSLER, MD, Department of Neurosurgery, Medical University of Vienna, Vienna, Austria

MICHAEL SCHULDER, MD, Associate Professor and Vice Chairman, Department of Neurological Surgery, New Jersey Medical School, Newark, New Jersey

A. GREGORY SORENSEN, MD, Co-Director, Athinoula A. Martinos Center for Biomedical Imaging, Department of Radiology, Massachusetts General Hospital, Boston; and Division of Health Sciences and Technology, Harvard-MIT, Boston, Massachusetts

ANDREAS STADLBAUER, PhD, Magnetic Resonance Centre of Excellence, and Department of Medical Physics, Medical University of Vienna, Vienna, Austria

GARNETTE R. SUTHERLAND, MD, Professor, Director, Seaman Family MR Research Centre, Division of Neurosurgery, Department of Clinical Neurosciences, University of Calgary, Calgary, Alberta, Canada

JOHN M. TEW, Jr, MD, Professor, Department of Neurosurgery, University of Cincinnati College of Medicine, Cincinnati, Ohio; and Mayfield Clinic, Cincinnati, Ohio

CHARLES L. TRUWIT, MD, Professor, Departments of Neurosurgery, Radiation Oncology, and Radiology, University of Minnesota Medical School, Minneapolis, Minnesota

RONALD E. WARNICK, MD, Professor, Department of Neurosurgery, The Neuroscience Institute, University of Cincinnati College of Medicine, Cincinnati; and Mayfield Clinic, Cincinnati, Ohio

CONTENTS

FORTHCOMING ISSUES

April 2005

Neuroendovascular Surgery: Techniques, Indications, and Patient Selection
Elad I. Levy, MD,
Lee R. Guterman, MD, PhD, and
L. Nelson Hopkins, MD, *Guest Editors*

July 2005

Intervential Neuroradiology
Arun Paul Amar, MD, and Sean Lavine, MD
Guest Editors

October 2005

Motion Sparing Surgery
Dean Chou, MD, and
Christopher Ames, MD, *Guest Editors*

RECENT ISSUES

April 2004

Peripheral Nerve Tumors: Diagnosis and Management
Eric L. Zager, MD, and Jason H. Huang, MD
Guest Editors

July 2004

Pain Treatment
Gary Heit, MD, PhD, *Guest Editor*

October 2004

Metastatic Spine Disease
Meic H. Schmidt, MD,
Daryl R. Fourney, MD, FRCSC, and
Ziya L. Gokaslan, MD, FACS, *Guest Editors*

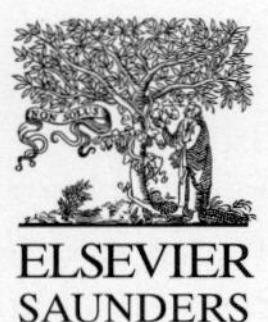

ELSEVIER
SAUNDERS

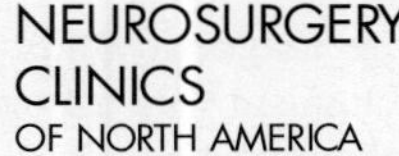

NEUROSURGERY CLINICS OF NORTH AMERICA

Neurosurg Clin N Am 16 (2005) xi–xiii

Preface

Intraoperative MRI Developments

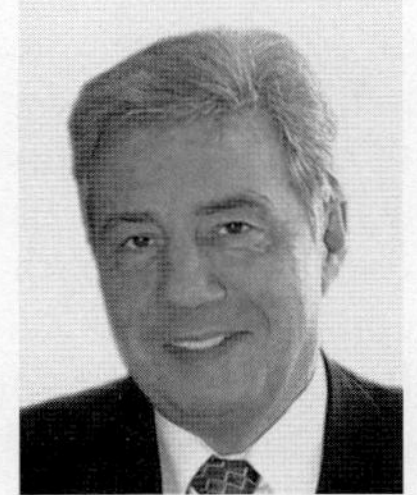

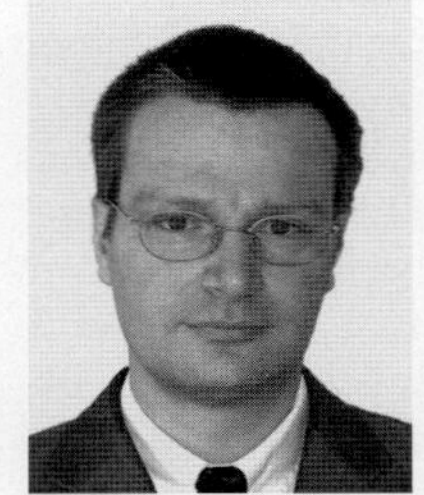

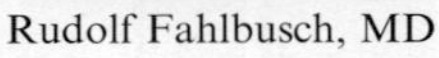

Rudolf Fahlbusch, MD Christopher Nimsky, MD
Guest Editors

MRI has become a routine pre- and postoperative imaging modality in the treatment of brain tumors and epilepsy. In the last 20 years, significant progress in scanning technology has resulted in high-resolution three-dimensional anatomic imaging of the brain. In addition to anatomic imaging, information on function and metabolism in the individual patient is available. Since the mid-1990s, even the intraoperative application of MRI has been possible and has opened new avenues in immediate intraoperative quality control.

In this issue of *Neurosurgery Clinics of North America*, we focus on current MRI developments with an impact on intraoperative use in neurosurgery and on the intraoperative application of MRI technology. This issue compiles the contributions from a variety of experts in their respective specialties.

In the first part, a general overview of MRI techniques is followed by focusing on current developments with a distinct impact on intraoperative application, ranging from functional imaging with fMRI, to investigation of metabolism with magnetic resonance spectroscopy, to diffusion tensor imaging.

In the second part, a comprehensive and state-of-the art overview of the intraoperative application of MRI technology is provided. Experts using different low-, middle-, and high-field MRI systems available from 0.12 to 1.5 T focus on different aspects, such as integration of navigation, glioma resection, pituitary adenomas, biopsies, epilepsy, and functional imaging, followed by a perspective outlook.

With the development of open MRI systems in the mid-1990s, the concept of intraoperative imaging, up to then only realized with CT and ultrasound, experienced a renaissance. The first designs were based on low-field magnets, with magnetic field strengths up to 0.5 T. The use of MRI scanners in the operating environment for nearly 10 years has proved to be safe and reliable as well as applicable to neurosurgical procedures, even if these procedures have to be adapted to the MRI environment to a certain extent. Nevertheless, the optimal solution for intraoperative imaging setups, combining excellent image quality with smooth operating room work flow integration and ergonomic comfort for the neurosurgeon, still does not exist. All installed systems are prototypes with certain drawbacks. There are different concepts with respect to scanner and operating room design; intraoperative imaging necessitates operating directly in a scanner with the drawback of restricted space for the surgeon or some kind of intraoperative transport of the patient or the scanner itself. There are different operating table concepts, ranging from patient transport with an air-cushioned operating room table to an adjacent operating room, to movement of the patient along the longitudinal axis of the scanner to reach the

1042-3680/05/$ - see front matter
doi:10.1016/j.nec.2004.07.012

fringe magnetic fields, to the use of some rotating mechanism with an operating room table adapted to the scanner. Also, the issues of MRI-compatible head fixation and coil design for intraoperative use have not yet been resolved without drawbacks. Regarding the overall operating room design, there are also different concepts, ranging from systems dedicated for intraoperative use only to hybrid systems combining intraoperative use with the application of the scanner for routine radiologic diagnostics.

To date, there is also no definite consensus as to which direction intraoperative MRI systems will develop. The current extremes range from low-field movable installations at 0.12 T up to concepts integrating ultrahigh-field strength imaging at 3 T in the operating room. Whether new scanner designs with larger and shorter bores or the application of different physical principles that allow flat MRI scanners (eg, below the operating table) will contribute to optimizing the intraoperative application of MRI technology further is not yet decided. Going to higher magnetic field strengths allows having a better signal-to-noise ratio, shorter scanning times, and a better resolution in certain modalities, such as functional imaging and spectroscopy. With regard to ultra-high-field MRI, however, there may be increased problems with artifacts as well as geometric image distortions and restrictions caused by the specific absorption rates, because the deposited radiofrequency energy must be considered in the sequence design to obtain the same performance as in 1.5-T setups. Conversely, imaging techniques in the direction of ultralow-field MRI, which could be based on taking advantage of certain contrast media effects relating to the Overhauser effect, do not seem to be an alternative to anatomic patient imaging yet, even though some early success has been achieved in small animal imaging. The optimal solution would be a nearly invisible imaging system giving online real-time feedback to the neurosurgeon without disturbing the surgical work flow.

Meanwhile, it is agreed that intraoperative anatomic imaging is not sufficient alone. Intraoperative imaging has to be combined with intraoperative guidance, implemented, for example, in the form of microscope-based navigation. There has to be the possibility to use intraoperative images for guidance, allowing so-called "updating" of the navigation, which compensates for the effects of brain shift. Furthermore, and of paramount importance, is the integration of functional data, such as functional MRI (fMRI) identifying eloquent cortical brain areas and diffusion tensor imaging data identifying major white matter tracts as well as magnetic resonance spectroscopy for data on metabolism. All these functional modalities should also be available during surgery, reflecting the current status of the brain with respect to anatomy, function, and metabolism. Increasingly, detailed brain mapping, rendering the whole brain as "eloquent," has to address the problem of information overflow for the surgeon in the operating theater. In addition, adequate functional paradigms have to be developed further and standardized, especially with respect to their intraoperative application. Even nowadays, speech mapping by fMRI is not yet standardized enough for reliable pre- and intraoperative localization. In addition to guidance maintained by navigation systems, integration of robotic devices is under development.

Another important aspect of intraoperative MRI is its acceptance in overall society. This seems to be no problem with regard to the patients benefiting from this technology; however, acceptance is still ambivalent among physicians, public opinion, and politicians as well as health insurance providers. Intraoperative imaging per se seems to be more and more accepted as immediate quality control during surgery. In the case of high-quality intraoperative imaging, early follow-up imaging (up to 3 months) is not necessary any longer. Intraoperative MRI is in competition with ultrasound and CT as an alternative intraoperative imaging modality, however. Recent technical developments, especially in the field of CT, allowing high isotropic resolution, may have the consequence that these imaging technologies have to be considered as alternative intraoperative imaging modalities in neurosurgery, especially if economic restrictions are considered. Detailed economic analyses exceeding previous preliminary cost-benefit analyses must address these aspects. Preliminary results presented recently by Hall et al [1] have to be extended and evaluated on a broader platform for industry, insurance companies, politicians, and physicians. Furthermore, the significance of MRI as an intraoperative imaging modality has to be seen in competition with other imaging modalities, especially in operating room setups designed for the simultaneous use by other surgical disciplines.

In the future, perhaps as an alternative to the expensive and highly advanced setups allowing the identical armamentarium for pre- and intraoperative diagnostics, it will be possible to have a less cost-intensive system for intraoperative imaging. Such a system, based on whatever imaging modality, must generate detailed anatomic information about the intraoperative situation in which preoperative data on function and metabolism have to be integrated applying advanced mathematical techniques, including nonlinear registration techniques as well as mathematical simulations and models. None of these techniques are yet robust and time-efficient enough that they can be applied for intraoperative use.

Intraoperative imaging is well established, especially with respect to the completion of surgical resections in complicated procedures; however, it is an open question as to which direction intraoperative imaging will take. The problem of the practicability of intraoperative MRI is under investigation, whether it is in the hands of neuroradiologists and performed by them or by neurosurgeons. Intraoperative MRI varies from simple image generation to advanced image processing at a high scientific level. The experts working on the latter level should be obliged to present their findings on the application of the method objectively.

Reference

[1] Hall WA, Kowalik K, Liu H, Truwit CL, Kucharezyk J. Costs and benefits of intraoperative MR-guided brain tumor resection. Acta Neurochir Suppl 2003;85:137–42.

Rudolf Fahlbusch, MD
Department of Neurosurgery
University Erlangen-Nuremberg
Schwabachanlage 6
91054 Erlangen, Germany

E-mail address: fahlbusch@nch.imed.uni-erlangen.de

Christopher Nimsky, MD
Department of Neurosurgery
University Erlangen-Nuremberg
Schwabachanlage 6
91054 Erlangen, Germany

E-mail address: nimsky@nch.imed.uni-erlangen.de

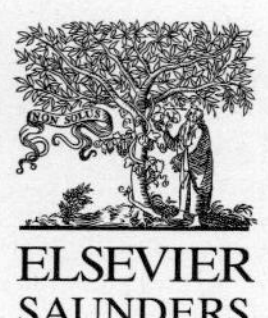

ELSEVIER
SAUNDERS

Neurosurg Clin N Am 16 (2005) 1–64

NEUROSURGERY
CLINICS
OF NORTH AMERICA

Basic principles of magnetic resonance imaging

Wendell A. Gibby, MD

Riverwoods Imaging Center, 280 West Riverpark Drive, Provo, UT 84604, USA

The discovery of nuclear magnetic resonance (NMR) by Purcell et al [1] and Bloch et al [2] first revolutionized analytic chemistry and then medical imaging. NMR imaging has taken us to yet another dimension of diagnostic imaging in which superior contrast resolution; multiplanar capabilities; and imaging of physiologic processes, such as blood flow, perfusion, diffusion, cortical activation, metabolite concentrations, and motion, have provided an entire new world of insight into the nervous system. It is an ironic historical curiosity that the name NMR imaging was changed to MRI because of the public's perceived fear of nuclear devices, because MRI uses no ionizing radiation.

The fundamental interaction of atomic particles and radiofrequency (RF) energy allows us to create spectacular MRI scans on a routine basis. Through recent discoveries in physics, we know that one of the most fundamental particles in nature is the quark [3]. A basic property of subatomic particles is that they possess spin and angular momentum. Within the proton, there are two quarks that spin parallel to each other and a third that spins opposite, giving a net unopposed spin. We also know that a proton has a net +1 positive charge. A moving charge produces a magnetic field. In fact, magnetism is defined by the force created by a specific quantity of moving charge. A tiny magnetic dipole is then created. Not only protons but any atom that has an odd number of protons or neutrons has a net unbalanced nuclear spin, and thus a nuclear magnetic moment. Electrons also possess spin and charge, and thus have a magnetic dipole associated with them. Elements containing unpaired electrons, that is, those in which the electrons are not paired in outer orbitals and in which spins are not canceled, also have an effective magnetic moment. The magnetic moment associated with an electron is approximately 1000 times greater than that of a proton.

In this article, no attempt is made to define rigorously with mathematic techniques the interactions of the nuclei with each other and with external energy. Rather, an attempt to explain these concepts through the use of simple physical models that speak a universal language is made. Of course, no physical model is able to explain the nature of subatomic particles completely, just as no single mathematic equation currently explains the dual nature of matter. A number of earlier articles on the basics of MRI [4–10] are included within the references for the interested reader. I recognize that this article may go into far more detail than the typical reader requires. Nevertheless, for those few brave, intrepid, and curious souls who really wish to know what is going on in the mysterious insides of an MRI scanner, I have tried to make this model as complete as possible. Having a basic understanding of these principles allows one to optimize image quality, reduce error, and improve conspicuity of pathologic findings. A cookbook approach gives mediocrity at best.

We are all familiar with the property of a magnet, which when placed within a magnetic field, aligns itself in such a way that its interaction with the magnetic field creates the lowest steady-state energy. For example, a compass aligns its "positive" pole with the South Pole of the earth, with opposites attracting. A compass can have any orientation with respect to an external magnetic field, and with it, any energy of interaction from zero to the maximum. Things are not quite as simple at the atomic level. By quantum theory, only certain energy states are allowed, which are discrete in value. The hydrogen nucleus having a spin quantum number of positive ½ and negative ½ gives dipole vectors that point 35.26° with and

E-mail address: wgibby@novarad.net

doi:10.1016/j.nec.2004.08.017

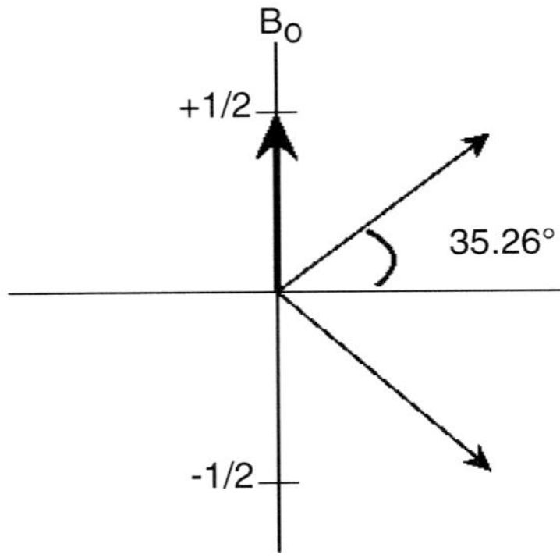

Nuclear Moment $= \sqrt{(S+1)S} = \sqrt{(1/2+1)1/2} = \sqrt{3/4}$

$$\sin\theta = \frac{y}{R} = \frac{1/2}{\sqrt{3/4}} = 35.26^\circ$$

Fig. 1. Hydrogen nucleus with spin quantum numbers of positive ½ and negative ½. The magnetic dipoles reside in energy states pointing with and against the magnetic field. The vectors pointing against the magnetic field are in a higher energy state.

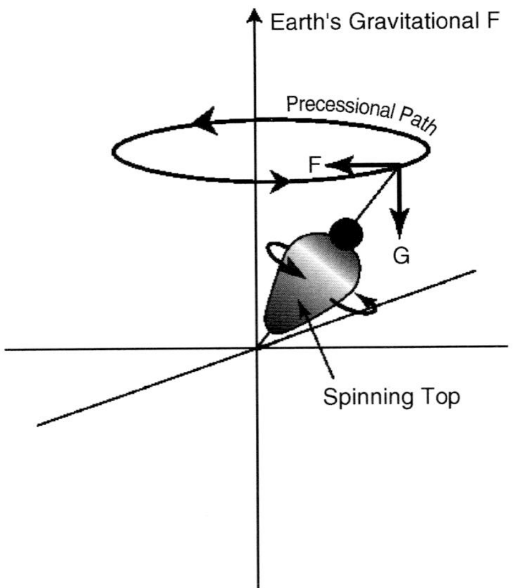

Fig. 2. A spinning top oriented off-axis with earth's gravitational field experiences two forces: the gravitational field, G, tending to pull the top toward the earth and an opposing centrifugal force, F, from the spin of the top. The result is a wobbling or precessional motion around earth's gravitational field. A similar motion occurs with spinning magnetic dipoles when placed within a magnetic field.

against the magnetic field [5] as illustrated in Fig. 1.

Precession

When first placed in a magnetic field, the off-axis proton dipoles begin to precess at a rate known as the Larmour frequency. The often-used analogy of a spinning top precessing under the force of the earth's gravitational field is illustrated in Fig. 2. An important point to remember is that the motion of the precessing magnetic dipole and the motion of the atom are completely independent. The small spinning dipole within the nucleus maintains its orientation relative to the magnetic field in spite of rapid molecular tumbling and translational motion caused by thermal energy within the lattice of the molecular structures.

There are only two things that influence the precessional rate (angular velocity) of the spinning dipole. Each different element, be it a single proton, a nucleus composed of many protons and neutrons, or an electron, has a different angular momentum, and thus a different precessional rate for a given magnetic field strength [5]. The precessional frequency of hydrogen in a magnetic field at 1.5 T is 63.866 MHz, whereas that for phosphorous is 25.876 MHz [11].

The second critical element in determining how fast a proton precesses is the net magnetic field that it experiences. A top that is precessing on the moon precesses at a different velocity than if it were spinning on the earth because of a difference in the gravitational force. Likewise, protons spinning in different magnetic field strengths precess at different velocities. This is given by the relation: Frequency $= \gamma \cdot \beta$, where γ equals the gyromagnetic ratio (for hydrogen, $\gamma = 2.6751978 \times 10^8 s{-}1T^{-1}$) and β equals the field strength in tesla [12]. Our model now describes an ensemble of precessing magnetic dipoles with their vectors pointed in the direction of the magnetic field.

Fig. 3. (*A*) The vectors oriented with B_0 spin in an opposite direction than those oriented opposite the magnetic field. Most of these cancel each other out. We are left with net vectors precessing around the *z*-axis oriented with the magnetic field (approximately 1 of 100,000 vectors). (*B*) The nuclear dipoles exchange energy with the surrounding molecular lattice. There is only a tiny energy difference between the up and down states, leaving a small net fraction of dipoles in the lowest energy state (pointing up).

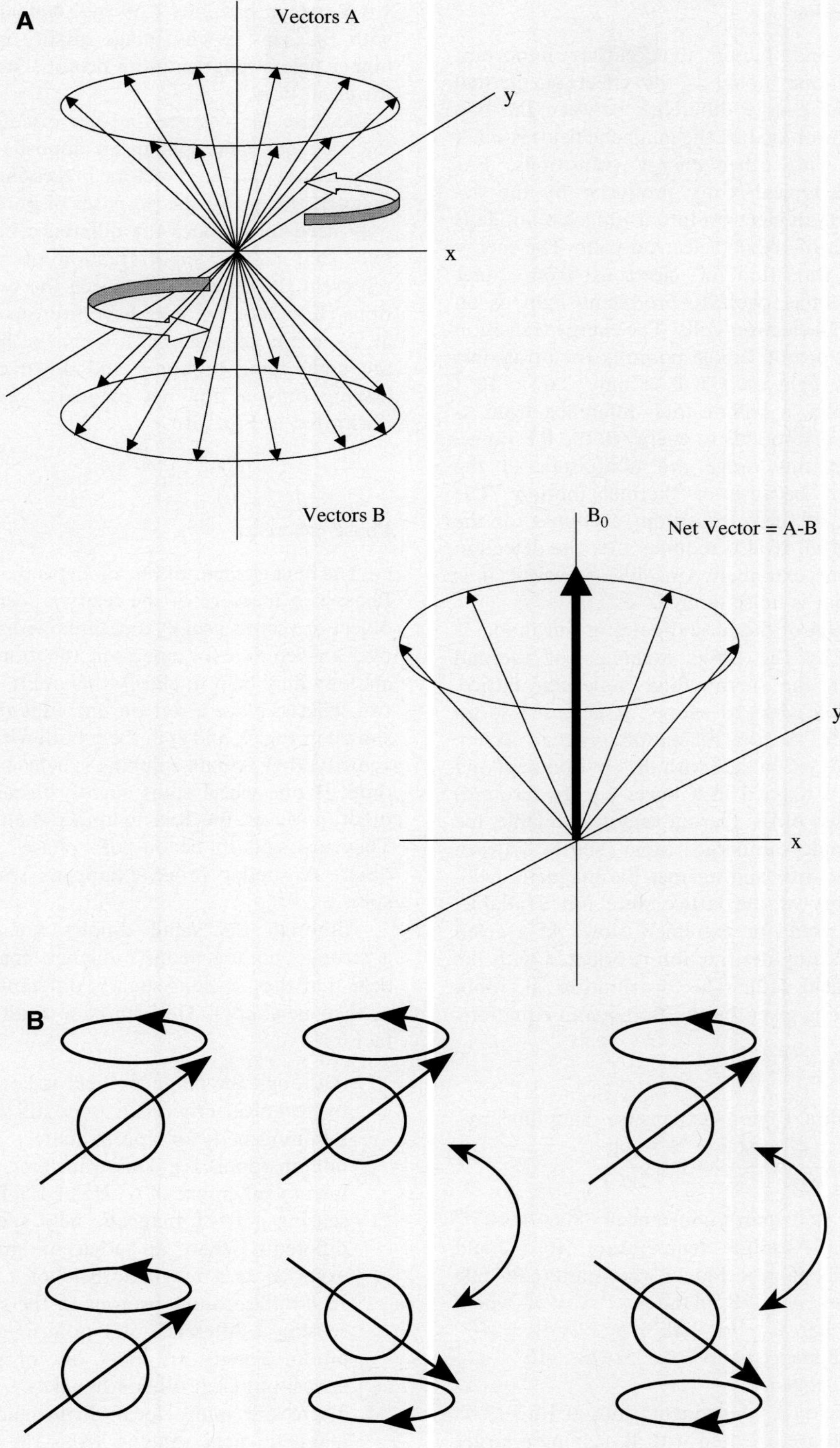
A
Vectors A
y
x
Vectors B
B_0
Net Vector = A-B
y
x
B

Thermal motion

The second factor that causes important changes in our model is the effect of thermal motion. The energy difference between the two states (ie, for or against the magnetic field) is small compared with other energy transitions. For example, a typical x-ray produced by the deceleration of an electron into a tungsten anode is on the order of 100,000 electron volts. The energy from the transition of electrons from outer orbitals to inner orbitals, producing light, is on the order of 4 electron volts. The energy transition for a small proton dipole pointing for or against a magnetic field at 1.5 T is only 2.6×10^{-7} electron volts, a trillion-fold difference from x-rays. This corresponds to energy in the RF range. Energies in this range are ubiquitous in the environment because of thermal motion. The low energy of these transitions accounts for the safety of MRI. It also requires that the detection apparatus be extremely sensitive, however. It is a system that is noise limited.

Thus, each of the little dipoles in our model is influenced by the rapid exchange of thermal energy with the surrounding molecular lattice. As the dipole absorbs energy, it is raised to an excited state. As the relaxation process occurs, this energy is exchanged with the environment and the dipole is aligned in a lower energy (ground) state. Because of the thermal energy available, the proton dipoles undergo rapid shifts between orientations with and against the magnetic field. If the energy of the lattice were not available, relaxation would be extremely slow. At a given time, only a tiny net fraction is oriented with the magnetic field [12]. The distribution at room temperature is given by the Boltzmann equation:

$$\frac{N+}{No} = e^{-\frac{\Delta E}{kT}}$$

which with a Taylor's expansion, simplifies to

$$\frac{N+}{N-} = 1 + \frac{\Delta E}{kT} \text{ or } \frac{N+}{N-} = 1 + \frac{h\gamma B}{2\pi kT}$$

where k = Boltzman's constant (1.38066×10^{-23} J K^{-1}); T = Absolute temperature; B_o = Field strength in Tesla; h = Planck's constant (6.062608×10^{-34}) J sec; $\omega = \gamma B_o$ in rad sec^{-1}; $\nu = \gamma \frac{B_o}{2\pi}$ where $\gamma = \frac{\omega}{2\pi}$ in hz; $E = h\nu$; $\Delta E = h\nu = h\gamma B_o = \frac{h\gamma B_o}{2\pi}$; γ = gyromagnetic ratio (2.6751978×10^{-8} s^{-1} T^{-1}) for hydrogen.

This is field (B_o) dependent; thus, at 1.5 T, 9.88 of 1,000,000 are oriented with B_o, giving a larger fraction of nuclei available for excitation than at 1.0 T, which has only 6.59 of 1,000,000 oriented with B_o. This is why image quality is better at higher field strengths; more protons are available for excitation.

Because the vectors that are oriented against the magnetic field spin in an opposite direction, they cancel out any vectors precessing with the magnetic field. For the purposes of our model, we only need to consider the difference between the two, that is, the small fraction of nuclei that represent the difference between the two populations (Fig. 3A). We now have protons precessing at a specific frequency in a magnetic field, which are undergoing rapid up and down transitions, leaving only a tiny net magnetic vector, as is illustrated in Fig. 3B.

Phase coherence

The next element of our model is that of phase. Phase is a measure of the relative position of an object or vector; usually measured with an angle ϕ over a given time for a periodic function. A simple analogy may help to clarify this point. If we take two wheels, place a dot on one edge of them, as shown in Fig. 4, and spin them both with the same velocity, they remain spinning synchronously over time. If one wheel spins slightly faster than the other, however, the dots no longer align over time. They are said to be out of "phase" with each other. A similar process happens with nuclear spins.

Although the small dipoles are placed in a strong "homogeneous" magnet, the magnetic field that they sense is slightly different than that of their neighbors. This can be a result of several factors:

1. Although the magnetic field is homogeneous by technical criteria, it may still contain an inhomogeneity of approximately 1 part per million (ppm) [7]. This translates into a frequency difference of 63 Hz at 1.5 T. A dipole sensing a 1.5-T magnetic field spins slightly differently than an adjacent proton that experiences a magnetic field of 1.500001 T. In 8 milliseconds, protons in the same voxel sensing a difference of 1 ppm magnetic field inhomogeneity are 180° out of phase and cancel out each other's signal.
2. There are many local disturbances to the magnetic field ranging from the molecular level up through the tissue level. For instance,

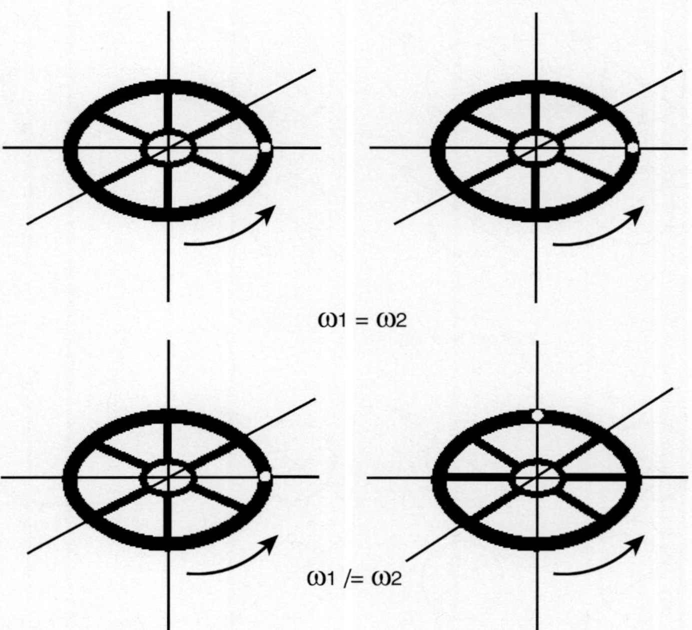

Fig. 4. A dot is placed on a spinning wheel. In the first case, the angular velocity of the two spinning wheels is equal and the dots stay synchronized with one another. They are said to be "in phase." In the second instance, the velocity of the first wheel is different from that of the second wheel. Over time, the relative position of the dots drifts "out of phase."

oxygen atoms, by their nature, are highly electronegative and tend to attract more of the shared electron cloud around themselves than does the adjacent hydrogen atom in a molecule like water. This causes the hydrogen nucleus to have less of a screening effect from the overlying electron cloud. It experiences a stronger local magnetic field than a proton attached to a fat molecule in that the protons are more shielded by valence electrons. Therefore, the spins of water hydrogen nuclei precess at a slightly greater frequency than those of fat.

3. Different substances have different permeabilities to the magnetic flux and can thus distort magnetic field lines. Most materials are diamagnetic, meaning that the magnetic flux lines would rather go through a perfect vacuum than through that substance. For example, at an air-bone or bone–soft tissue interface, the magnetic flux lines are distorted. Some materials, such as iron, are ferromagnetic and concentrate magnetic flux lines. All these make the local magnetic field different for adjacent nuclei, causing them to precess at slightly different rates. Because they precess at slightly different frequencies, they rapidly become out of phase with respect to each other, and coherence is lost.

Our model now consists of small nuclear magnetic dipoles rapidly precessing in space, each with a slightly different angular velocity, out of phase with respect to adjacent dipoles, and rapidly exchanging energy with the environment such that their dipole orientations are flipping back and forth in restricted quanta of energy for and against the magnetic field. One may then wonder how any useful information can be extracted from these weak signals, precessing at different velocities and completely out of phase with each other.

Net vector

At this point, a short diversion is necessary to understand signal generation. Each of the individual spinning nuclear dipoles can have only one of two orientations with respect to the magnetic field. If we average the orientations of these, we can obtain a net vector that can have any orientation with respect to the magnetic field. This averaging of the individual directions is illustrated in Fig. 5. This net vector can be thought of as a larger single dipole. For example, if sufficient RF energy is given

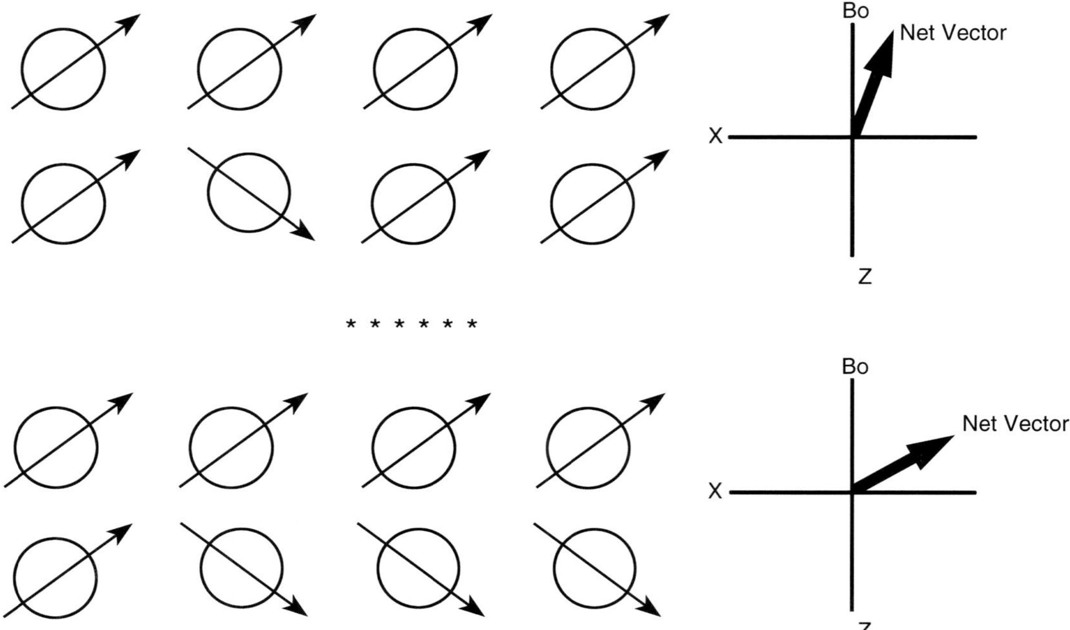

Fig. 5. The concept of a net vector. Each of the individual nuclear dipoles is added. Now, rather than pointing at 35.3° for or against the magnetic field, the net vector is the sum of the positions of all the vectors.

to a sample of spinning hydrogen nuclei, a fraction of them can be rendered into the excited state and the net vector tipped from 0° through perhaps 90°. This would reflect a 90° RF pulse. By convention, the axes used in MRI are *x*, *y*, and *z*. The *z*-coordinate is taken along the main magnetic field, and the protons process around *z* in the *x-y* plane. We remember that if a magnetic dipole spins, an electrical current can be induced in a coil oriented perpendicular to this, just as the converse is seen with a coil-conducting current that induces a magnetic field. This is shown diagrammatically in Fig. 6.

Signal formation

The key to obtaining any useful information from the precessing protons is to establish coherence, that is, having a large portion of the dipoles all spinning together with a net vector precessing in the *x-y* plane, where signal can be generated in a suitably oriented coil. How then is phase coherence established and signal generated? RF waves are electromagnetic radiation that have time-varying magnetic fields propagated through space. These time-varying magnetic fields can interact with the oscillating magnetic field of the spinning hydrogen dipole.

To understand how phase coherence is achieved, we must first understand the B1 field created by the transmitting RF coil. In Fig. 7, a loop of wire is fed an oscillating RF current. As we remember from our basic college physics, current flowing through a wire induces a magnetic field perpendicular to the flow of current according to the right hand rule. If the current is oscillating, as occurs with a RF pulse, a sinusoidal oscillation of the B1-induced magnetic field of the

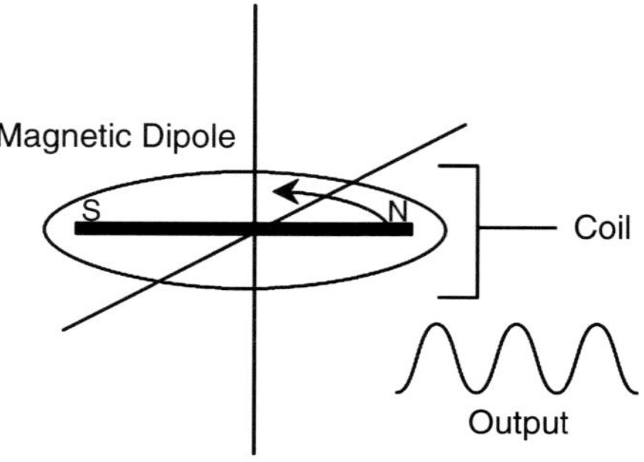

Fig. 6. An electromagnetic pickup coil oriented perpendicular to the spinning dipole acts as a tiny generator in which an oscillating electrical current is created.

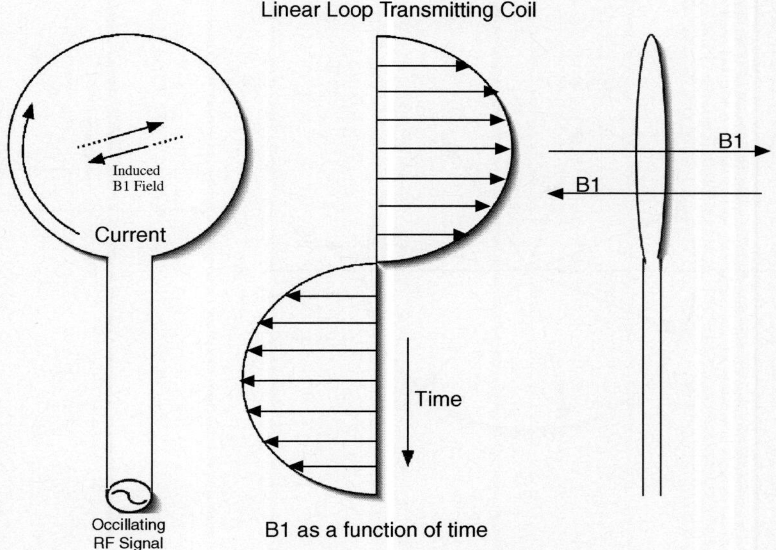

Fig. 7. Passing an oscillating current through a coiled wire creates an oscillating magnetic field (B1) perpendicular to the coil that moves in and out perpendicular to the face of the coil as a function of time.

coil is created. The transmitting coil creates a magnetic vector perpendicular to its face, which increases and decreases and then reverses over time as a function of the RF oscillation. If one thinks back to our spinning wheel analogy, the magnetic vector would be going in and out over time along the axis of the spokes (Fig. 8). Most RF transmitters use a circularly polarized transmitting coil, which creates a wave of an oscillating B1 magnetic field that rotates around the sample with a B1 vector going in and out perpendicular to the *z*-axis (Fig. 9).

The next thing to understand is spin locking. If we looked at only the vectors in the *x-y* plane from our net vector in Fig. 3B, it would look like Fig. 10. The vectors are precessing in the *x-y* plane all out of phase with respect to each other.

Spin locking or synchronization of the vectors occurs as the spin dipoles are "pushed" together by the synchronized B1 field of the RF transmit coil. Some authors use a rotating frame of reference, a mathematic trick in which the observer rotates around the vectors to describe a classic model of the interaction with the spinning vectors. I prefer to view this from a more linear approach. In Fig. 11, the circular motion of a given vector of the spinning nucleus observed from one point of the transmit coil can be viewed as a series of vectors of increasing and then decreasing sinusoidal intensity over time. In other words, the vector pointing at the coil is doing exactly the same thing that the oscillating transmitted RF wave is doing by creating a vector that goes in and out perpendicular to the *z*-axis. Think of the component of the vector facing the coil as something like a piston that oscillates in and out perpendicular to the axis of a fly wheel. The B1 vector acts like a piston opposing or reinforcing the motion of the spinning hydrogen vector (Fig. 12). The B1 vector created by the oscillating magnetic field of the RF wave quickly brings the vector of the nucleus into synchronization; however, this does not occur instantly. The time constant for this process is called $T1_{rho}$. If we think of an ensemble of nuclei spinning in a voxel in different phases, the B1 vector moves coherently in a circularly polarized fashion around the spinning nucleus, with all the B1 vectors in phase from the oscillating RF transmit coil. This quickly synchronizes all the opposing vectors, bringing them into coherence much like independent pistons working with or against a large coherently operated crank shaft with synchronized pistons (Fig. 13).

Thus, with the tiny individual magnetic dipoles in phase, we can add each of them together, giving a large single magnetic dipole. With coherence now established and a net dipole vector precessing in the *x-y* plane, a signal is generated in the coil or antenna. This signal represents a free induction

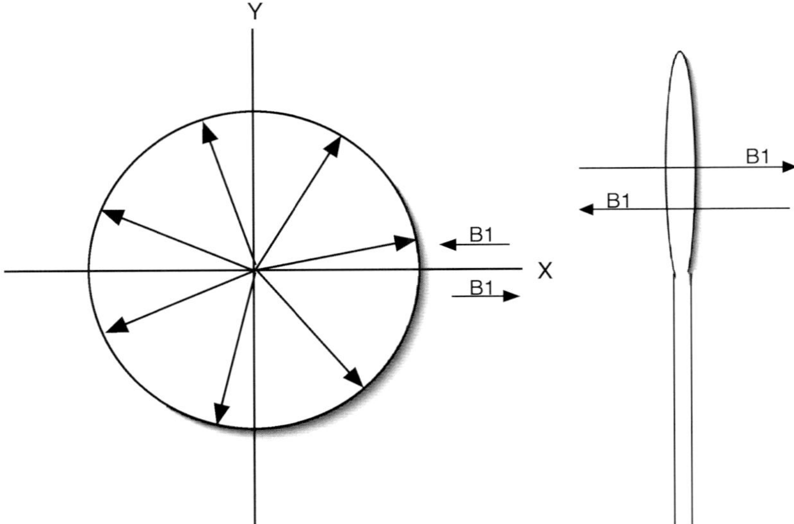

Fig. 8. The transmitting coil creates an oscillating B1 field over time that moves in and out perpendicular to the spokes of the turning wheel, which would be the representation of the precessing vectors in the *x*-*y* plane.

decay (FID). Of course, this does not last long. Because the precession rate for the nuclear dipoles varies with magnetic field differences, phase coherence is lost and the signal rapidly decays, as demonstrated in Fig. 14. The length of time the signal persists is a measure of how rapidly phase coherence is lost.

By applying RF energy, a two-part change has occurred within the system. First, a certain fraction of the nuclei were inverted into the excited state against the main magnetic field, giving us a net magnetic vector that is not oriented with the longitudinal *z*-coordinate. Second, phase coherence that had not previously been present was established. Over time, the system returns to its natural random state.

T1 relaxation

The rate at which the proton dipoles relax back into the aligned state with B_o (lowest energy) is constant over time for a given substance at a given field strength. As more of the protons relax, however, a smaller percentage of nuclei are in the excited state; thus, fewer are available overall to relax. This describes a typical exponential relaxation curve, as illustrated in Fig. 15. At a time of 1 T1, 64% of the longitudinal

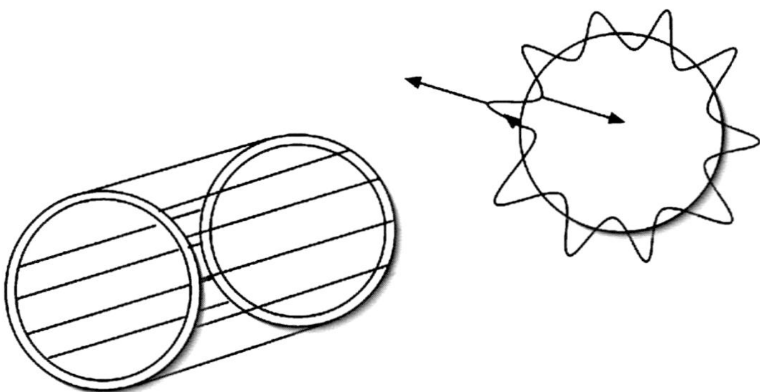

Fig. 9. A circularly polarized transmit coil creates an oscillating B1 field that moves in and out perpendicular to the *z*-axis that rotates around the sample.

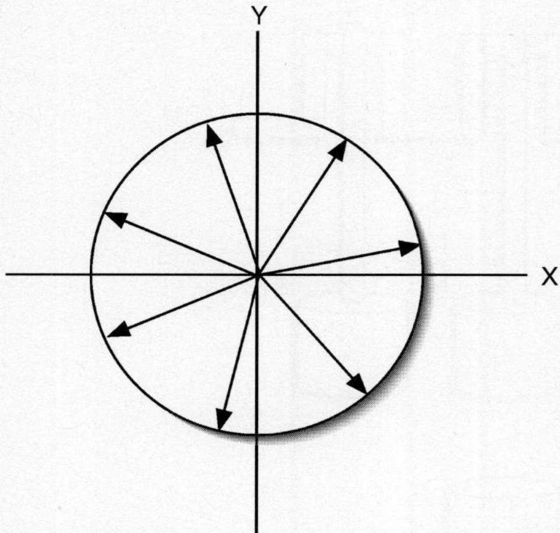

Fig. 10. Top down view of Fig. 3 demonstrates the precessing *x-y* component of the vectors spinning around randomly completely out of phase with respect to each other.

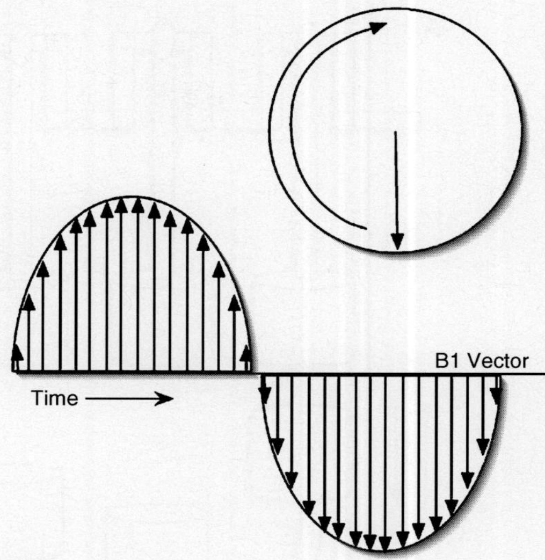

Fig. 11. If one stands at a given vantage point watching the precessing nuclear dipole, the vector increases and then decreases in a sinusoidal oscillating function over time.

magnetization has recovered. By four T1, 98% of the longitudinal magnetization vector has been recovered. The process of changing from an excited to a nonexcited orientation in the magnetic field involves an energy exchange, the energy of which is precisely equal to the Larmour frequency of the spinning nuclear vector. What MRI is really seeing inside the body is energy—the energy of precessing nuclear dipoles.

As previously noted, these energies of exchange can be obtained from molecular motions and vibrations in the molecular lattice. For this reason, T1 is commonly referred to as the "spin lattice relaxation time." From quantum theory, only a discrete energy value is allowed to induce this transition. Energy is related to frequency, υ, by the equation $E = h\nu$, where h is equal to Planck's constant [13]. An important concept is that the excited magnetic dipole can relax only if it can transfer its discrete energy into the surrounding molecular lattice. These molecular energy states are present in the form of rotational and vibrational motions of the molecules. Certain types and structures of molecules are far more efficient in accepting these energies, because their vibrational and rotational energies correspond more closely with the Larmour frequency. Frequencies that are too high or too low do not efficiently interact with the nuclear dipole; thus, T1 relaxation is slowed [14].

For example, water molecules are small. They rotate and vibrate quickly and have a relatively

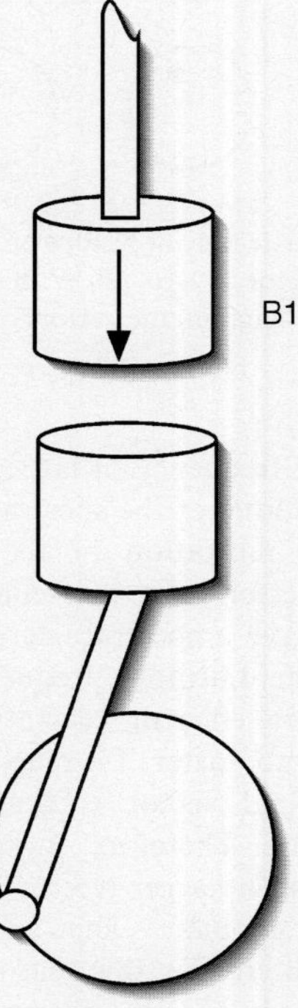

Fig. 12. The oscillating B1 vector exerts a force on the spinning proton nuclear vector much like two opposing pistons in a cylinder.

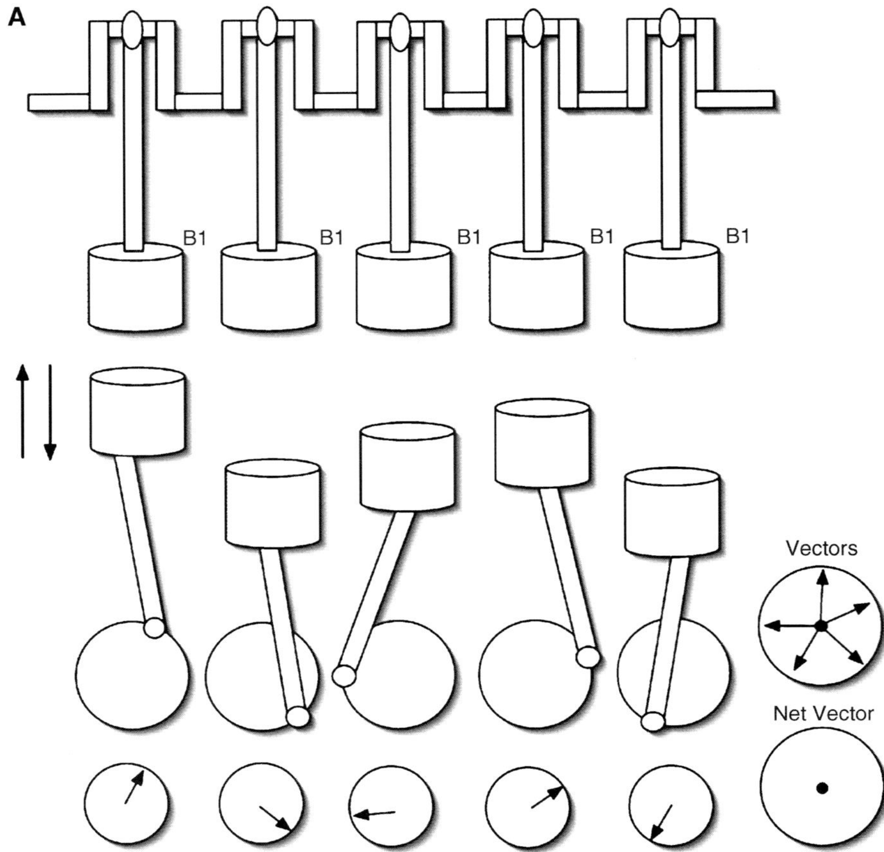

Fig. 13. (*A*) An assembly of pistons on the bottom row represents each of the different proton vectors at different phases, creating a net vector of zero. (*B*) With the application of the synchronized force of B1 represented by an array of pistons at the top of the diagram, the vectors of the precessing protons are rapidly brought into synchronization, giving a strong net vector.

higher spectral frequency of lattice energies. Pure water contains little of the spectral energy needed to induce T1 relaxation of the small nuclear dipoles. Conversely, fat molecules that tumble more slowly have a spectral energy more closely matched to the Larmour frequency and hence allow for more efficient relaxation. When the protons undergo faster T1 relaxation, more of their longitudinal vector is available for each succeeding pulse. Therefore, more signal is generated, because a larger vector is available to precess in the *x*-*y* plane. That substance appears relatively brighter. For this reason, fat is bright on T1-weighted (T1W) images (images that accentuate differences in the T1 of tissues) and water is dark (Fig. 16). Likewise, myelin, which has a slowing effect on the motion of adjacent water, is relatively bright on T1W sequences [15]. Nevertheless, this can be pushed too far. Extremely large solid-like structures, such as bone or proteins (eg, ligaments and other highly ordered proteins), have protons that are relatively immobile. They give little signal on T1W imaging, because the rotational and vibrational frequencies have been slowed to the point that they are no longer optimal for relaxation [12,16]. Similarly, protons on cholesterol and lipid membranes have relatively poor mobility and have longer relaxation times as opposed to adipose tissue (storage fat), which has molecules that are in an oil (liquid) state, are more mobile, and relax more quickly. Paramagnetic materials also improve T1 relaxation, as can nonparamagnetic calcium salts [17].

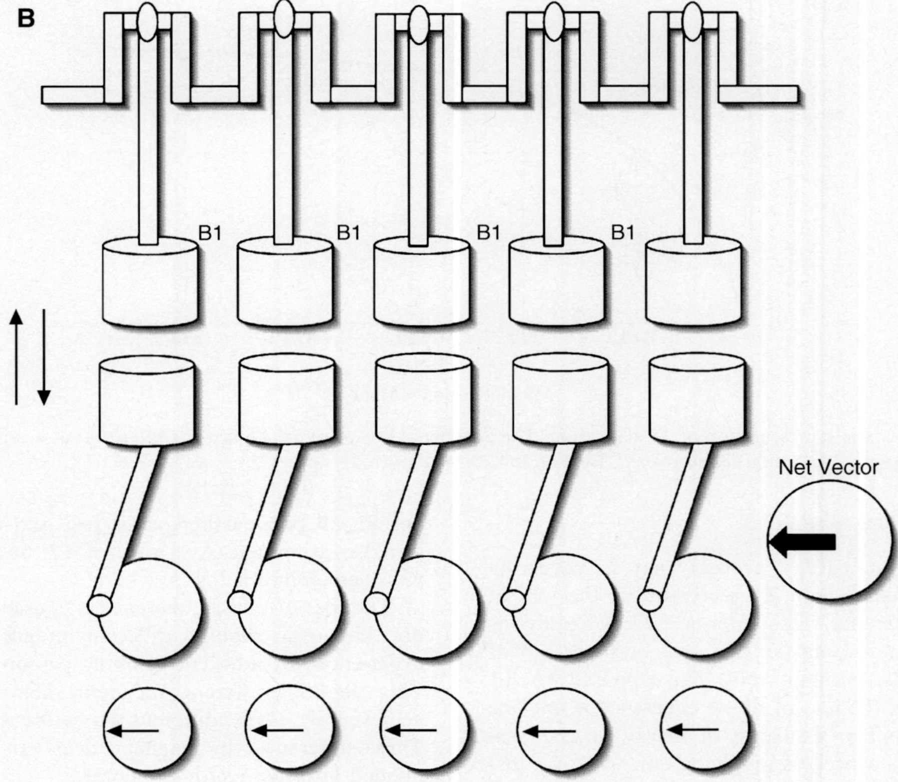

Fig. 13 (*continued*)

By the same token, the relaxation of biologic material is more or less efficient depending on the strength of the magnetic field. T1 relaxation is field strength dependent [18,19]. Table 1 gives data comparing T1 relaxation times of selected tissues at 24 and 2.5 MHz [105].

In general, T1 relaxation is more efficient for lower frequency (field strength is proportional to frequency) over the range of magnetic field strengths used clinically. Thus, shorter repetition times (TRs) can be used for a 0.35-T magnet versus a 1.5-T magnet to achieve equal T1 relaxation (and hence T1 contrast between tissues).

T1 relaxation is a thermodynamic process involving enthalpy, in that an energy exchange occurs. The surrounding lattice must be able to accept the precise quanta of energy emitted by the relaxing nuclear dipoles. The difference in relaxation between small, intermediate and large molecules is illustrated in Fig. 17. T1 can be measured by sampling the system at various time intervals to see how much longitudinal magnetization is present after a given amount of time. To measure T1 accurately, the TR (ie, the time before the system is re-excited) must span values above and below T1. The TR is varied, and signal intensity is plotted as a function of TR. The slope of the curve is related to T1: Signal = M_o $(1 - e^{-TR/T1})$ [20].

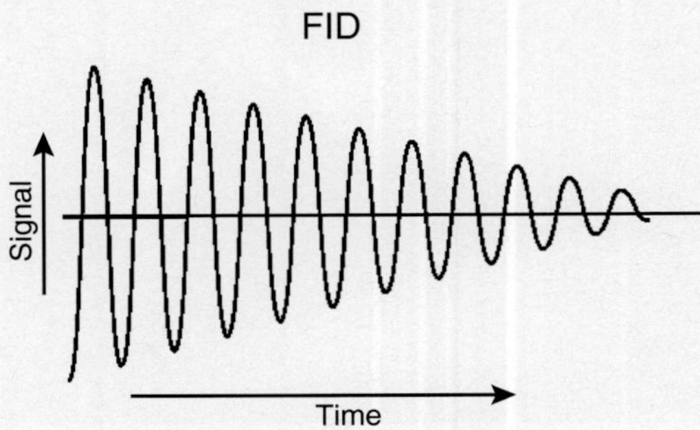

Fig. 14. When all the vectors are spinning in synchrony, the maximum signal intensity is generated in the coil. Over time, however, these vector dephase, and there is rapid loss of signal intensity. This represents free induction decay (FID).

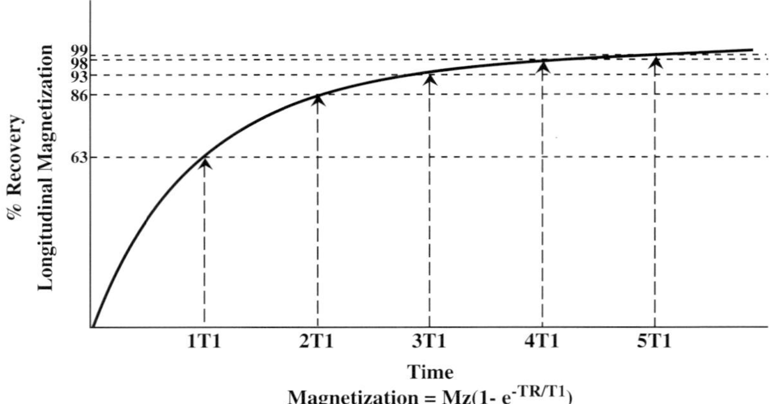

Fig. 15. Graphic representation of T1 relaxation. The exponential recovery of T1 demonstrates that at a time of 1T1, 63% of the signal intensity has recovered. By 5T1, 99% has recovered.

T2 relaxation

The other decay process that is occurring simultaneously with T1 relaxation is the loss of phase coherence. This is termed *T2 relaxation* or *spin-spin dephasing* (ie, one spin becomes out of phase with another spin). As opposed to T1 relaxation, the loss of phase coherence is not one that requires an exchange of energy. In chemical terms, it is a process involving entropy, or a disordering of an ordered state. This also occurs at an exponential rate [20] (there is more signal to dephase early on): Signal $= M_o\, e^{-(TE/T2)}$. As the spins dephase, the magnetic vectors precessing in the *x-y* plane gradually fan out. After a certain period, all phase coherence is lost and no more signal is generated. At a time of T2, 64% of the phase coherence is lost.

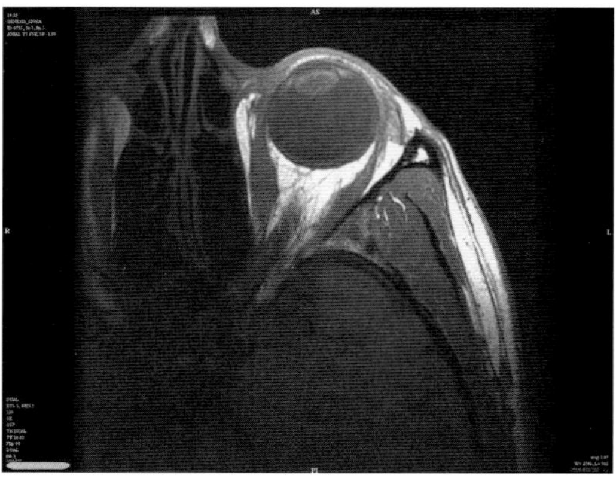

Fig. 16. Orbital MRI scan with T1 weighting. Fat is bright, bone is dark, muscles are low signal, and vitreous humor is dark. Note that the lens is slightly brighter than the vitreous fluid, because the water is bound to proteins, which slows its motion.

The loss of phase coherence is caused by only one thing—a slightly different magnetic field experienced by adjacent spinning proton dipoles. This slightly different magnetic field can be achieved by many different processes, however. These differences in magnetic field can be subdivided into two major categories.

Static magnetic fields

Static magnetic fields vary in intensity over space but not over time during image acquisition. Examples of this would include magnetic field inhomogeneities by the magnet itself, perturbation of the local magnetic field by materials that have different magnetic permeability, such as bone, air, or stationary paramagnetic or ferromagnetic materials. Because these magnetic field

Table 1
T1 relaxation values

	24 MHz (milliseconds)	2.5 MHz (milliseconds)
Clotted white blood	867	404
Serum	1590	820
Gray matter	644	332
White matter	469	264

From Ling CR, Foster MA, Hutchison JMS. Comparison of NMR water proton T1 relaxation times of rabbit tissues at 24 MHz and 2.5 MHz. Phys Med Biol 1980;25:748; with permission.

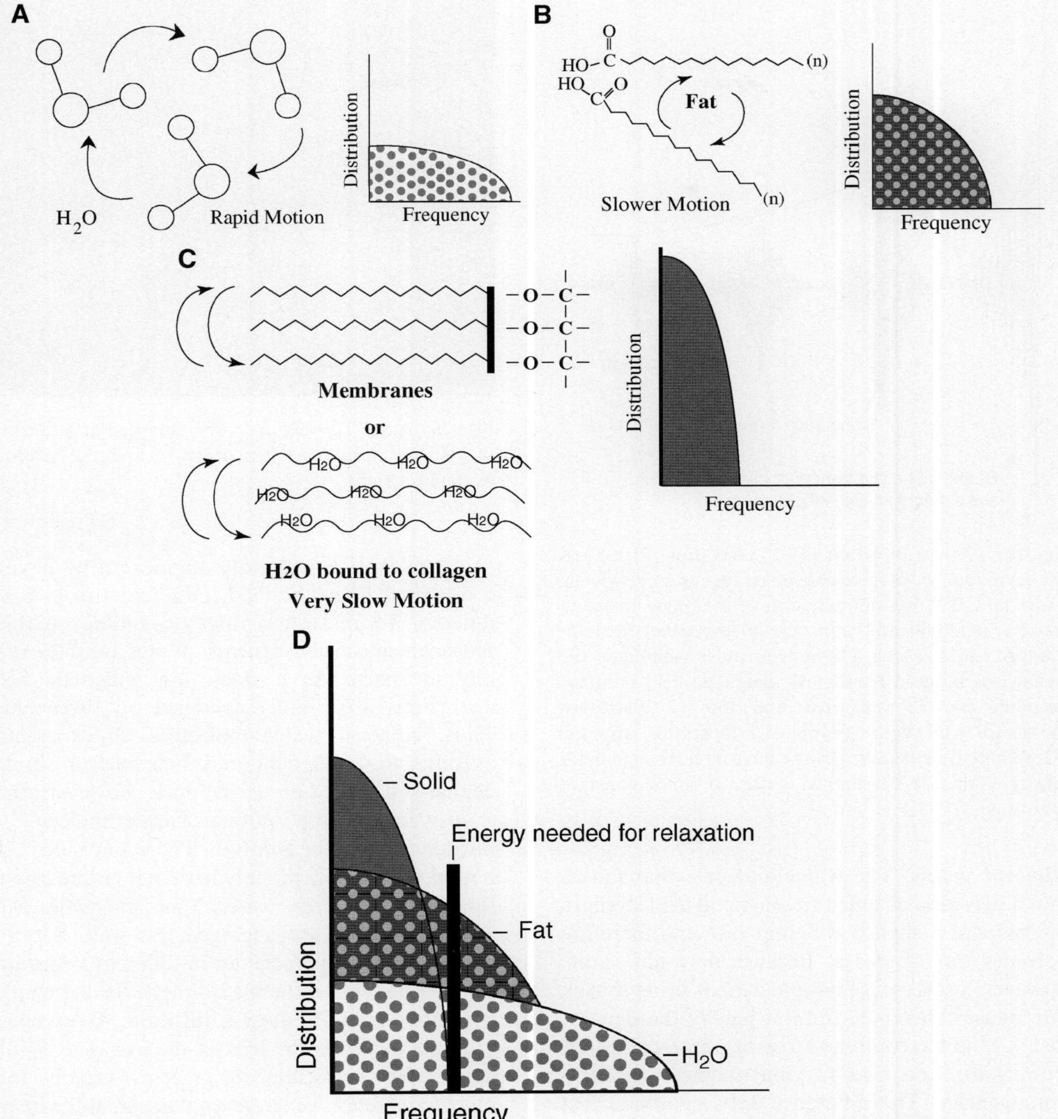

Fig. 17. (*A*) Water molecules tumble rapidly and have a large population of high frequency vibrational and tumbling energy states. As a result, T1 relaxation is inefficient. (*B*) Fat molecules, on the other hand have a larger proportion of motional states correlating with the energy needed for relaxation. (*C*) Complex molecules such as membranes or water bound to large protein molecules exhibit very slow motion resulting in low frequency components that are below the energy needed for relaxation. (*D*) A composite figure demonstrates that fat will have better efficiency at relaxation than eigher water or solid materials. This is the result of the quantum requirement for discrete energy transitions which can be supplied only with certain molecular vibrational and rotational states.

inhomogeneities are constant in time, the signal loss from dephasing can be recovered by the use of a second 180° pulse, which rephases the nuclear spins (more about this in the section on pulse sequences).

Time-varying magnetic fields

Water molecules, for instance, can move rapidly through space and across membranes and can randomly bounce around within and between

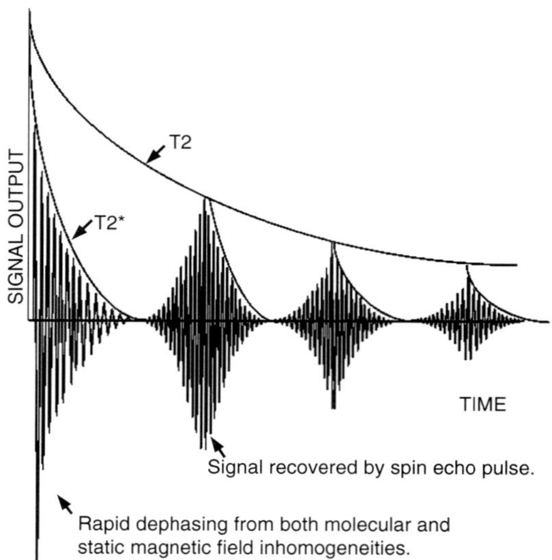

Fig. 18. T2 relaxation versus T2* relaxation. Phase loss occurs in two ways: reversible phase loss and irreversible phase loss. T2* is a combination of the phase losses of static (reversible) and nonstatic (irreversible) field inhomogeneities. Using a spin echo pulse technique, the signal loss induced from static magnetic field inhomogeneities can be recovered and the T2 relaxation measured. This figure graphically illustrates why the T2-weighted sequences always have greater signal intensity than a T2*-weighted sequence for a constant echo time.

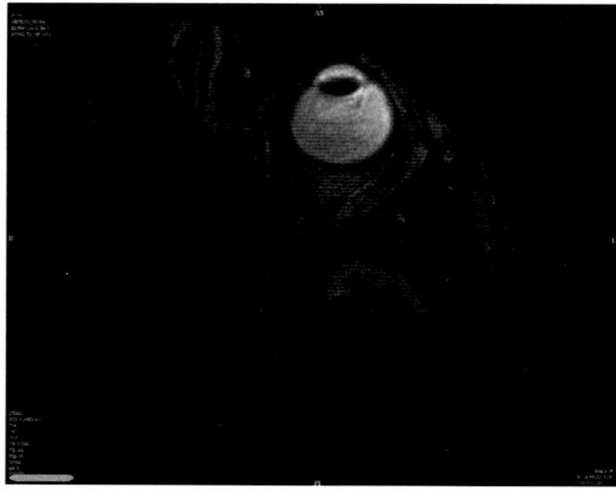

Fig. 19. Axial T2-weighted orbit image. Fat is darker, the lens is dark (complex protein), and the vitreous (water) is bright.

adjacent voxels. The water molecule that moves into a new area of different magnetic field strength precesses at a slightly different rate and therefore becomes out of phase. Because it is not static, however, a reversal of its spin cannot bring it back into phase coherence, and this part of the signal is lost. T2* is the combined loss of phase coherence from static and time-varying magnetic field inhomogeneity. The difference between phase lost from static and time-varying magnetic field inhomogeneities is shown diagrammatically in Fig. 18.

Phase loss can occur not only between adjacent voxels or imaging points in our data set but within a voxel as well. For example, fat and water precess at slightly different frequencies. The hydrogen of a water molecule, being less shielded by the electron cloud of its oxygen neighbor, experiences a higher magnetic field strength and thus precesses at a faster rate. If a voxel contains equal quantities of fat and water, they are exactly out of phase with each other at certain times causing the signal to cancel.

T2 relaxation is greatly augmented by having a distorted magnetic field. Different tissues have different T2 relaxation rates depending on their physiochemical constituents. Water tumbles rapidly in space. As it does, any magnetic field distortions are rapidly averaged out over time. Thus, adjacent water molecules all experience a similar magnetic field, and their nuclear dipoles dephase slowly. Let us suppose, however, that a protein or large polysaccharide molecule is introduced into the solution. The water molecules bound to the biologic polymer rotate more slowly than adjacent free water, and magnetic field inhomogeneities are averaged less well. Because of this, the water molecules in different hydration states experience different magnetic field strengths over the period of image acquisition. An excellent example of this is the lens of the eye. The rigidly held water molecules in proteins rapidly lose phase coherence, generate a small signal for imaging, and thus are dark on T2-weighted (T2W) images. Fat, being a much larger molecule than water, is held more rigidly in space over time and thus loses phase coherence more rapidly than free extracellular water; fat darkens relative to water with increased T2 weighting (Fig. 19).

If water molecules are adjacent to or within voxels containing materials that cause distortions of the magnetic field, they likewise rapidly lose phase coherence. For example, iron deposits in the basal ganglia destroy phase coherence, giving little signal on T2W images. Likewise, the injection of magnetite, a ferromagnetic substance that causes strong local field inhomogeneities,

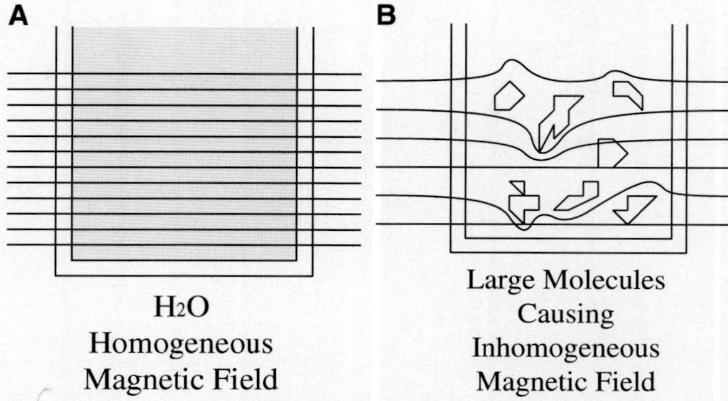

Fig. 20. Comparison of a small versus large molecules on magnetic field homogeneity. (*A*) The rapid tumbling motion of water molecules evens out micro magnetic distortions giving a homogeneous magnetic field. (*B*) Large solid or semi-solid molecules do not tumble as rapidly. Therefore, small perturbations of the local magnetic filed occur.

destroys phase coherence and gives dark signal on T2W images. Materials that are more solid move more slowly and thus have a more inhomogeneous local magnetic field. Fig. 20, illustrates how a semisolid material distorts the local magnetic field compared with a rapidly tumbling small molecule. For most substances, phase is lost much more quickly than restoration of proton dipole alignment with the *z*-axis (ie, T2 relaxation is much shorter than T1 relaxation). A comparison of various substances is given in a qualitative way in Table 2.

Table 2
T1-weighted and T2-weighted appearance of various body tissues

	Appearance on sequences	
	T1-weighted	T2-weighted
Rigid molecules		
Bone		
Fibrocartilage		
Ligaments	Dark	Dark
Scar		
Hemosiderin		
Watery substances		
Cerebrospinal fluid	Dark	Bright
Cysts		
Free water		
Intermediate molecules		
Fat	Bright	Intermediate
Proteinaceous material	Intermediate to bright	Intermediate to bright depending on water content
Hyaline cartilage	Intermediate	Intermediate to dark
Lens of eye	Bright	Dark

Recovery of magnetization vector to ground state (T1 relaxation)

Let us return to our model briefly. After an RF pulse is given, a magnetization vector is established that is precessing coherently in the *x-y* plane. Suppose that a sample contains a variety of substances that have different T1 relaxation values (A, B, and C for short, intermediate, and long T1s, respectively). Given a long enough time, all the magnetization vectors of the various substances return to an equilibrium position along the *z*-axis. If we excite the system at an intermediate time, those voxels with short T1s will have already relaxed, with their magnetization vectors oriented parallel to the *z*-axis before the next excitation. Tissues with longer T1s will be somewhere in between. Their relative positions are shown in Fig. 21. If the sample is given a repeat 90° RF energy pulse at this point in time, the entire vector of the short T1 substance labeled A can be rotated into the *x-y* plane and is available for generating signal. Those substances with intermediate and longer T1s (B and C, respectively) have less magnetization available to precess in the *x-y* plane and generate less signal in our receiver. Thus, maximum signal is obtained by waiting a longer period for full longitudinal magnetization recovery to occur or by speeding the T1 relaxation of the slower substances through the use of paramagnetic agents. Differential intensity between voxels of different T1s can be achieved by selecting a TR close to the T1 of the tissue of interest. To repeat, the brightest tissues on T1W pulse sequences are those that have the shortest T1 and thus have the most available longitudinal magnetization available for inversion into the *x-y* plane

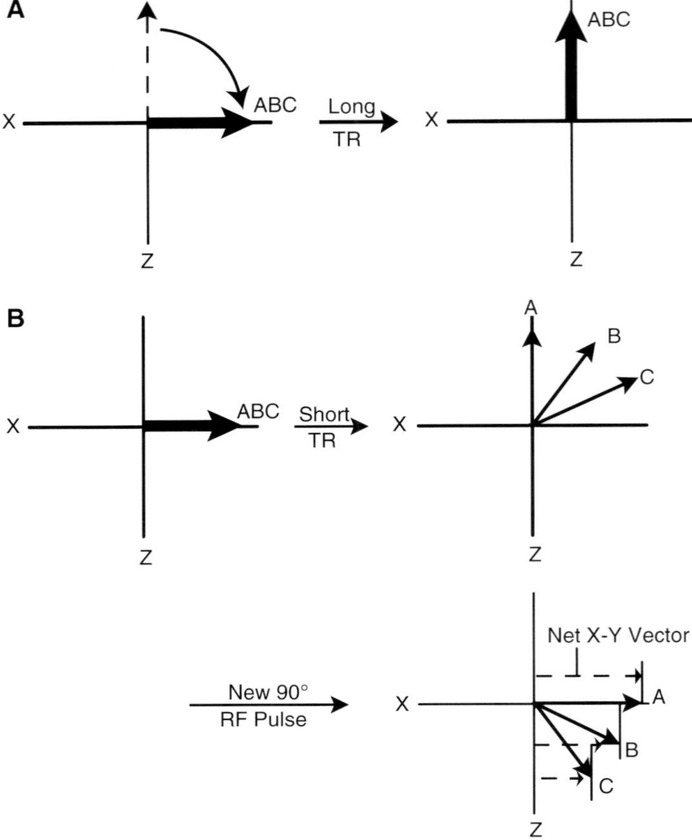

Fig. 21. Comparison of T1 relaxation between substances with short, intermediate, and long T1s. (*A*) In the first instance, vectors A, B, and C are excited into the *x-y* plane. A long time follows before the pulse is repeated. At such time, TR, repitition time, all the vectors will be back to their ground state and ready for full excitation into the *x-y* plane. (*B*) A similar experiment is performed, except that a short TR is used. At the time that a new 90° radiofrequency (RF) pulse is delivered, substance A with a short T1 will be tipped fully into the *x-y* plane, giving the largest signal. Its net vector is larger than that of a substance such as C, which has a long T1 relaxation time that has not fully relaxed before excitation, yielding a smaller net vector in the *x-y* plane.

at the beginning of each pulse repetition. Table 3 gives the values of T1 for various tissues. Remember, T1 relaxation is field strength dependent; therefore, it is not possible to use values obtained at high field strength to compare with low field measurements and vice versa. One should also know that there is considerable variability in the measurement of T1 between different instruments and different investigators. As such, the T1 relaxation of a tissue is not useful as an absolute comparison with other disease processes. Field strength, equipment type, temperature, selection of the sampling sequence, TR [21], and slice thickness all influence the obtained value.

How fast tissues lose coherence

Paradoxically, tissues that have a short T2 have the least signal. This is easily understood by the fact that as phase is lost, signal is destroyed and image intensity is decreased. Substances like free water, which maintain phase coherence for a longer period, have relatively greater signal than tissues with a short T2 if the data sampling (related to echo time [TE]) is taken at longer and longer times after excitation. Almost all pathologic processes (eg, tumors, inflammatory disease, infections, trauma) result in increased water content and edema. For this reason, they are best seen on

Table 3
T1 Relaxation values for various tissues

Brain	1.5 T	4.0 T
Gray matter	850 [21]–1023 [23]	1724 [77]
White matter	550 [21]–710 [23]	1043 [77]
Cerebrospinal fluid	3200 [21]	4550 [77]
Fat (adipose)	200 [106]	
Muscle	800 [106]	

T2W images. The optimum TE should be that closest to the T2 of the tissue of interest [22]. For instance, a cyst or area of edema may have long T2 times; sampling is best done at long TEs to distinguish the affected area from adjacent tumor tissues. If one wishes to distinguish between gray and white matter (Fig. 22), such long TEs are not advantageous, because a significant amount of signal is lost; the tissue is sampled long after the optimum difference between the signal intensities is observed. If one wishes to view only cerebrospinal fluid (CSF), a long T2 of 200 milliseconds provides a myelographic effect (Fig. 23). Such relative signal intensity for different substances as a function of TE is illustrated in Fig. 24. Table 4 gives T2 relaxation values for various biologic tissues and fluids. T2 relaxation, unlike T1 relaxation, is not field dependent. Equipment variances and differences in sampling techniques have led to wide variations in reported T2 values of different tissues. Again, these cannot be used to compare absolute values. However, on a given MRI machine, the reproducibility of T1 and T2 measurements is excellent, ranging from 5% to 9% variance [23].

Initially, it was hoped that different pathologic processes could be differentiated on the basis of characteristics T1 and T2 signatures [24,25]. Unfortunately, there is a wide overlap between benign and malignant processes [26–28], yielding

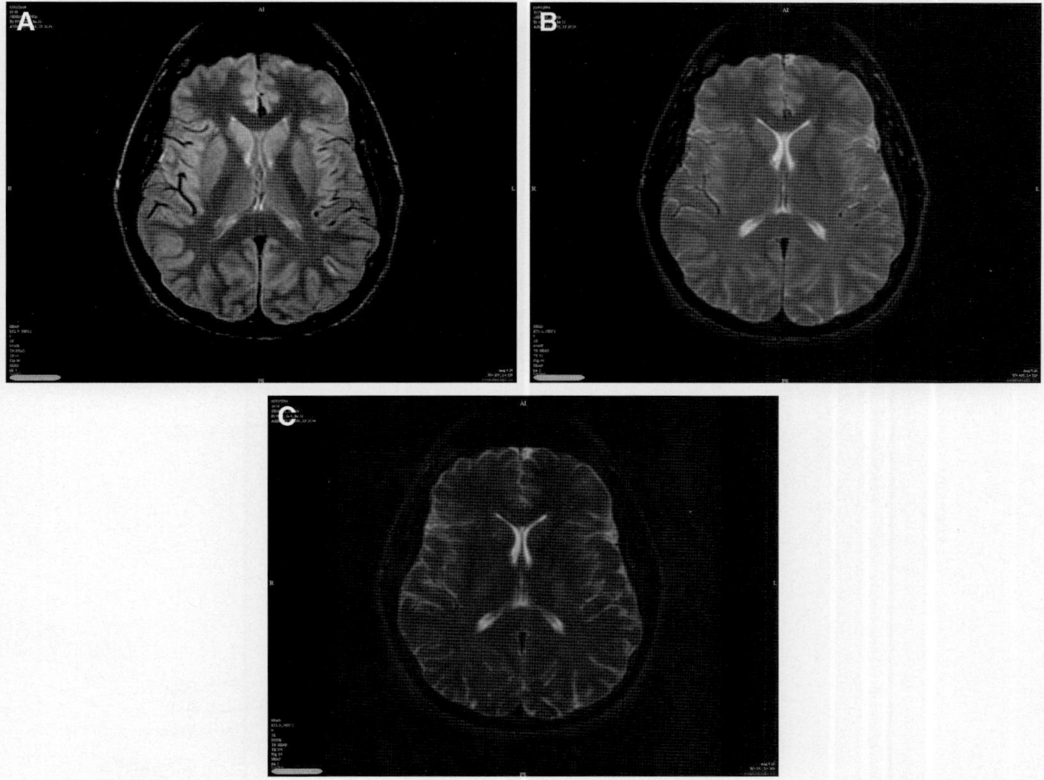

Fig. 22. A patient studied with Carr-Purcell-Meiboom-Gill sequence, multiecho, T2-weighted images with echoes at 31, 81, and 160 milliseconds. (*A*) At the lower echo time (TE; 31 milliseconds), the best gray/white differentiation is achieved. Notice that the white matter is relatively dark compared with the gray matter at a TE of 81 milliseconds (*B*) and 160 milliseconds (*C*). With an extremely long TE, however, the cerebrospinal fluid is prominently displayed, but there is loss of the gray/white differentiation.

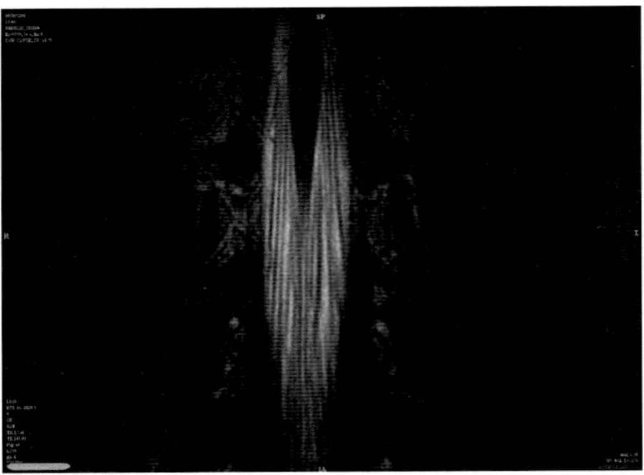

Fig. 23. Fast spin echo (FSE), heavily T2-weighted, coronal, lumbar MRI scan demonstrating excellent contrast between the cerebrospinal fluid of the subarachnoid space and the conus medullaris (*arrows*). All other structures are relatively dark. (FSE repetition time = 8000 milliseconds, echo train length = 16 milliseconds, echo time = 192 milliseconds, 24-cm field of view, 4-mm slice, 512 × 384 matrix, number of excitations = 2).

little benefit to measuring T1 or T2 of a given disease. Furthermore, the characterization of pathologic processes is complex by relaxation measurements and changes as the pathologic process develops [29].

Table 4
T2 Relaxation values for various biologic tissues and fluids

	T2	Frequency (MHz)
White matter	65 [106]–75 [23]	60
Grey matter	105 [106]–85 [23]	60
Cerebrospinal fluid	2000 [107]	25 [107]
Blood	250	20
Fat	200	60
Muscle	63	63

Data from different experiments and under different conditions.

From Bottomley PA, Foster TH, Argersinger, Pfeifer LM. A review of normal tissue hydrogen NMR relaxation times and relaxation mechanisms from 1–100 MHz: dependence on tissue type, NMR frequency, temperature, species, excision and age. Med Physic 1984;11(4): 425–48; with permission.

How much hydrogen is available to image

A third important parameter of signal intensity is that of the hydrogen spin density. Substances that contain more hydrogen atoms have more signal than those with fewer hydrogen atoms (eg, water versus bone). An obvious fact is that if the hydrogen atoms move out of the plane of interest

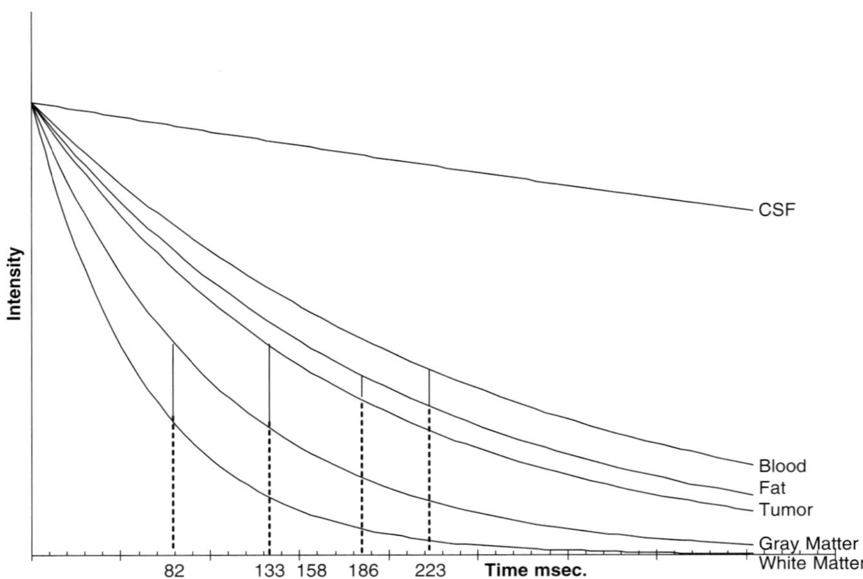

Fig. 24. Hypothetic T2 decay curves for various biologic substances, such as white matter, gray matter, cysts, and tumors. Notice that the best time to sample the data (echo time [TE]) depends on what one is looking for [ie, if one wishes to distinguish between gray and white matter, a TE of 65 milliseconds is chosen; if one wishes to distinguish between gray matter and cerebrospinal fluid, a TE of 145 milliseconds is chosen]).

during signal acquisition, signal is again lost. This can be illustrated by the flow void seen with flowing vessels.

We can combine these concepts into a single equation that should not be difficult to understand [22]. The signal intensity (I) for a given sample is related to the number of hydrogen atoms (ie, hydrogen spin density) given by S and to two exponential decay components: the T1 relaxation given by $1 - e^{-(\frac{TR}{T1})}$ and the T2 relaxation given by $e^{-(\frac{TE}{T2})}$; therefore, $I = S \times [1 - e^{-(\frac{TR}{T1})}]\ [e^{-(\frac{TE}{T2})}]$. For signal to be acquired, the magnetization vector must precess within the *x-y* plane and must be coherent.

To summarize our model thus far, the spinning of small subatomic particles creates a small magnetic dipole. The energy of interaction with an externally applied magnetic field can exist only in discrete energy states (quantum levels). For the hydrogen proton, there are two allowed. In a magnetic field, these nuclear dipoles precess around the *z*-axis. A thermal equilibrium is established with populations of dipoles spinning with and against the applied magnetic field. When suitable energy is given in the form of RF, a small fraction of these hydrogen nuclei can be excited and brought into phase coherence, precessing in the *x-y* plane. Over time, their orientations reestablish equilibrium with the magnetic field (B_o) at a rate given by the exponential time constant T1. They lose phase coherence with an exponential time constant known as T2. Their precessional rate is only dependent on the net local magnetic field experienced by the nucleus. T1 relaxation is thus governed by how quickly the nuclei exchange energy with the lattice or surrounding molecules, and T2 relaxation is governed by local magnetic field inhomogeneities.

Basic pulse sequences

I have purposely been vague up to this point as to the exact pulse sequences and gradients that are needed to establish this. So far, we have only given the example of a 90° RF pulse causing an FID.

A "bewildering" array of pulse sequences is available for MRI [30]. Slight variations on these sequences have led to various acronyms. Some pulse sequences are nearly synonymous with or identical to others but have been given different names by different authors. Spin echo (SE), inversion recovery (IR), short time inversion recovery (STIR), gradient-recalled acquisition in the steady state (GRASS), steady-state free precession (SSFP), Carr-Purcell-Meiboom-Gill (CPMG) sequence, to name only a few, are included in the current literature. On top of that, with each new pulse sequence modified by variations of gradients and acquisition times, equipment manufacturers have coined acronyms for their own particular use (Box 1).

We now examine the standard SE sequence that is at the heart of most conventional MRI. Other pulse sequences, such as IR and fluid-attenuated inversion recovery (FLAIR), are explained. Gradient-recalled echo and limited flip angle techniques that are variations of the SE pulse are also introduced. I limit discussion of the pulse sequences in this article based only on their ability to discriminate different tissue signal characteristics, including T1 and T2 relaxation. The length of this primer does not allow one to cover the breadth of MRI pulse sequences. Modifications of these sequences are also used to measure flow, phase, diffusion, and perfusion as well as to reduce artifacts and perform functional imaging. The interested reader is referred to the textbook *Neuroimaging, Clinical and Physical Principles* [31].

Table 5 is a summary of some of the most common pulse sequences used in MRI today. A basic understanding of the pulse sequences used to generate signals in the NMR experiment is necessary, because this lies at the heart of the data recorded. The pulse sequence can be thought of in three phases:

1. A preparation pulse to excite the tissue. The manner in which the tissue is excited, whether it is a short flip angle or large flip angle, has a significant impact on T1 contrast.
2. A time interval between excitation of the tissue and acquisition of the data. This is the period during which dephasing (T2 relaxation) occurs. A longer time increases T2 effect.
3. The overall time between data sampling, or TR. A long TR allows samples to recover, minimizing T1 contrast, whereas a short TR accentuates T1 contrast.

Spin echo pulse

A SE sequence is established as follows. RF energy is given to the system at the Larmour frequency with enough intensity to flip the magnetic vector into the *x-y* plane. This is the so-called "90° pulse." The vector then precesses in

Box 1. Acronyms

3D FASTER	Three-dimensional field echo acquisition with a short repetition time and echo reduction
3D GRE	Three-dimensional gradient echo
3D MPRACE	Three-dimensional magnetization prepared rapid gradient echo
ADC	Apparent diffusion coefficient
BASE	Basis imaging with selective inversion-prepared
bEPI	Blipped echoplanner imaging
BMS	Bulk magnetic susceptibility
BOLD	Blood oxygenation level-dependent contrast
BOSS	Bimodal slice select radiofrequency pulse
BP MR	Biphasic MRI
BW	Bandwidth
CBF	Cerebral blood flow
CBV	Cerebral blood volume
CE-FAST	Contrast-enhanced Fourier acquired steady-state technique
CNR	Contrast-to-noise ratio
CP	Cross-polarization
CPMG	Carr-Purcell-Meiboom-Gill (measurements of T2)
CSF	Cerebrospinal fluid
CSMEMP	Contiguous slice multiecho multiplanar
DIGGEST	Direct imaging of local gradients by group echo selection tomography
DISE	Driven inversion spin echo
DMSSFP	Double-mode steady-state free precession
DOPING	Double pulse interfaced echo imaging
DPSF	Diffusion perfusion snapshot flash
DSC	Dynamic susceptibility contrast
DWI	Diffusion-weighted imaging
EPC	Echo phase correction
EPI	Echoplanar imaging
EPISTAR	Echoplanar imaging and signal targeting with alternating radiofrequency
ETL	Echo train length
FAcE	Free induction decay acquired echoes
FAISE	Fast acquisition interleaved spin echo (which is the same as fast spin echo)
FAST	Fourier-acquired steady-state technique
FATS	Fat-suppressed acquisition with echo times and real times shortened
FC	Flow compensation
FE	Field echo, frequency encode
FEER	Field even echo rephasing
FFE	Fast field echo
FFF	Fast Fourier flow
FFP	Fast Fourier projection
FID	Free induction decay
FIRFT	Fast inversion recovery Fourier transform
FISP	Fast imaging with steady-state precession
FLAG	Flow-adjusted gradients
FLAIR	Fluid attenuation inversion recovery
FLASH	Fast low-angle shot
fMRI	Functional MRI
FONAR	Field focusing nuclear magnetic resonance
FOV	Field of view

FR	Frequency encode
FSE	Fast spin echo (turbo spin echo)
FT	Fourier transform
FWHM	Full-width at half-maximum
G	Gauss
GARP	Globally optimized alternating phase Rectangular pulse
GATORCIST	Respiratory gated imaging
Gd	Gadolinium
GINSEST	Generalized interferography using spin echoes and stimulated echoes
GMN	Gradient moment nulling
GMR	Gradient moment rephrasing
GRASE	Gradient spin echo
GRASS	Gradient acquisition in steady state
GRE	Gradient echo imaging
GREAT	Ghost reduction by equalized acquisition triplets
GROPE	Generalized compensation for resonance offset and pulse length errors
HASTE	Half-Fourier acquisition single-shot turbo spin echo
IR	Inversion recovery
IR-EPI	Inversion recovery echoplanar imaging
IVIM	Intra voxel incoherent motion
LFA	Limited flip angle
MAST	Motion artifact suppression technique
MBEST	Modulus blipped echoplanar single-pulse technique
MBS-MRA	Minimum basis set magnetic resonance angiography
MEMP	Multiecho multiplanar
MESS	Multiple echo single shot
mFISP	Mirrored fast imaging with steady-state precession
MIP	Maximum intensity projection
MOTSA	Multiple overlapping thin slab acquisition
MPGR	Multiplanar gradient recalled
MPIR	Multiplanar inversion recovery
MPRAGE	Magnetization prepared rapid gradient echo
MR	Magnetic resonance
MRA	Magnetic resonance angiography
MRI	Magnetic resonance imaging
MS-EPI	Multishot echoplanar imaging
MSIT	Multiple slab imaging technique
MT	Magnetic transfer
MTC	Magnetization transfer contrast
MTR	Magnetization transfer ratio
MTSA	Multiple thin slab acquisition
NEX	Number of excitations
NMR	Nuclear magnetic resonance
NSA	Number of signal averages
PAIR	Partial volume-sensitized inversion recovery
PC	Phase contrast
PE	Phase encoding
PEDD	Proton-electron dipole dipole
PEG	Phase encode grouping
PGSE	Pulsed gradient spin echo
PIETIR	Prolonged inversion and echo time inversion recovery

(*continued on next page*)

POMP	Phase-ordered multiplanar
PPG	Peripheral pulse gating
PPM	Parts per millions
PRE	Proton relaxation enhancement
PRFT	Partially relaxed Fourier transform
PSIF	Mirrored fast imaging with steady precession
PT2	Preferential T2
QCSI	Quantitative chemical shift imaging
QMRI	Quantitative MRI
QUIPSS	Quantitative imaging of perfusion using a single subtraction
RACE	Real time acquisition and evaluation of motion
RAM FAST	Rapid acquisition matrix Fourier acquired steady-state technique
RARE	Rapid acquisition relaxation enhanced
RARE	Rapid acquisition with refocused echoes
RASE	Rapid acquisition spin echo
RBC	Red blood cell
rCBF	Regional cerebral blood flow
RF	Radiofrequency
RF-FAST	Radiofrequency Fourier-acquired steady-state technique
ROI	Region of interest
ROPE	Respiratory ordered phase encoding
RUFIS	Rotating ultrafast imaging sequence
SAAV	Simultaneous acquisition of artery and vein
SAR	Specific absorption rate
SAT	Saturation pulse
SD	Standard deviation
SE	Spin echo
sEPI	Spiral echoplanar imaging
SIMUSIM	Simultaneous multislice imaging
SIP	Saturation inversion projection
SMART	Simultaneous multislice acquisition using rosette trajectories
SmaRT	Simulataneous multislice acquisition with arterial-flow tagging
SMI	Simulataneous multislice imaging
SNR	Signal-to-noise ratio
SPACE	Spatial and Chemical-shift encoded excitation
SPAMM	Spatial modulation of magnetization
SPECT	Single photon emission computed tomography
SPGR	Spoiled gradient recalled (spoiled gradient acquisition in steady state)
SPIR	Selective population inversion recovery
SS	Slice select gradient
SSFP	Steady-state free precession
SSP	Section-sensitivity profile
STE	Stimulated echo
STIR	Short tau (inversion time) inversion recovery
STREAM	Suppressed tissue with refreshment angiography method
T	Tesla
T2 FFE	T2 fast field echo
T2 PEDD	T2 proton electron dipole dipole interaction
T2 PRE	T2 proton relaxation enhancement
TCF	Time correlation function
TD	Trigger delay
TE	Time delay between excitation and echo maximum

TEI	TE interleaved
TFE	Turbo field echo
TI	Time following inversion pulse
TMR	Topical magnetic resonance
TOF	Time of flight
TONE	Tilt optimized nonselective excitation
TOSS	Total suppression of sidebands
TPPI	Time-proportional phase incrementation
TR	Time to repetition
TRICKS	Time-resolved imaging of contrast kinetics
TSE	Turbo spin echo
TSR	Total saturation recovery
Turbo FLASH	Turbo fast low-angle-shot
URGE	Ultra rapid gradient echo
USPIO	Ultra small superparamagnetic Iron oxide
VAS	Variable angle spinning
VEMP	Variable echo multiplanar
VENC	Velocity encoding value
VIGRE	Gradient echo
VINNIE	Velocity encode cine imaging
VOI	Volume of interest
VPS	Views per segment
WATERGATE	Water suppression pulse sequence
WEFT	Water-eliminated Fourier transform

the *x-y* plane in a coherent fashion. Over a short period, the individual nuclei comprising the net vector drift out of phase. The signal rapidly decays as an FID. If the receiver coil were turned on at this time, a sinusoidal wave of rapidly decreasing intensity would be produced (ie, an FID). A certain time later (1–100 milliseconds in imaging), a second RF pulse is given, which now corresponds to a 180° pulse. The vectors are inverted, which causes them to spin in the opposite direction. Fast-spinning protons are now behind the slower protons, and phase coherence can be re-established for those protons that became out of phase because of static magnetic field inhomogeneities. Fig. 25 displays the SE pulse sequence in which the magnetization is deflected into the *x-y* plane, loses phase coherence and is then inverted by a 180° pulse, changes rotational direction, and is rephased. Over a period equal to the time between the 90° and 180° pulses, phase coherence is re-established and signal is generated as an echo. The data are then acquired. The total elapsed time from the 90° pulse to the echo is called the TE, or "time to echo." This is the prototype SE, or Hahn echo [32], described only a few years after the discovery of NMR.

The entire pulse sequence is repeated many times in a typical experiment. Several averages or number of excitations (NEXs) may be obtained to increase the signal-to-noise ratio. Multiple phase-encoding steps are taken to achieve spatial localization. The time for which the pulse sequence is repeated is called the TR, or "time of repetition." Fig. 26 shows the entire pulse sequence. Image contrast is a function of the timing parameters chosen, TE, TR, and tissue-specific properties [33–35]. All image contrast has some effects from T1, T2, and proton density; therefore, sequences are designated as being "weighted" toward a given parameter.

Proton density weighting

Consider first the consequences of altering the TR. Assume that the TE is taken to be as short as possible to reduce T2 or dephasing effects. If a long TR is used, all the magnetization will have returned to the *z*-axis. At the start of the next pulse train, it will be available for deflection into the *x-y* plane. This gives maximum signal, and the relative signal intensities of tissues are based not on the relative T1 relaxation characteristics but on how much hydrogen there is (ie, proton density),

Table 5
Common pulse sequences used in MRI

Acronym	Pulse sequence	TE	Range	TR	Range	Flip	TI	Contrast effect
SE	Spin-echo	Short Short Long	5–20 10–20 40–200	Long Short Long	200–600 2000–4000 2000–4000	90° 90° 90°	None	T1W Proton T2W
CPMG	Multi-echo	Short Long	20–60 80–200	Long >2000 milliseconds	2000–4000	90°	None	Proton and T2W
GRASS	Gradient echo	Short Long Short	2–20 5–40 5–10	Short Short Long	10–50[a] 10–50 400–800	45° <20° 45E–90°	None	Proton/steady state T2*W/steady state T1W
SPGR	Spoiled grass	Short	2–10	Short	5–500[a]	45–90	None	T1W
IR	Inversion recovery	Minimum Short	10–20	Long >2000 milliseconds	2000–4000	180°	Medium 600 milliseconds	Heavy T1W
STIR	Short time inversion recovery	Long	50–120	Long >3000 milliseconds	2000–4000	180°	170 milliseconds Short	T1W and T2W are additive, suppresses fat
FLAIR	Fluid-attenuated inversion recovery	Long 150 milliseconds	80–200	Very long 6000 milliseconds	4000–8000	180°	2000 milliseconds Long	T2W with attenuation of free water

[a] Depends on flip angle.

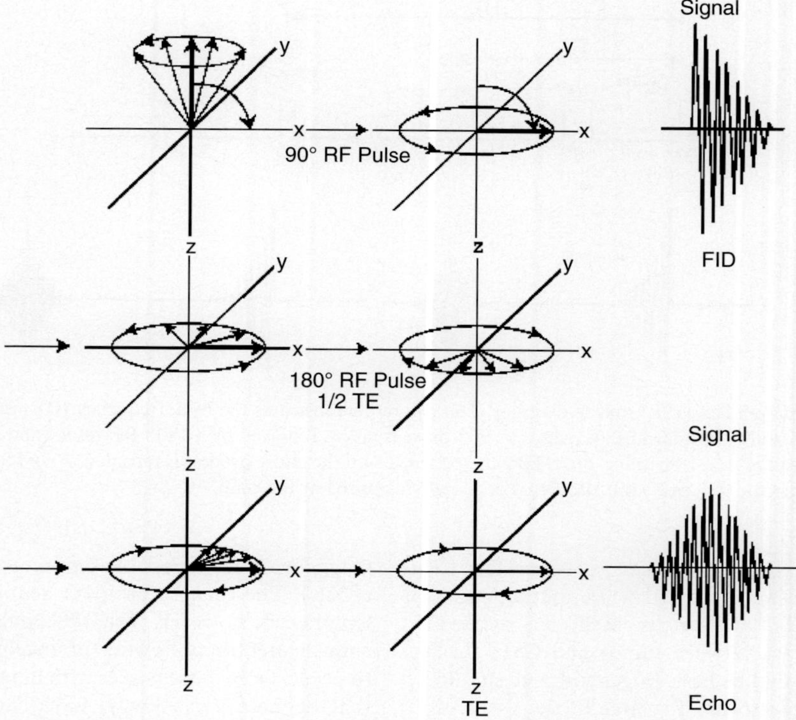

Fig. 25. Magnetic vector diagram of standard spin echo sequence. The incoherent precessing vectors are brought into coherence, and the net vector is tipped into the *x-y* plane. A free induction decay (FID) occurs. After a short time, the vectors begin to dephase. A 180° radiofrequency (RF) pulse is then applied, inverting the vectors and reversing their direction. After a period of time has elapsed (echo time [TE]), the vectors rephase and an echo is produced.

as illustrated in Fig. 27. Proton density contrast is often misunderstood or ignored. Wehrli et al [36] demonstrated that most of the contrast seen between gray and white matter on T2W SE sequences can be ascribed to differences in proton density: gray matter has more water protons than white matter. Furthermore, to achieve maximum tissue contrast, the selection of pulse sequence to be used is highly dependent on hydrogen spin density. As the ratio of spin densities increases between two substances, SE becomes a better pulse sequence than IR [37].

T1 weighting

Suppose, however, that only a short time is allowed for the magnetization to recover to the *z*-axis. Only those substances that have extremely short T1s will have achieved their full potential magnetization before being pulsed with a repeat pulse, as illustrated in Fig. 28. The pulse sequence then becomes T1W, allowing for differential intensities to be observed between substances that have differing T1 values. The equation describing just the recovery of longitudinal magnetization as a function of time is: Magnetization $= Mz\ (1 - e^{-TR/T1})$, where Mz is the total net magnetic vector in the *z*-axis before 90° excitation, TR is repetition time, and T1 is a constant for each tissue. The time for complete relaxation is infinity. For 99% recovery, one must wait 4.6 times T1, as shown previously in Fig. 15. Obviously, most of the relaxation occurs within the first 2.0 times T1. Different tissues and substances have characteristic relaxation rates specific to that individual material. Furthermore, as was discussed earlier, T1 relaxation is also dependent on magnetic field strength. To optimize tissue contrast between voxels containing elements of different T1 relaxation values, one should thus know what the relaxation rate for a given tissue is. In Fig. 29, a family of curves of tissues with

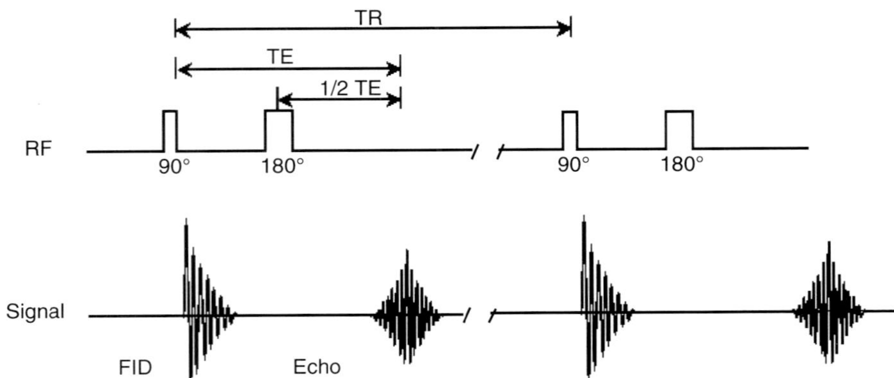

Fig. 26. Standard spin echo (SE) timing diagram. This figure demonstrates the radiofrequency (RF) pulse timing and associated signal from a standard SE sequence. A 90° pulse is given, followed by a 180° RF refocusing pulse at ½ echo time (TE). A period of time (repetition time [TR]) then elapses, and the entire process is repeated. An FID (free induction decay) occurs after the 90° pulse but the signal is actually acquired at the echo.

different T1 relaxation values is illustrated to discriminate between fat and white matter which have short T1s, a short is used. To achieve maximal contrast between tumor and CSF, then a longer TR would be best. In general, one should select a TR close to the T1 value of the tissue of interest. This ensures the widest possible separation between tissues with close T1 values.

T2 weighting

The SE sequence can also be used to acquire T2W data. In this instance, the TR between pulses is set quite long so that as much of the longitudinal magnetization as possible can recover (ie, no T1 effects). The time before data acquisition is now lengthened, however. The 180° pulse is given at a much later time, allowing for increased dephasing to occur. Only those tissues with long T2s (ie, those that dephase very slowly) have enough residual phase coherence available so that when the 180° pulse is applied, they can be brought back into phase. Because of phase losses incurred from non-static magnetic field inhomogeneities, only a fraction of the initial magnetization vector can be recovered. By necessity, less and less signal is acquired as TEs are lengthened and images become noisier. Fig. 30 illustrates this pulse sequence.

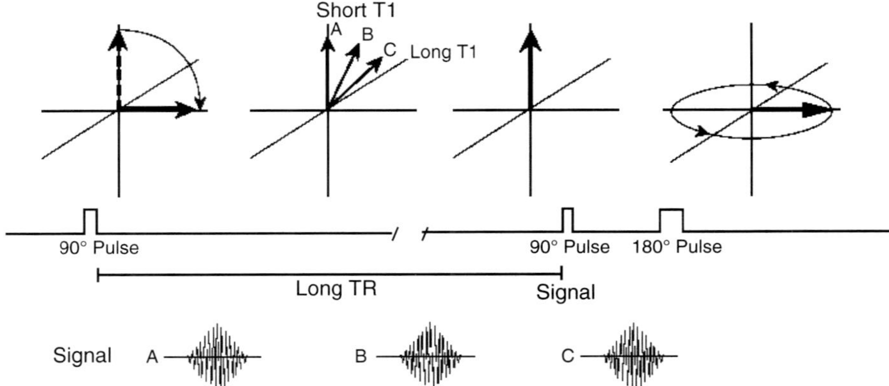

Fig. 27. Proton-weighted sequence. A 90° radiofrequency pulse is given. A long time (repetition time [TR]) elapses, and all the tissues (A, B, and C) relax to the ground state. When the next 90° pulse is given, 100% of the magnetization is available to tip again into the *x-y* plane. Therefore, maximum signal is achieved. Only if the materials have a different proton density (ie, quantity of available mobile hydrogen) is there a difference in signal between the three tissues.

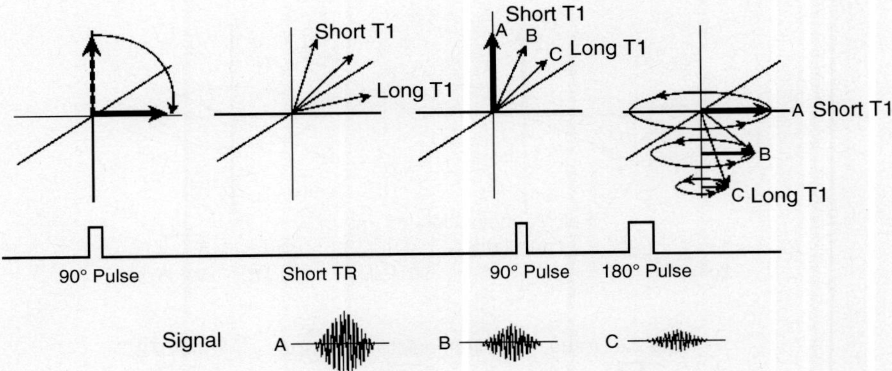

Fig. 28. T1-weighted pulse sequence. A 90° radiofrequency pulse is given, and a short time elapses before repeating the process. Tissue A with a short T1 has relaxed to the ground state, giving a maximum vector when reflipped into the *x-y* plane. Tissue C with a long T1 has not relaxed to the ground state, however. When the tissue is given a new 90° pulse, only a small vector is produced, creating substantially less signal intensity. In this pulse sequence, tissues with a short T1 relaxation time (TR) are the brightest.

Substances that have prolonged T2 values include free water, such as CSF, edema, cysts, and most pathologic processes in which tissue injury has occurred. T2W images, although having a lower signal-to-noise ratio than T1W images, are still the most useful for diagnostic neuroimaging [36].

Carr-Purcell-Meiboom-Gill sequence

The CPMG sequence [38,39] is a commonly used variation of the SE pulse sequence. In fact, most T2W SE sequences use this technique to acquire proton and T2W images simultaneously. The first part of this pulse sequence is exactly like

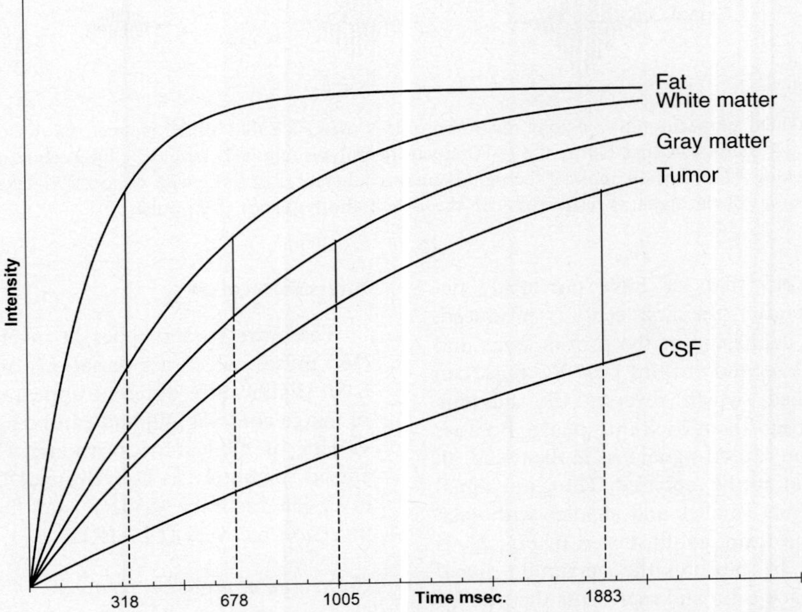

Fig. 29. Relaxation curves for different tissues, A through E. The optimal time to discriminate between fat and white matter would be at 318 milliseconds. In other words, a short repetition time (TR) is best to discriminate between tissues of short T1 values. A longer TR would be better to discriminate between tissues of longer T1 values, such as tumor and cerebrospinal fluid; in this case, 1883 milliseconds at 1.5-T field strength. CSF, cerebrospinal fluid.

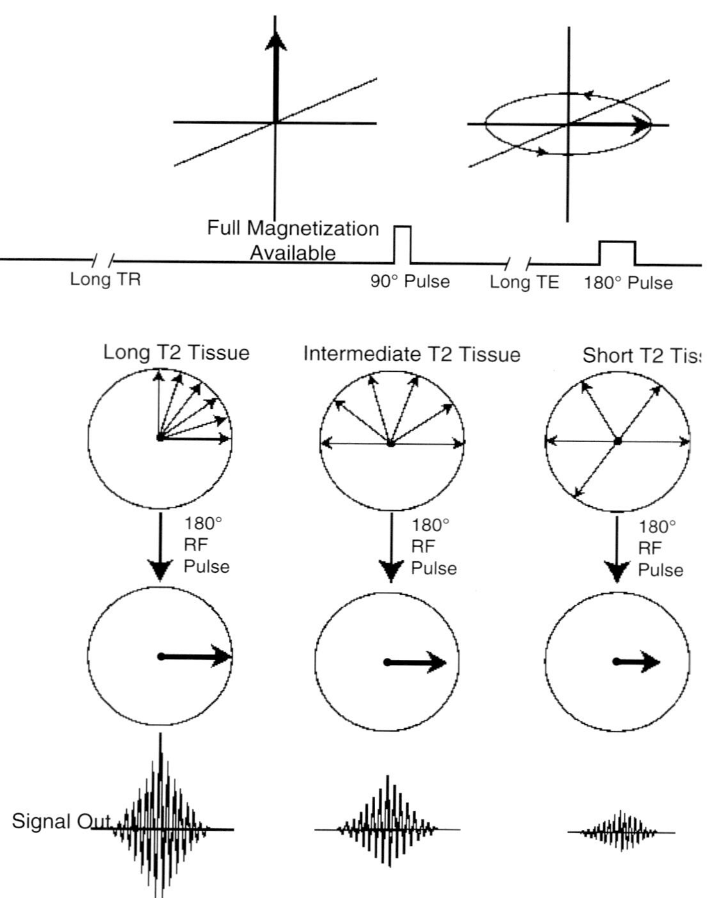

Fig. 30. T2-weighted spin echo pulse. A long repetition time is used such that all the magnetization is available before tipping into the x-y plane. The time before the 180° refocusing pulse is relatively long (ie, a long echo time [TE] is used). For tissues with long T2 relaxation, most of the signal remains coherent. For those with a short T2 relaxation time (TR), only a small amount of the signal is recovered with the 180° radiofrequency (RF) pulse.

the SE sequence that we have previously described. Soon after the first echo is produced, there is rapid dephasing of the proton spins and signal is lost. A second or third 180° RF pulse can then be applied, which reverses the spinning vectors and brings them back into phase. Because of T2 relaxation caused signal loss in the tissue, all of the signal cannot be rephased. Thus, our signal progressively gets smaller and smaller with each echo. This echo train, as illustrated in Fig. 31, is a curve fitted by plotting the maximum signal intensities at each echo and represents the true T2 relaxation curve for the tissue. The rapid T2 decay for the FID of each echo is the result of true tissue T2 and dephasing from static magnetic field inhomogeneity. Together, these are called T2*.

Inversion recovery

There are several types of inversion recovery (IR) pulses, which are variations on a theme but have significantly different appearances in terms of image contrast [40] and can be used for a wide variety of clinical applications. These are discussed separately as conventional IR, short-time inversion recovery (STIR), and fluid-attenuated inversion recovery (FLAIR).

Conventional inversion recovery

In the usual IR pulse sequence [34], a 180° pulse is given, which rotates the magnetization vector into the negative z-direction, as shown in Fig. 32. Note that this requires twice the RF power

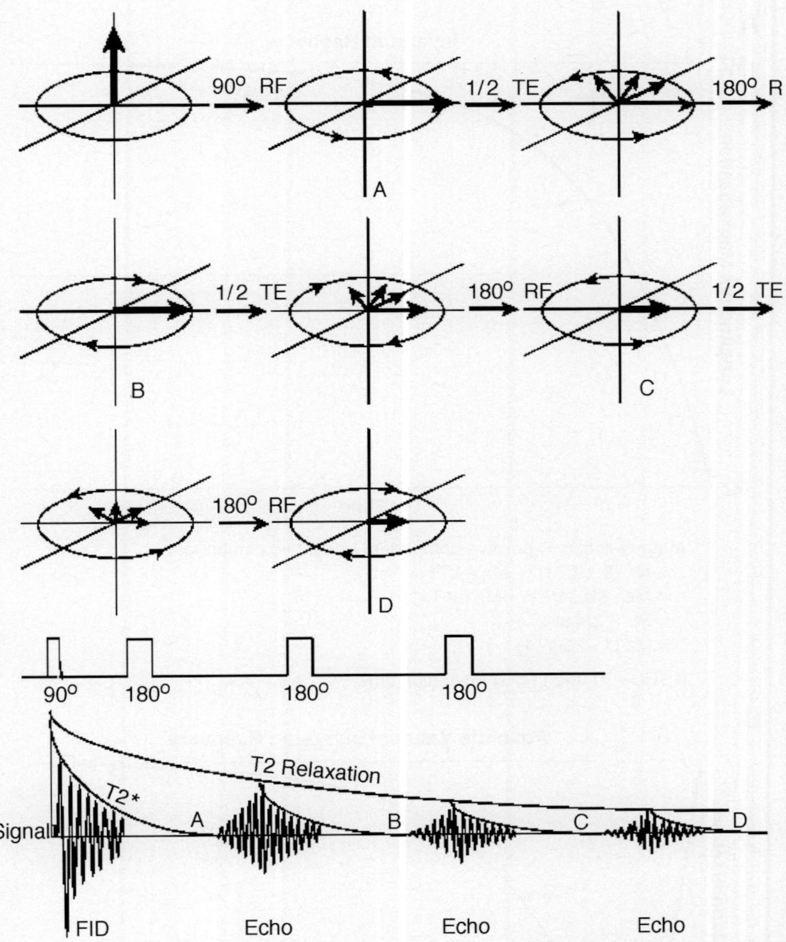

Fig. 31. Carr-Purcell-Meiboom-Gill sequence. This sequence applies a series of refocusing 180° radiofrequency (RF) pulses with repeated echoes. A curve of signal decay can be traced, giving the T2 relaxation of the substance. FID, free induction decay; TE, echo time.

and that it also requires a longer time to recover to the steady-state positive *z*-direction. This is governed by the exponential decay time constant, T1. If TR is assumed to be extremely long relative to T1, the equation describing T1 relaxation can be shown to be: Signal = $S_o (1 - 2e^{TI/T1})$, where S_o is the total *z*-component of the magnetic vector, TI is the time to inversion, T1 is the familiar relaxation constant (which is tissue dependent) [33], and TR is repetition time.

Fig. 33 shows the typical way in which the signal intensity from an IR pulse sequence is plotted as a function of time. After inversion, as the magnetization vectors begin returning to the *z*-axis, those with short T1s do so first. At a time called TI, a 90° pulse is given. If this is performed

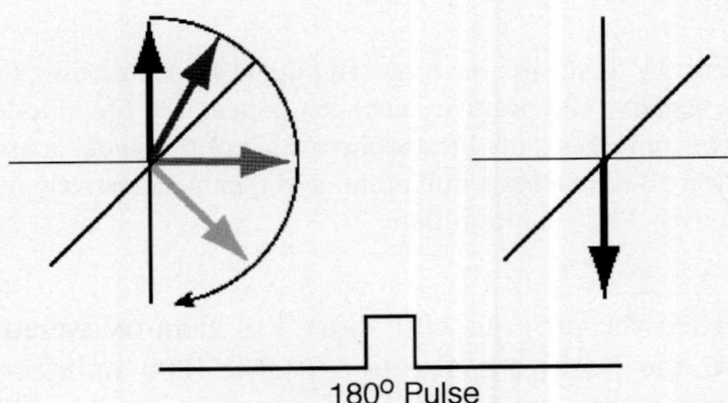

Fig. 32. Inversion recovery pulse sequence. With a 180° radiofrequency pulse, the magnetization vector is rotated 180° to the negative *z*-direction.

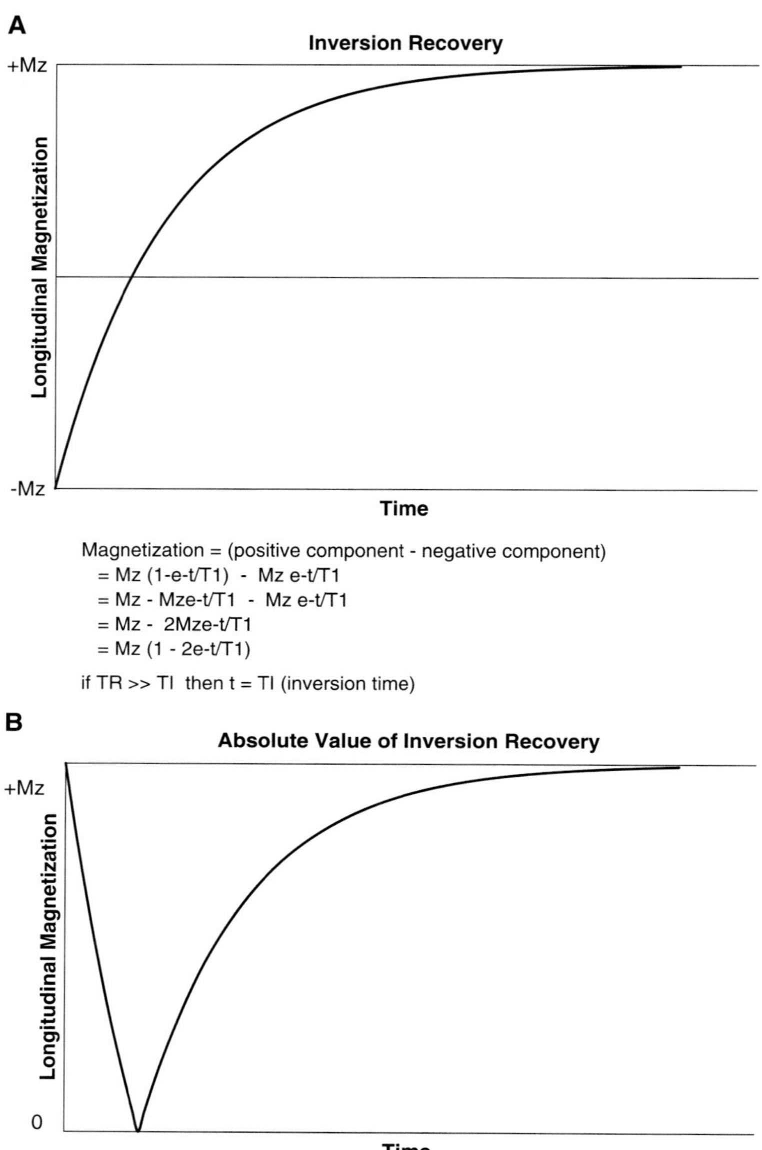

Fig. 33. Inversion recovery (IR) signal reconstruction. (*A*) Exponential recovery of magnetization after IR pulse. IR has a negative and positive signal component. (*B*) Magnitude reconstruction of the IR pulse. When the data are analyzed by the computer, only the absolute value of the signal is usually taken. Thus, signal intensity for a given substance initially decreases, reaches a null point, and then progressively returns to full magnetization when the vector reaches the positive *z*-axis. TR, repetition time.

when the protons with short T1s have recovered to the positive *z*-direction (~500–1000 milliseconds), they are then flipped into the *x-y* plane to produce signal. The net vector of the slower relaxing nuclei (which has perhaps only recovered to the *x-y* plane at the time of the 90° pulse) is returned to the negative *z*-direction and produces no significant signal in the FID. Thus, only protons with short T1s have recovered and are brought into the *x-y* plane to have their signals sampled. Sampling occurs by using another rephasing 180° pulse just like the SE technique, and

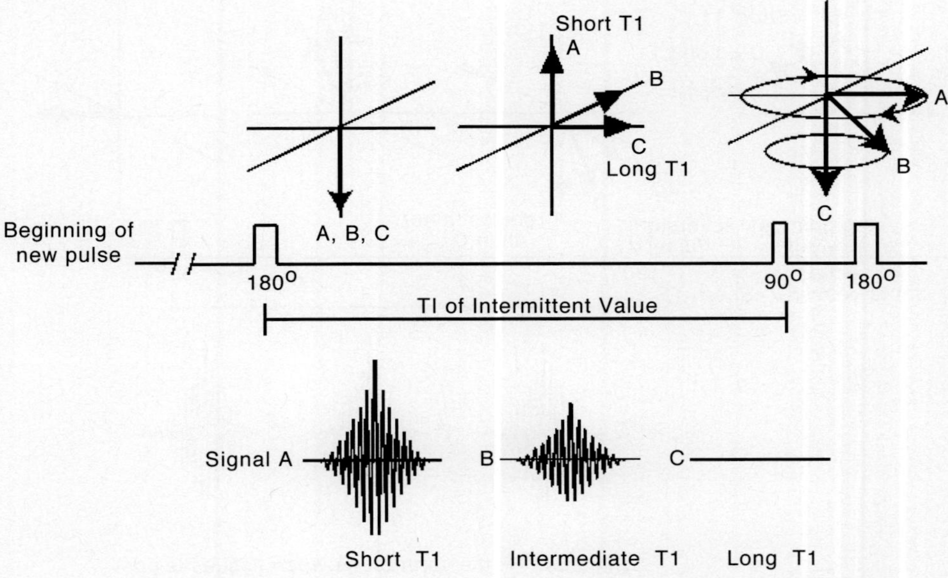

Fig. 34. Conventional T1-weighted inversion recovery pulse sequence. A 180° radiofrequency (RF) pulse is given, inverting the vectors of tissues A, B, and C. After a period called the time to inversion (TI), tissues with short T1s, such as those labeled A, have largely returned to the *z*-axis. Tissues with long T1s, such as those labeled C, are now in the *x-y* plane. A 90° RF pulse is applied, followed in short succession by sampling of the echo with a 180° pulse. The effect of this is to rotate the vectors of tissue A into the *x-y* plane and give maximum signal intensity. Those tissues with longer T1s, such as those labeled C, give little signal intensity.

the echo is then sampled a short time (½ TE) later. This is sometimes called an inversion recovery spin echo pulse sequence [41]. In general, for a T1W sequence, parameters are chosen such that the TI is approximately equal to the T1 of the tissue of interest. This ensures that most of the dipoles have recovered to the *z*-axis; if you wait too long, all the vectors recover, yielding no contrast. For brain, the T1 of white matter is ≈500 to 600 milliseconds at 1.5 T. A minimum TE is used to reduce T2 weighting. This pulse sequence is illustrated in Fig. 34. The second 180° pulse is given to rephase the protons and recover signal lost from static field inhomogeneity. It also facilitates data collection, because the necessary phase-encoding and frequency-encoding gradients needed for two-dimensional (2D) image reconstruction can be applied.

If a long TE is chosen (ie, the sample is allowed to dephase for a significant time before the second 180° pulse is given), the sample becomes T1W and T2W. This has self-negating effects. The tissues are sampled such that only protons that have short T1s are detected; they are then dephased, giving low signal.

Inversion recovery imaging with a repetition time that is short

For T1 contrast to be achieved, a fairly long TR is needed. Consider, for instance, what happens if not enough time is allowed before the process is repeated. Let's assume that after all the pulses, the vectors with short T1s are now beginning to align with the *z*-axis. Those with longer T1s are precessing just above the *x-y* plane, however. If these protons are reirradiated with a 180° pulse, as illustrated in Fig. 35, the vectors with short T1s are inverted to the negative *z*-axis. Those with longer T1s are now precessing in the *x-y* plane. After a period, the short T1 protons will have caught up with the longer T1 protons, they will both be in the *z*-plane at the time the next 90° pulse is given, and both will be inverted into the *x-y* plane and give signal. Thus, no contrast is achieved. With IR, the TR must long.

As discussed in later sections, the TR is a major determinant of total imaging time. Although spectacular T1W images can be obtained using IR, the imaging time required is significantly longer than with SE technique. The T1W IR

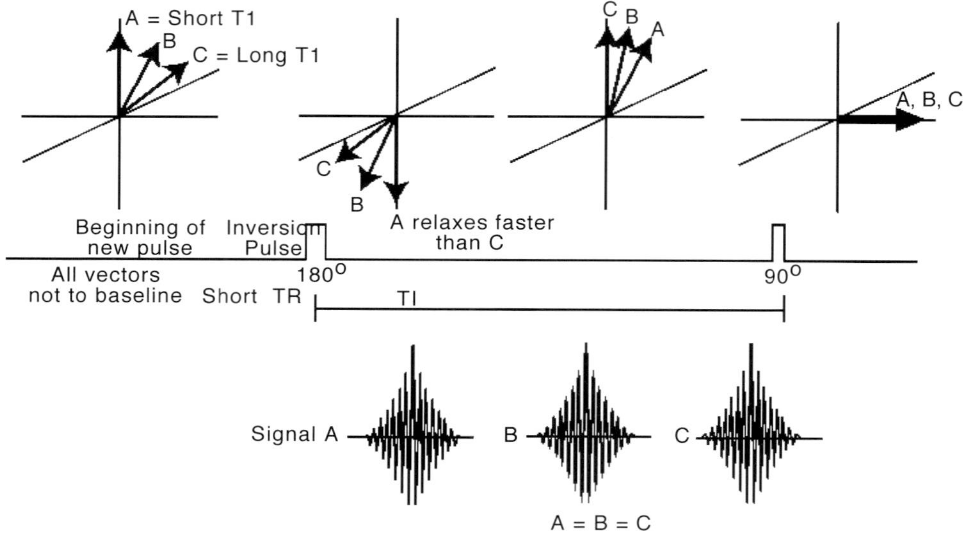

Fig. 35. Inversion recovery (IR) with a short repetition time (TR). What happens if the TR is too short? At the beginning of the sequence, the tissues have not fully relaxed. When they are inverted, the slower relaxing tissues have not fully relaxed. When they are inverted, the slower relaxing tissues, such as those labeled C, are ahead of those with a short T1. When the tissues are sampled at the time to inversion (TI) with a 90° pulse, there is no contrast between them. For this reason, the TR must be long with IR sequences.

image of the brain illustrated in Fig. 36 required 17 minutes, whereas the SE T1W image of the same patient illustrated in Fig. 37A took only 5 minutes for the same NEX. Fig 37B shows an IR fast sequence with a multiecho acquisition that took only 2 minutes. Consequently, IR sequences are rarely used for routine T1W imaging unless they are used in conjunction with newer fast SE technology. They find special application in the imaging of myelination of the brain in young infants and other areas in which optimum T1 contrast is desired. They are useful in evaluating multiple sclerosis plaques for neuronal dropout (holes). No other pulse sequence routinely gives such excellent T1W contrast [42]. The dramatic T1 contrast achieved in IR results from the fact that a full range of 180° is available in which to spread out the longitudinal magnetization rather than just 90° as in SE (ie, there is more dynamic range for T1 contrast) [43].

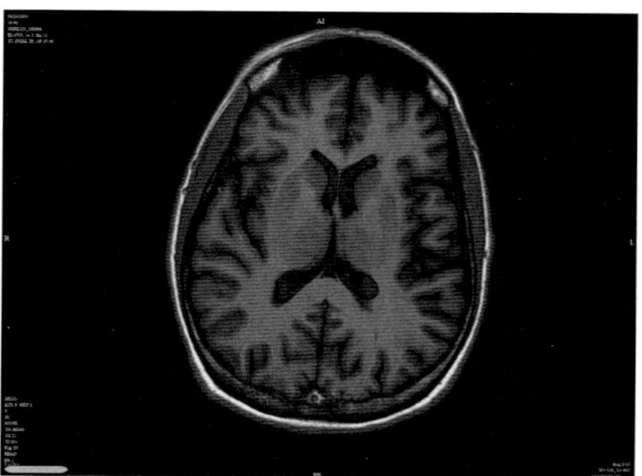

Fig. 36. T1-weighted inversion recovery image of the brain (17 minutes).

Short time inversion recovery imaging

STIR imaging allows only a short time between the 180° pulse and the second 90° pulse. In this variant of IR, the second 90° pulse is applied when a tissue of interest has reached the null point. At short inversion times, all the magnetization vectors precess in the negative *z*-direction. When the 90° pulse is given, bringing them into the *x-y* plane, signal is generated. The fact that the vectors are in the positive *z*- or negative *z*-direction before the 90° pulse is of no consequence, because the computer registers magnitude only and not the sign of the signal. Note, however, that for a tissue with a given T1, at a certain time

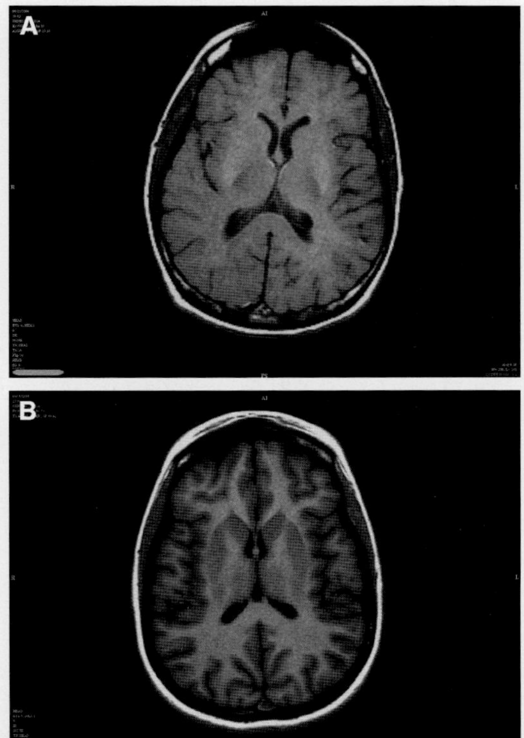

Fig. 37. (*A*) T1-weighted (T1W) spin echo (SE) image of the brain (5 minutes). (*B*) T1W fast inversion recovery image of brain with fast SE technology required only 2 minutes.

(when TI = T1 × 0.693), it will have recovered to the *x-y* plane just as the second 90° pulse is given: Signal = $S_o (1 - 2e^{-TI/T1}) = 0$. This is illustrated in Fig. 38 for the tissue labeled A. When this occurs, it now precesses in the negative *z*-direction without transverse magnetization; hence, no signal is generated. The signal of A is then effectively nulled.

In STIR imaging, the inversion pulse is chosen such that a material with a short T1 is nulled; by this means, the signal from that substance can be suppressed. To suppress fat, for instance, a TI of 173 milliseconds (at 1.5 T) is chosen (0.693 × 250 milliseconds [T1 of fat]). If an appropriate TE is chosen for data collection, the effect of T1 and T2 on lesion detection can be additive. The T1 and T2 of most pathologic lesions are prolonged [44]. A longer TE is used before data collection; therefore, only those substances that have long T1s and long T2s are bright (hence, additive contrast effects). This can be used to significant advantage in areas like the orbit [45–47], where the adjacent bright fat can obscure detection of lesions of the optic nerves. Fig. 39A is a normal STIR image of the orbit demonstrating excellent fat suppression. Notice that the optic nerve is of lower signal intensity than the extraocular muscles. The STIR image of Fig. 39B from a different patient demonstrates the effectiveness of this pulse sequence to show optic neuritis. The bright signal of the conal fat is well suppressed, whereas the edema of the optic nerve is seen. Fig. 39C shows optic nerve enhancement, confirming the diagnosis of optic neuritis. STIR can also effectively suppress fat within the vertebral bodies so as to evaluate bony lesions, such as metastasis (Fig. 40). Newer chemical saturation pulse sequences are also highly effective at suppressing fat [48]. Furthermore, STIR not only suppresses fat but any short T1 substance, such as hemorrhage or gadolinium enhancement [49].

Fluid-attenuated inversion recovery

One of the most exciting pulse sequences to be applied to neuroradiology in the past several years is FLAIR. FLAIR is really a variation of STIR imaging. It might be considered a long time inversion sequence with a long TE. A 180° RF inversion pulse is applied. Before the next 90° pulse is applied, a long time is given to allow substances, such as fluid, with long T1s to recover to the *x-y* plane (Fig. 41). When the 90° pulse is given, substances with long a T1, such as free water, are inverted to the negative *z*-axis. Substances with short a T1 have recovered completely before this pulse and thus give maximum signal when data sampling occurs. As such, this sequence effectively nulls out free water much as a STIR sequence can be used to null out fat.

This sequence can be particularly helpful in evaluating periventricular white matter lesions (Fig. 42). Water bound to complex macromolecules within plaques has a relatively shorter T1 than the free water within the ventricles [50]. The long inversion time effectively suppresses free water; therefore, the CSF is nulled. Lesions that contain complex partially bound water (which is less mobile) have a shorter T1 than free water and are not nulled. These protons are analogous to water bound to proteins. Furthermore, a fairly long TE is used. This results in a heavily T2W sequence. As a result, the sequence becomes additive for contrast effects of tissues with

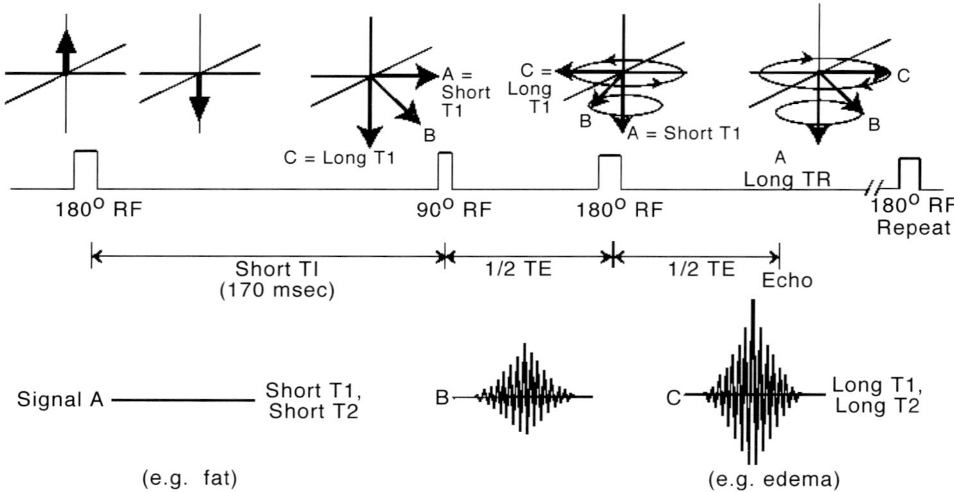

Fig. 38. Short time inversion recovery (STIR) sequence. In this case, a 180° radiofrequency (RF) pulse is given. A relatively short time is allowed for the tissues to relax. At this point, tissues with short T1s, such as those labeled A, are in the *x-y* plane. The 90° pulse given at the end of the inversion time now rotates substances with short T1s into the *z*-axis, which gives no signal from tissue A and maximum signal from tissue C when sampled by the 180° refocusing RF pulse. In this sequence, the contrast effects of T1 and T2 are additive. A long T1 and a long T2 produce maximum signal intensity. TE, echo time; TR, repetition time.

prolonged T2 and shortened T1 (eg, white matter lesions). Long inversion times of 2000 milliseconds or greater require long TRs of 6000 milliseconds or greater. This technique is prohibitively long for most conventional imaging; however, coupling this sequence with a fast image acquisition technique [51–53] results in good-quality images in a reasonable period of 2 to 3 minutes.

FLAIR is effective at highlighting lesions like demyelination [54], stroke, ischemic gliosis [55–57], and tumor. It is a highly sensitive technique (more so than SE) [51]; however, it is nonspecific. Even normal partially myelinated white matter tracts are highlighted. The protein-rich pituitary stalk is also normally bright on FLAIR [58]. In Fig. 43, an example of FLAIR in a patient with venous infarcts of the thalami from cerebral vein thrombosis demonstrates its dramatic and positive contrast compared with fast SE T2W images. FLAIR is more sensitive for the detection of acute infarcts. In addition, old infarcts with areas of cystic encephalomalacia can be distinguished from acute infarcts [59]. The suppression of free water greatly augments the ability of the viewer to detect underlying lesions. FLAIR has also been used effectively in evaluating subarachnoid hemorrhage by removing interfering CSF signal.

In an elegant comparative clinical study, Hittmair et al [50] concluded that the fast STIR sequence was clearly superior to other techniques, such as conventional SE, fast SE, and FLAIR, for the detection of cervical cord multiple sclerosis plaques. This is somewhat surprising, given the high sensitivity of FLAIR for evaluation of multiple sclerosis in the brain. In the cervical spine, CSF flow artifacts and incomplete suppression of CSF signal, combined with poor lesion contrast, reduce the utility of FLAIR, however. A STIR study with a TR of 2200 millisecond, effective TE (TEeff) of 50 millisecond, TI of 110 millisecond, echo train length of 8, and NEX of 6 was determined to be the most effective.

Notice that in contradistinction to the STIR sequence, positive contrast is additive for tissues with short T1 and long T2 in this sequence in comparison to STIR, in which long T1 and long T2 tissue contrast is augmented. This means that the FLAIR sequence is more sensitive for lesions in which bound water is highlighted. It might be thought of as a situation in which the cup is half empty or half full. Overall, pathologic tissues have longer T1s than normal tissue; however, a subcomponent of the lesion has T1s that are shorter than the free water within the lesion. When the

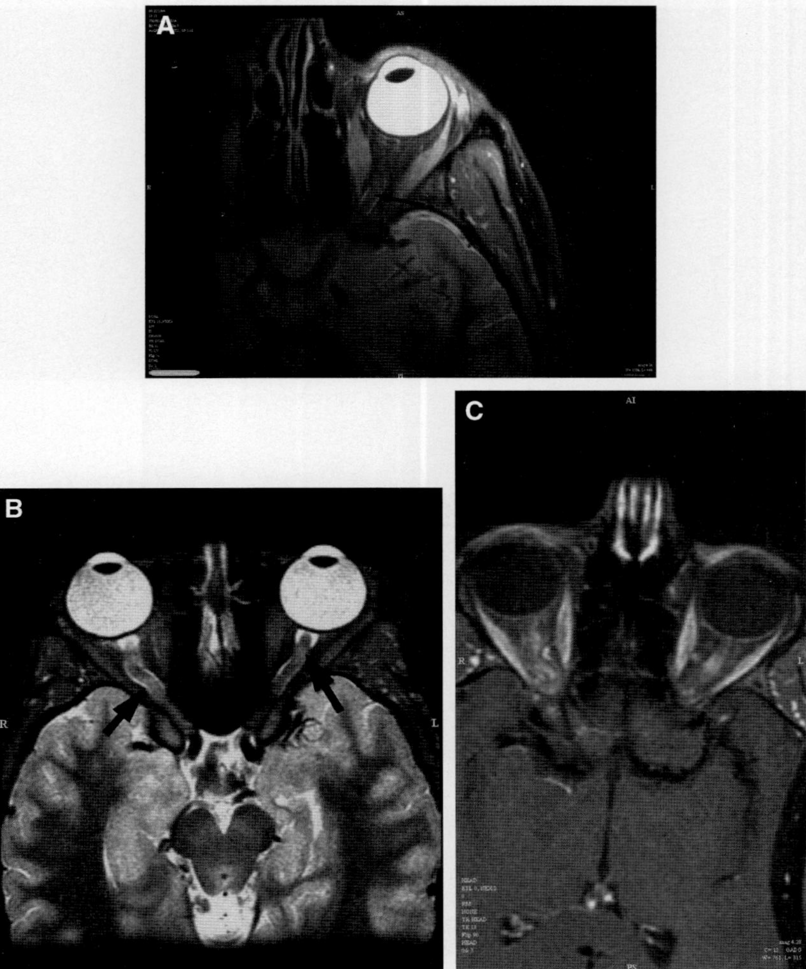

Fig. 39. (*A*) Normal optic nerve (*arrows*) with short time inversion recovery (STIR) has signal intensity less than muscle (*arrowheads*). (*B*) In a different patient with bilateral optic neuritis, there is increased signal intensity in the optic nerves bilaterally. Note that the signal intensity of the optic nerves exceeds that of the extraocular muscles (*arrows*). (*C*) Same patient as in Fig. 39B. Axial T1-weighted, fat-suppressed, gadolinium-enhanced images of the orbits reveal bilateral optic nerve enhancement, confirming the diagnosis of optic neuritis. The STIR images are complimentary, showing edema of the optic nerves. Notice that the STIR images in Fig. 39B give excellent suppression of the orbital fat.

additive effect of T2 contrast is present, highly structured water, such as that in normal brain, rapidly decays, whereas the gliotic lesions remain bright, giving relative high signal intensity. A model of this is given in Fig. 44. A gliotic lesion is represented by an interstitial matrix of loosely associated water and glial cells as well as increased free water content. After application of the long IR sequence, the free water is suppressed, whereas the bound water still has signal. FLAIR sequences give a brighter signal than adjacent brain while suppressing unwanted signal from CSF. FLAIR can be helpful in discriminating dilated perivascular spaces (free water) from white matter lesions (gliosis with bound water) (Fig. 45).

Chemical selective saturation

We have just seen how the pulse sequence can be designed to null the signal of a given tissue based on its relaxation characteristics. There is a second powerful technique that allows

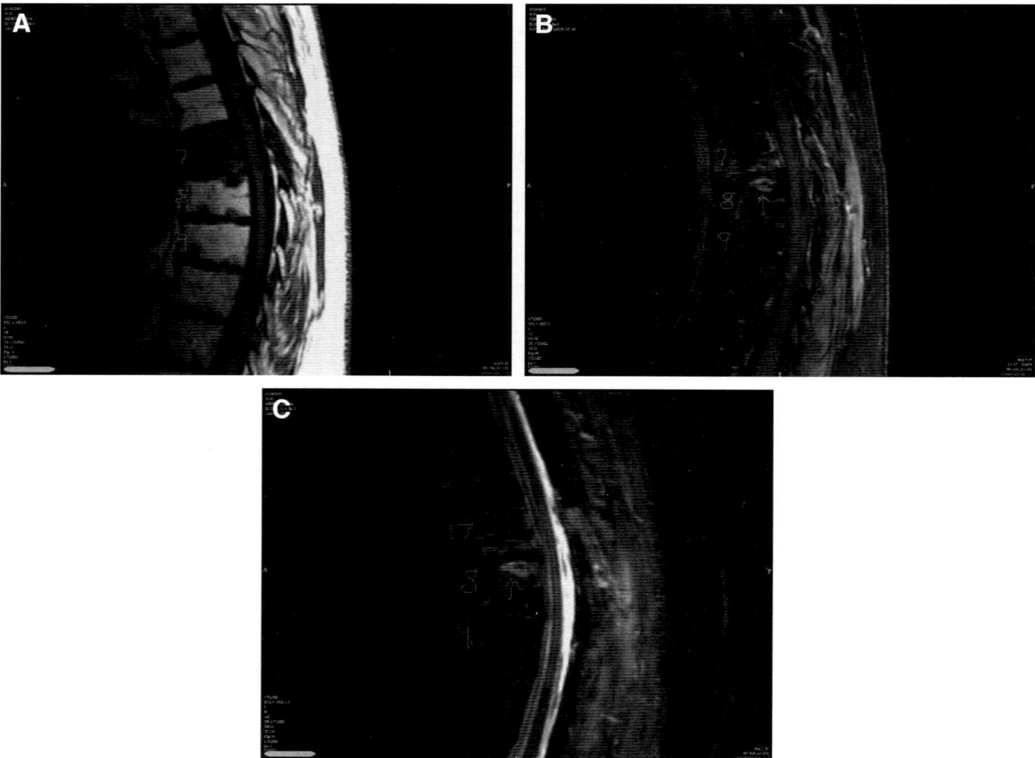

Fig. 40. Comparison of short time inversion recovery (STIR) fat-suppressed images and chemical fat suppression in metastatic disease of the thoracic spine. Sagittal phased-array MRI in a patient with cancer. (*A*) T1-weighted (T1W) spin echo (SE) image without fat suppression demonstrates normal brightness to the subcutaneous and paravertebral fat. The spinal cord is unremarkable. There is diffuse replacement of the normal fatty marrow with low signal intensity in the T7 vertebral body. (*B*) Sagittal T1W, gadolinium-enhanced, fat-suppressed SE image demonstrates pathologic enhancement of a lesion which is T8 (*arrows*) not as well demonstrated on the other pulse sequences. In addition, there is heterogeneous vertebral body involvement of T7. (*C*) Sagittal STIR image of the thoracic spine illustrates the additive effects of contrast with this sequence. Fat is suppressed in the vertebral bodies and the adjacent paravertebral fat. The increased water content of the metastatic lesion in T8 is more conspicuous than on the unenhanced T1W image.

suppression of unwanted tissue signal based on selective chemical saturation [60,61]. If one were to take an NMR spectra of a given voxel of tissue, it is readily apparent that the proton resonances vary slightly depending on the chemical constituencies. A hypothetical and simplified spectrum of several substances is given in Fig. 46. Suppose that a standard SE pulse sequence is used. By applying a narrow frequency pulse and exciting only one of the chemical constituents, such as fat, before the SE sequence is begun, the signal from the fat can be eliminated by saturating it. An example of this is given in Fig. 47. A narrow frequency pulse is applied to the tissue of interest, exciting only fat molecules. Now, when the SE sequence is applied, the proton vectors of the fat molecules are already in the *x*-*y* plane. When the 90° pulse is applied for the SE sequence, they are inverted along the negative *z*-direction and generate no signal during the FID or after the 180° refocusing pulse. A similar strategy may be used to suppress silicone (eg, in the evaluation of silicone breast implant rupture) and to suppress water associated with complex proteins (eg, magnetization transfer).

Fat suppression with chemically selective pulses, although generally a useful technique, must be interpreted with caution at times. The saturation only works in a highly uniform field. This means that tissue situated well away from the isocenter of the magnet, asymmetric anatomy, and areas in which there is distortion of the

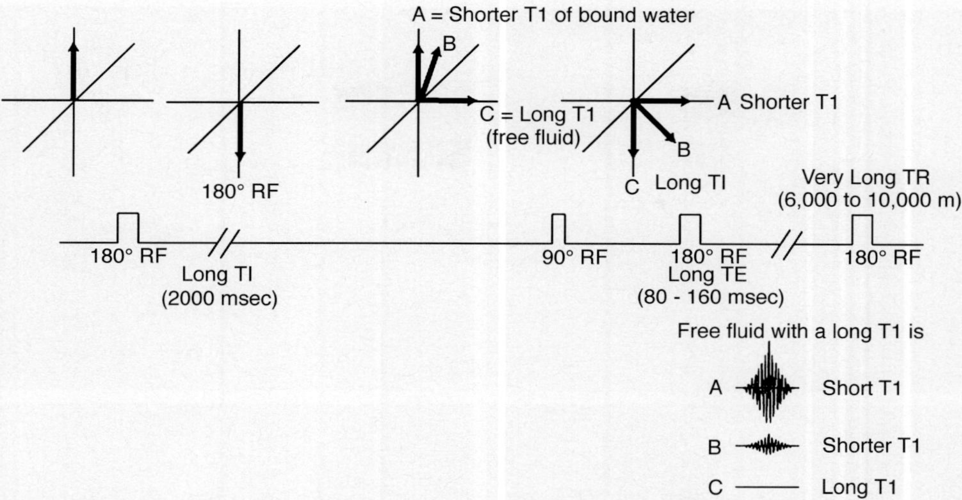

Fig. 41. Fluid-attenuated inversion recovery (FLAIR) sequence. A 180° radiofrequency (RF) inversion pulse is given. A long time to inversion (TI) is allowed before the 90° RF pulse is performed. By this time, substances with a shorter T1, such as bound water, have returned to the *z*-axis. Free fluid represented by tissue C, which has a long T1, is now at the *x*-*y* plane, however. When the second 90° pulse is given, substances, such as tissue C, with a long T1 are inverted into a negative *z*-direction. At the echo, no signal is obtained. Tissues with a relatively shorter T1, such as those with bound water, give maximum signal in the *x*-*y* plane. Note that an extremely long repetition time (TR) is needed (6000–10,000 milliseconds) to allow complete recovery of the tissues with long T1s back to baseline before the pulse sequence is begun again. A fairly long echo time (TE) is then used for data sampling. This sequence therefore highlights substances that have a relatively short T1 and a long T2.

magnetic field from metal artifact, for example, yield poor fat saturation and, at times, confusing signal intensities. Fig. 48 gives an example of how fat suppression can be used to evaluate a brain lesion.

Pulse preparation

The second form of pulse sequence modification seen extensively in MRI is that of a pulse preparation. In this case, various things are done to the proton vectors that affect their later tissue contrast. For example, in diffusion-weighted imaging, strong gradients are applied after tissue excitation to emphasize differences in microscopic motion of protons. Spoiler gradients are commonly applied in conjunction with fast gradient echo imaging techniques to reduce residual and unwanted transverse magnetization between each pulse sequence. Finally, the intrinsic tissue contrast can be altered by applying special preparatory RF pulses before initiation of the main pulse sequence. Examples include magnetization-prepared rapid gradient echo and magnetization-prepared IR sequences.

Gradient echo imaging

Gradient-recalled acquisition schemes (eg, GRASS, fast low-angle shot, fast imaging with steady-state precision) are similar to the SE pulse sequence except that the 180° refocusing RF pulse is not used. Additional gradients may also be added. One of the reasons why the proton spins undergo rapid T2 phase decay is the application of encoding gradients during data acquisition. To obtain phase coherence, these gradients must be reversed in the second half of the pulse sequence so that all the protons are brought back into phase during data acquisition. This reversal of the encoding gradients forms its own natural echo from what little transverse magnetization is remaining. Areas that are dephased by the slice-encoding and frequency-encoding gradients are brought back into phase by reversing the gradient polarity, which makes the faster spinning vectors slower, as shown in Fig. 49. The precessional direction of the vectors does not change as it does with SE, however. Note that in this case, we are working with T2* relaxation, which occurs much more quickly than T2 relaxation. Therefore, TEs used must be much shorter if any signal is to be

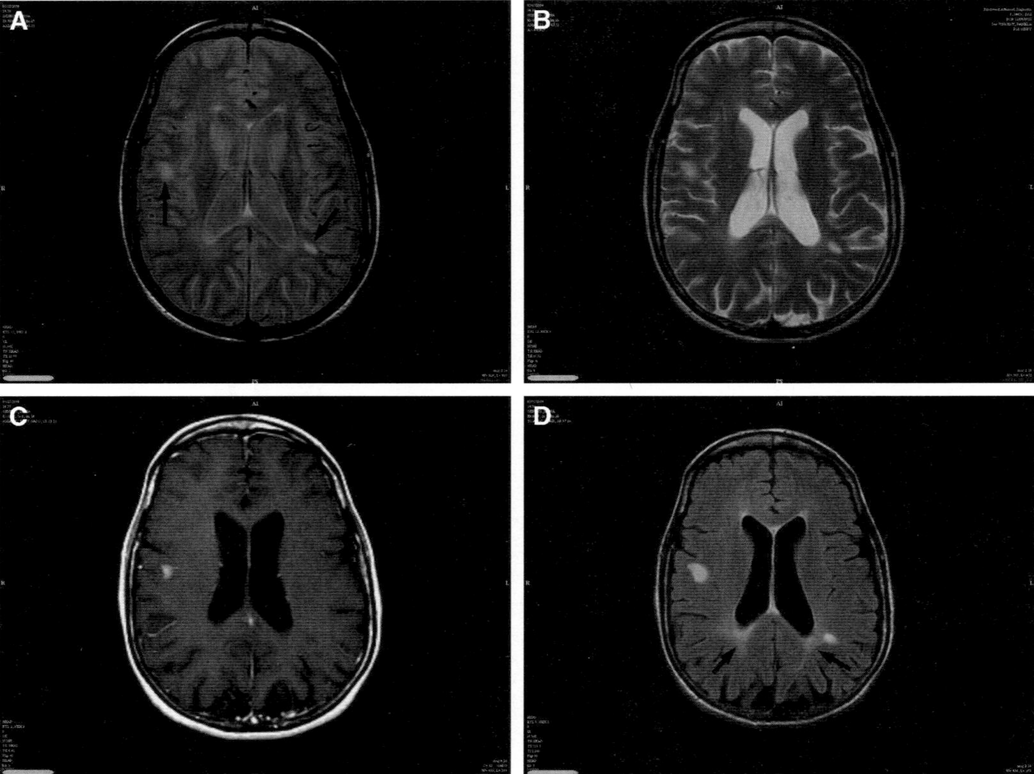

Fig. 42. Imaging in a multiple sclerosis patient demonstrates the utility of fluid-attenuated inversion recovery (FLAIR). (*A*) Proton-weighted T2-weighted (T2W) fast spin echo (FSE) image at the level of the lateral ventricles demonstrates several periventricular white matter lesions (*arrows*). These are fairly well seen, although smaller lesions can be missed (repetition time [TR] = 3150 milliseconds, echo time [TE] = 10.9 milliseconds). (*B*) T2W FSE (TR = 3150 milliseconds, TE = 98 milliseconds). The periventricular demyelination is less observable because of adjacent cerebrospinal fluid in the sulci. (*C*) Axial T1-weighted gadolinium-enhanced (TR = 416 milliseconds, TE = 8.4 milliseconds) spin echo sequence demonstrates an enhancing plaque lesion in the posterior right frontal lobe. Although this sequence is excellent for showing areas of blood-brain barrier breakdown, many of the plaques are not active and hence not visible. (*D*) Axial fast FLAIR images (TR = 8800 milliseconds, TE = 123 milliseconds, time to inversion [TI] = 2200 milliseconds) reveal the plaques previously identified with the proton-weighted sequence with a much greater degree of conspicuity. In addition, the periventricular white matter disease in the periatrial areas is much more evident (*arrows*). Also notice the area of vasogenic edema in the posterior right frontal-temporal cortex. The vasogenic edema is larger than the area of blood-brain barrier breakdown seen on the contrast-enhanced images.

received. Furthermore, because there is not a reversal of the direction of the spinning vectors from a 180° RF pulse, phase loss caused by static field homogeneities cannot be recovered. These images tend to be more artifact prone, particularly at tissue interfaces, where diamagnetic effects are present, and in regions where there is ferromagnetic or paramagnetic material. Fig. 50 demonstrates the differences between SE and gradient echo sequences. They are also prone to chemical shift artifacts. The major advantage to gradient-recalled acquisition imaging is that the second 180° RF pulse need not be used. This means less RF power deposition within the patient over a given time and the ability to image faster. It also means that there is less saturation (ie, loss of the longitudinal magnetization) and less cross-talk from excitation of adjacent slices. As a result, thinner and faster slices can be obtained.

Limited flip angle imaging

This technique is most often used in conjunction with gradient echo imaging [62]; however,

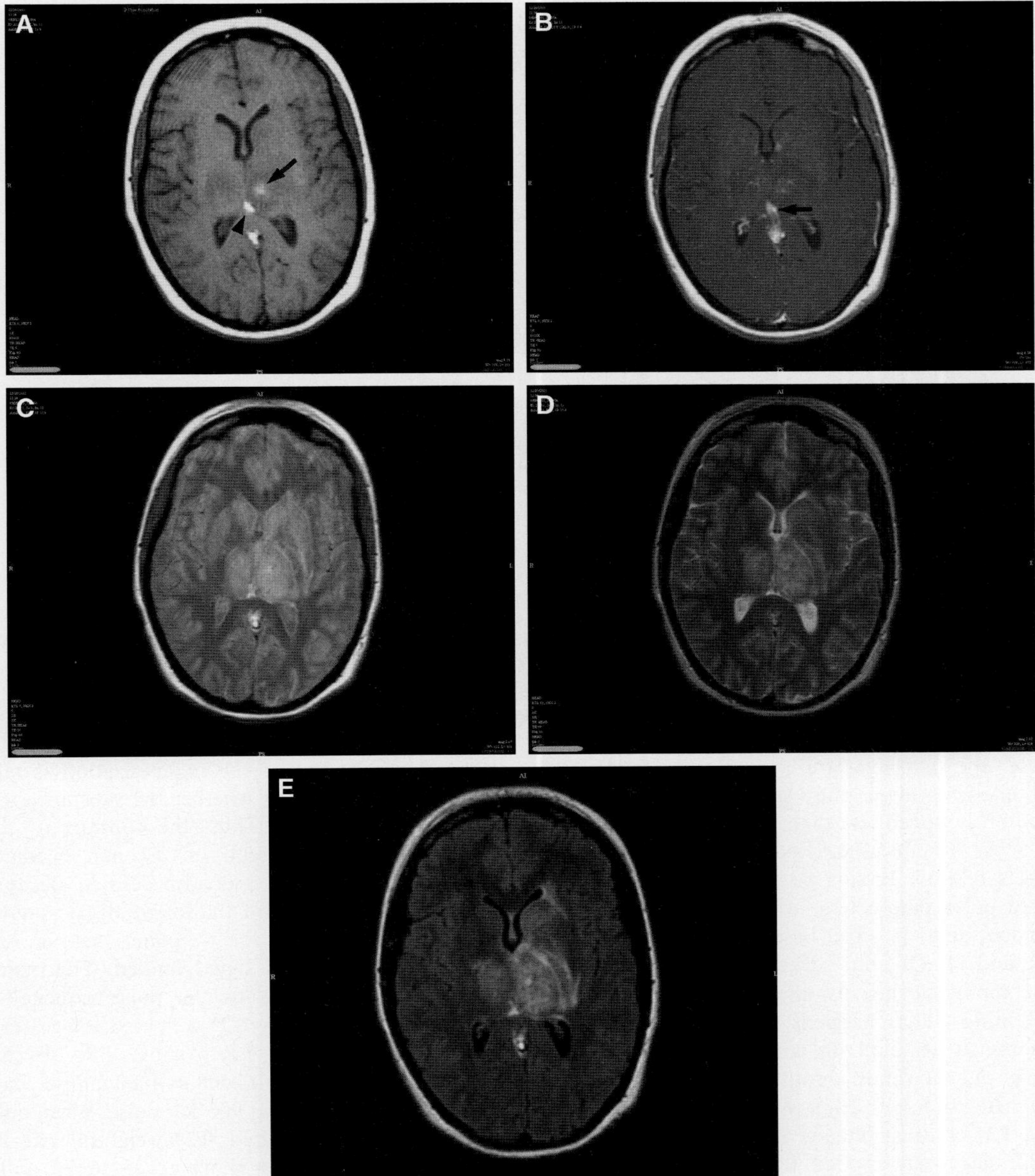

Fig. 43. A 23-year old patient with an internal cerebral vein and straight sinus thrombosis causing recent venous infarcts. The dramatic sensitivity of FLAIR sequences compared with other spin echo (SE) techniques is demonstrated. (*A*) Axial T1-weighted SE image through the level of the thalami demonstrates a small amount of high signal intensity in the left thalamus consistent with a recent hemorrhage in the Met-hemoglobin form (*arrow*). There is also high signal intensity just posterior to this in the great vein of Galen consistent with thrombosed Met-hemoglobin (*arrowhead*). (*B*) After gadolinium enhancement, there is some minimal enhancement of congested veins of the thalami and left basal ganglia as well as slow flow in the vein of Galen (*arrow*). (*C*) Proton-weighted fast SE image yields little contrast between the areas of venous infarction and surrounding brain. (*D*) Axial T2-weighted (T2W) SE image demonstrates swelling of the thalami bilaterally, more so on the left side. (*E*) Axial T2W FLAIR image dramatically highlights the extent of the vasogenic edema in the left caudate nucleus and the thalami bilaterally as well as in the internal capsule on the left.

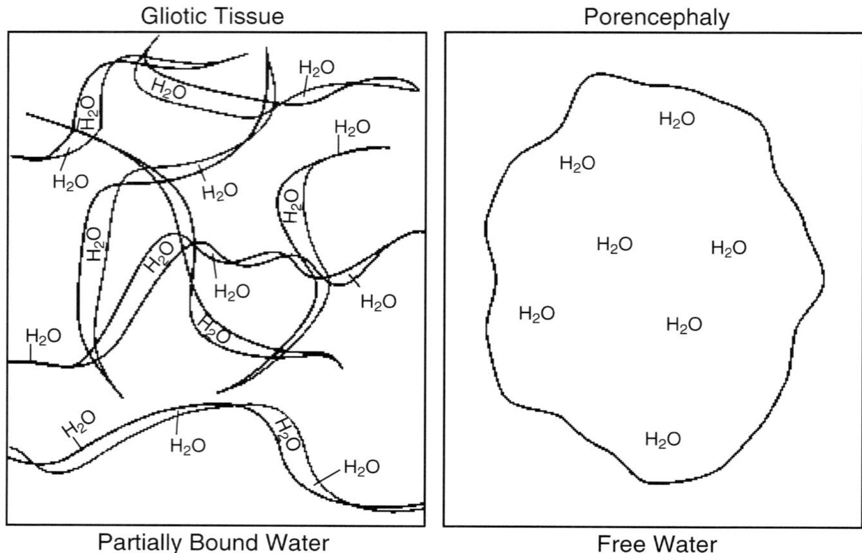

Fig. 44. Gliotic lesion versus porencephaly. Gliotic tissue is represented by a matrix of proteinaceous strands and debris to which water is loosely bound. This slows the molecular motion of the water, shortening its T1. On a fluid-attenuated inversion recovery (FLAIR) image, this water is not suppressed and remains relatively bright. Such a lesion is bright because of the decreased T1 of the water and the relatively long T2 of loosely associated water. Conversely, water in a porencephalic cyst undergoes rapid rotational movement and has poor relaxation efficiency. The water with the long T1 in the FLAIR sequence is effectively suppressed, and signal is not seen.

these are two separate imaging principles. In a limited flip angle pulse sequence, the *z*-magnetization is tipped less than 90°. Typically, values of 5° to 40° are used, depending on the contrast effects desired. In this pulse sequence, there are three pulse parameters, which are operator dependent and can affect tissue contrast: flip angle, TR, and TE. Of course, these are not independent. The flip angle heavily affects the degree of T1 weighting. What happens is that T1 effects are eliminated at small flip angles because you are using only a small amount of the longitudinal magnetization with each pulse. Only spin density and T2* contrast remain. In Fig. 51, an 18° RF pulse has been applied to our system. The *z*-magnetization is tipped only a short distance. Because of this, the net *x*- and *y*-vectors are smaller. These begin to dephase as expected. When the spins are brought back into alignment, an echo is generated. Because limited flip angle sequences use gradient reversal, only those phase losses caused by the earlier applied gradient in the opposite direction can be recovered. Because only a small portion of the longitudinal magnetization is used each time, the tissue is not as saturated as if a 90° or 180° RF pulse had been applied. Unless the TR is extremely short (which saturates the sample), most of the magnetization is still available regardless of whether the substance has a short or long T1. Thus, the contrast of the images does not depend on T1 and becomes dependent on T2* or hydrogen density. Because only a small amount of the longitudinal magnetization is flipped into the *x*-*y* plane, these images tend to be noisy and signal limited. The major reason for wanting to use this pulse sequence is that of speed. Heavily T2*-weighted images can be obtained even at fairly short TRs. In SE imaging, we had to wait 2500 to 4000 milliseconds before applying the next 90° RF pulse. When only a small flip angle is used, T2* weighting can be achieved with TRs as short as 25 to 75 milliseconds. Because this sequence is virtually always used with the gradient reversal acquisition technique rather than being T2W, these are T2* weighted. This means that rather than seeing true T2 decay of a tissue, we see the effects of tissue T2 and static local field inhomogeneity.

Summary of our model to this point

The basic SE pulse sequence and its variants have been introduced. The incoherent spinning nuclei are brought into coherence by a 90° RF

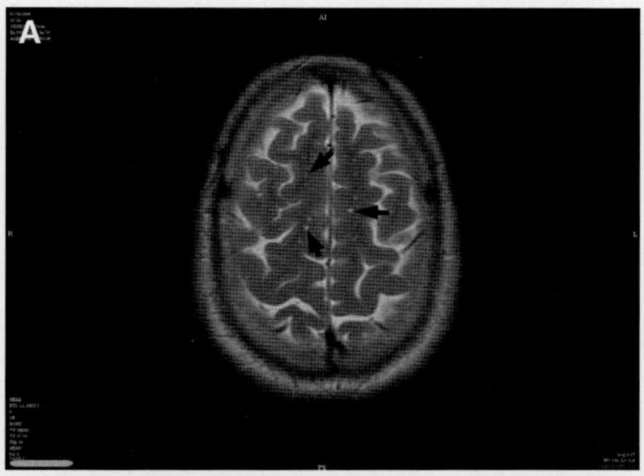

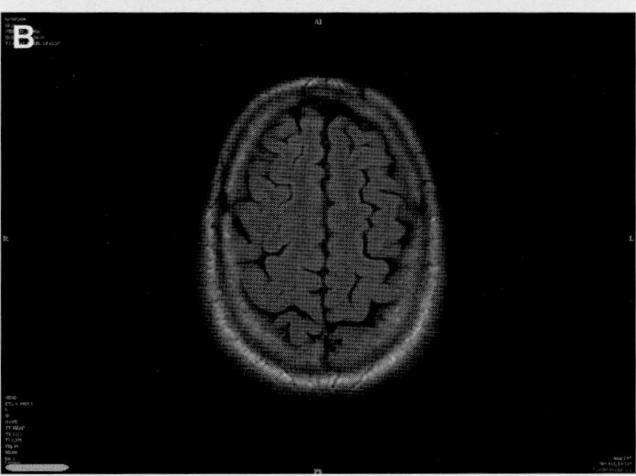

Fig. 45. Fluid-attenuated inversion recovery (FLAIR) sequence demonstrating the difference between état criblé and white matter lesions. (*A*) Axial heavily T2-weighted (T2W) fast spin echo image over the vertex of the brain demonstrates multiple areas of increased signal abnormality in the subcortical white matter (*arrows*). (*B*) FLAIR image through this same location shows no evidence of signal abnormality. The increased signal in the T2W image is caused by free water in dilated perivascular spaces, which are suppressed by the FLAIR sequence. Therefore, these are not true white matter lesions.

pulse. Time is allowed to elapse, and a second 180° pulse is administered, inverting the spinning vectors and bringing them into phase coherence again. This creates a second signal, or "echo." The echo occurs at time to TE (time to echo). The shorter the TE, the less decay of signal there is; hence, the best signal-to-noise ratio is obtained with short echo sequences. For this reason, most T1W and proton-weighted sequences give the highest anatomic detail. Most pathologic processes exhibit prolonged T2 values, however. By using long TEs, the discrimination of normal versus abnormal tissue is enhanced. The IR family of pulse sequences has been introduced, each with unique capabilities. Traditional IR yields beautiful T1W sequences. STIR images can be used to suppress short T1 substances, such as fat. FLAIR is a unique T2W sequence that suppresses free water, such as CSF, but highlights bound water, such as myelin plaques.

Forming an image: spatial encoding

With a basic understanding of nuclear magnetic relaxation and pulse sequences, we are now ready to tackle some of the most difficult concepts involved in MRI. The concept of spatially encoding the MRI signals was first devised by Lauterbur [63] in 1973. A myriad of different techniques have been devised to localize and acquire the NMR signals spatially point by point [63–65], line by line [66–68], plane by plane [69,70], or even three dimensionally [71,72]. The technique described in this article is essentially that of spin warp imaging, first described by Kumar et al [70] and modified by Edelstein et al [73]. Many investigational groups, such as those headed by Mansfield [69], Lauterbur [63], Crooks [68], Hinshaw [74], and Pykett [66], made substantial contributions to the development of the techniques required for rapid signal acquisition.

Spin echo, single-slice, two-dimensional data acquisition

This technique encompasses most currently used data acquisition schemes for MRI (if one includes the modification of fast SE). At the end of this section, I briefly discuss other techniques, such as gradient echo imaging and three-dimensional (3D) data acquisition.

When the body is placed in a strong homogeneous magnetic field, the protons align for and against the magnetic field. A net vector of magnetism exists, directed along the *z*-axis. Each of the individual nuclei is out of phase, and the net vectors of each voxel are pointed only toward the *z*-direction, as is illustrated in Fig. 52. The task now at hand is to excite and record information from only one voxel. A voxel is a small volume of tissue equal to the pixel size times slice thickness. A pixel is the size of a single point in a slice. In the technique described by Damadian et al [65], the magnetic field was shaped with gradients such that only one point in the center was homogeneous and was thus sensitive to the spinning nuclei of the given frequency. The sensitive point or field-focusing NMR method required the physical movement of the object within the gantry. The

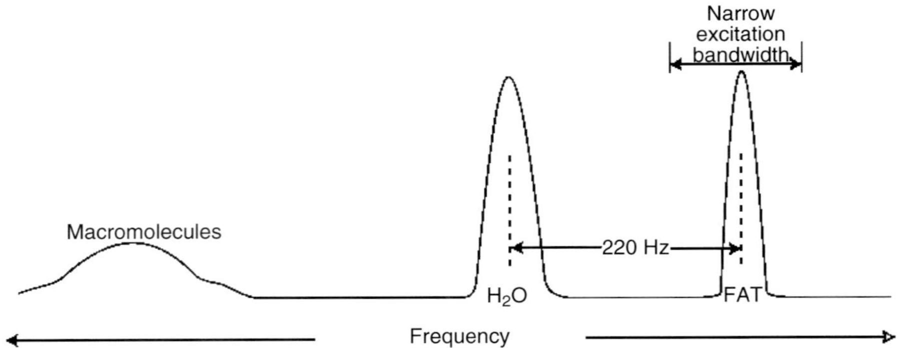

Fig. 46. The protons of fat, water, and macromolecules precess at slightly different frequencies. At 1.5 T, the separation between fat and water is 220 Hz.

data were acquired point by point, with the rather crude image requiring longer than 20 minutes, because each voxel must be recorded independently. The success of current imaging schemes relies on simultaneous acquisition of many of these points; otherwise, imaging times would be far too long for practical use.

Selective excitation

The heart of NMR imaging is the fact that the hydrogen nuclei precess at different frequencies, depending only on the local magnetic field strength. By applying a magnetic field gradient across the static magnetic field, the nuclei at one location can be made to precess at a different frequency than those in another location. This is diagrammatically shown in Fig. 53. The hydrogen nuclei are represented by circles, with the larger circles being those spinning at higher frequencies. We also know that for nuclear excitation to occur (ie, to tip the spins from alignment with the magnetic field to alignment against the magnetic field), an energy input that is exactly equal to that of the Larmour frequency is required. The Larmour frequency is the frequency at which

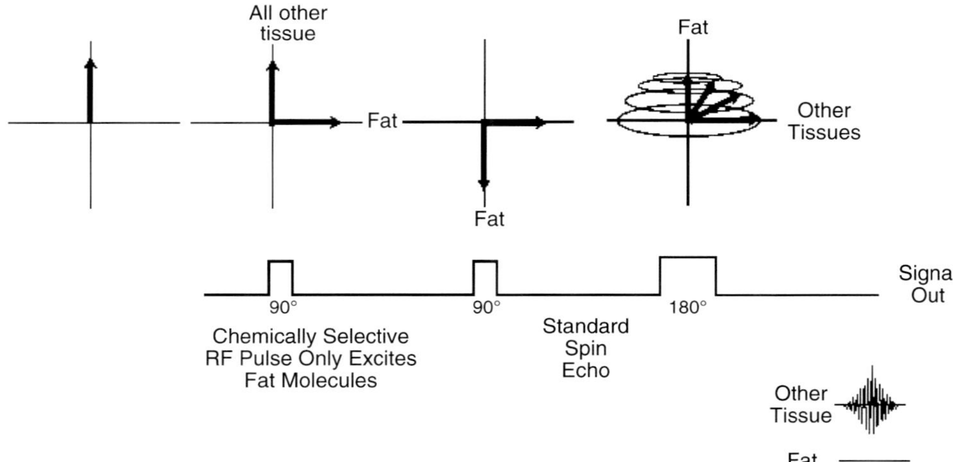

Fig. 47. A chemically selective 90° radiofrequency (RF) pulse (for fat in this case) is applied just before the standard spin echo sequence. This has the effect of rotating the proton vectors for the fat molecules into the *x-y* plane. When the next 90° pulse is given, the fat is inverted into the negative *z*-axis and all other tissue precesses within the *x-y* plane. A standard 180° refocusing RF pulse is given, which has the effect of returning fat back into the positive *z*-direction. As such, it has no net vector in the *x-y* plane and does not yield signal.

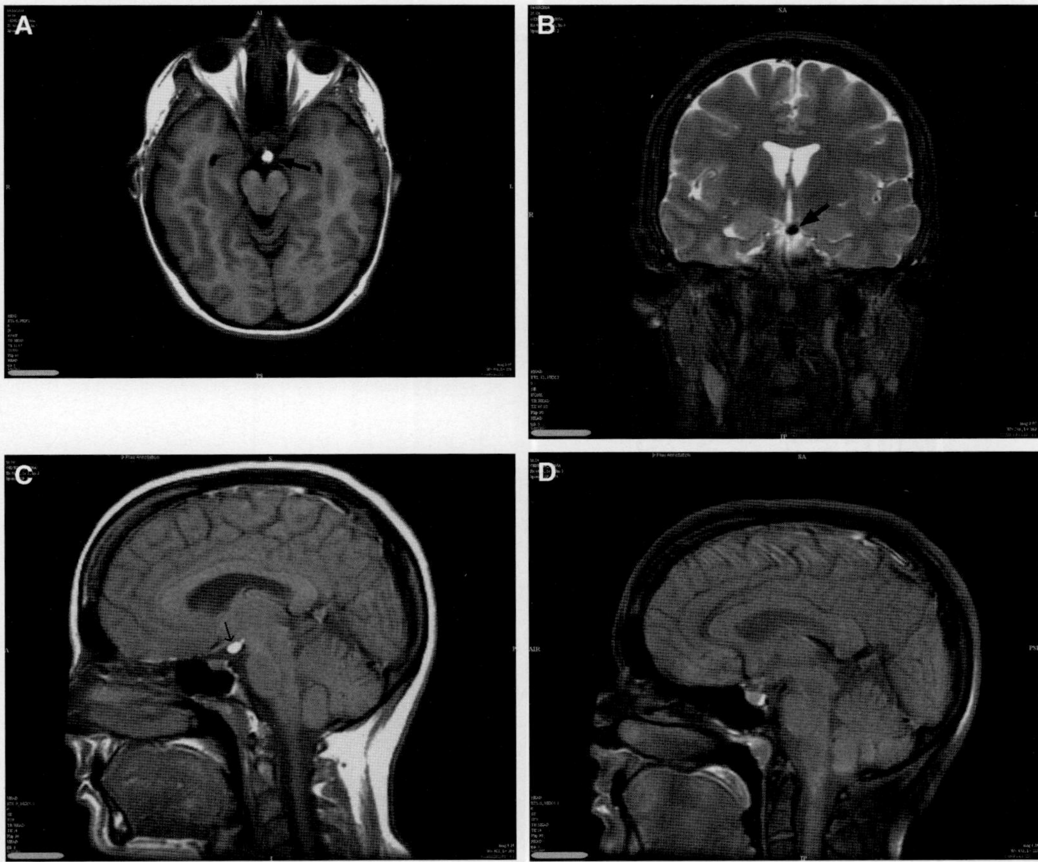

Fig. 48. Small lipoma of the interpeduncular cistern just ventral to the basilar artery. (*A*) Axial T1-weighted (T1W) inversion recovery image reveals a small, round, high signal intensity lesion ventral to the midbrain and behind the pituitary gland in the interpeduncular cistern (*arrow*). (*B*) Coronal spin echo (SE) image demonstrates that the lesion darkens considerably on a heavily T2-weighted image (*arrow*). (*C*) Sagittal T1W SE image also reveals the high signal intensity lesion just above and behind the pituitary fossa in the interpeduncular cistern (*arrow*). (*D*) The key diagnostic images are the sagittal fat-suppressed T1W images, which reveal that the lesion is completely suppressed after the application of a chemically selective saturation pulse. This confirms the diagnosis of benign fat as opposed to tumor, hemorrhage, or other lesion.

the protons precess at a given field strength ($\nu = \gamma \cdot G/2\pi$).

Suppose that our system has a static magnetic field of 1.4565 T, which corresponds to protons spinning at 62 mHz. If a small magnetic gradient is applied (0.0235 mT) on the *z*-axis, those on the left side spin at 62 mHz, whereas those on the right side spin at 62.001 mHz. This difference is 0.001 Hz. Shown diagrammatically in Fig. 54 is a volume of tissue with the gradient applied and the various nuclei spinning at different frequencies depending on their location. If the sample is now irradiated with a 90° RF signal that has a broad bandwidth (ie, 62 mHz ± 1000 Hz), all the protons are excited. If a narrow bandwidth is given, however, corresponding, for example, to 62.0050 mHz ± 10 Hz, a narrow slice of nuclei can be excited. All of the other nuclei on either side of the slab of interest are not excited and thus do not contribute to signal later on in the imaging process. This means that we have reduced a 3D object to a 2D object in terms of spatial localization.

Selective excitation is a first and important step in the process of image formation. Notice that the RF is delivered while the *z*-gradient is turned on for the 90° or 180° pulse. This means that the *z*-gradient must be turned on, time must allowed for

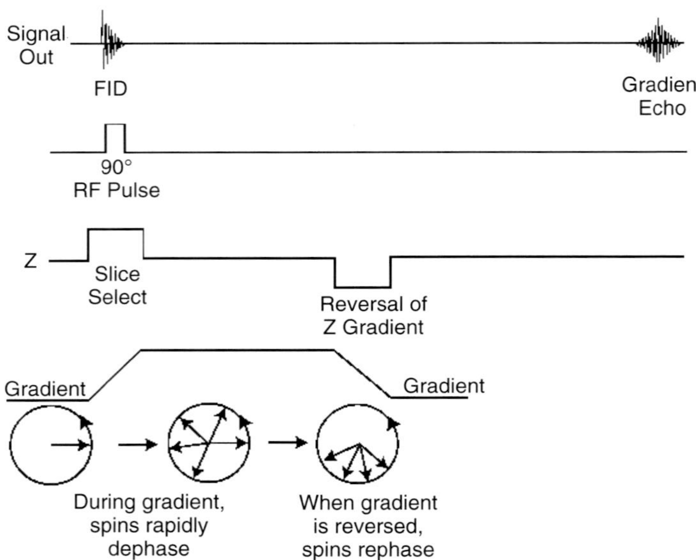

Fig. 49. Gradient echo sequence. A 90° radiofrequency (RF) pulse is given. When the slice selection gradient is turned on, there is rapid dephasing of the spins because of the gradient. Those in the region of higher gradient strength spin more quickly than those in the region of lower gradient strength. When the *z*-slice select gradient is reversed, the spins are rephased. The vectors that were previously spinning in the higher gradient strength are now spinning in the lower gradient strength. This is a simplified diagram showing only the *z*-slice select gradient. A similar reversal of the *x*-gradient must occur simultaneously. Note that a spin echo would not occur in a traditional spin echo sequence unless a gradient echo was also present. FID, free induction decay.

it to stabilize, and the 90° or 180° pulse must then be applied. The *z*-gradient is then switched off.

Prescanning

In SE imaging, a 90° pulse is initially delivered, that is, the average vector of each voxel is rotated into the *x-y* plane. How is this accomplished? Depending on the size of the structure the RF permeability is, and the tissue type, there are different amounts of RF absorption. This varies with the slice thickness, patient size, and coil loading, for example. This also changes as a function of field strength. The body is less "permeable" to RF at higher frequencies, resulting in nonuniform RF tip angles as a function of depth from the skin, especially at greater than 30 MHz [75]. How can we know how much RF energy to deposit into the tissues to exactly tip the average vector of each voxel into the *x-y* plane to achieve maximum signal return? This is done by prescanning. The prescan is part of the setup for each pulse sequence. During this process, a RF pulse is given to the center slice (or, depending on the system, the entire area) of the region to be imaged. A FID is then measured for amplitude, and the process is repeated with greater or smaller RF energy until a maximum FID is observed. At this point, the "tip angle" is 90°.

Phase encoding

After selective excitation of a single plane, our 3D object has now been reduced to a 2D object. Phase encoding is the next step in uniquely identifying each voxel of information. Immediately after the application of the 90° RF pulse with the *z*-gradient turned off, all the spins in the selected plane are precessing at the same angular velocity and each has an identical phase. This plane of spins precessing in the *x-y* plane is diagrammed in Fig. 55. These spins rapidly become out of phase, and the FID signal generated is quickly lost. For the sake of simplicity, however, let us assume that the spins remain precessing in phase. If a gradient is now applied along the *x*- or *y*-direction for a brief period, the *y*-axis in this example, the following events occur.

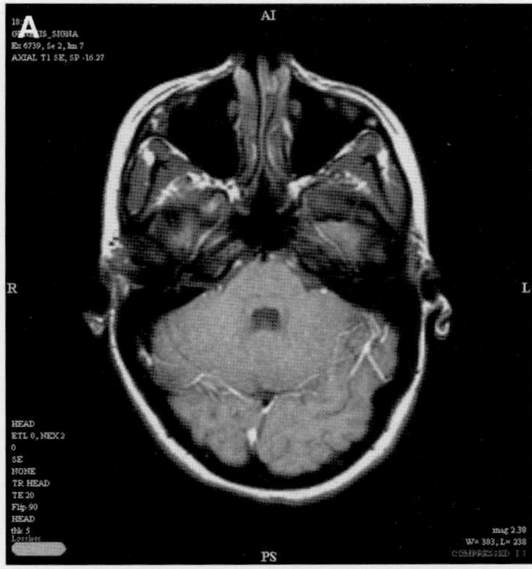

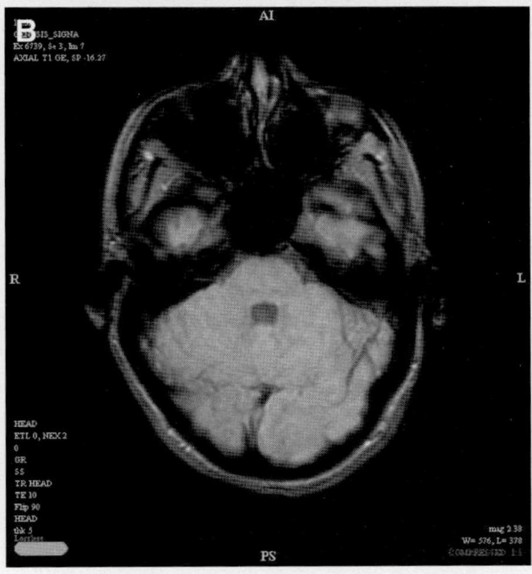

Fig. 50. (*A*) A standard T1-weighted (T1W) spin echo image was obtained through the posterior fossa and paranasal sinuses in the axial plane. (*B*) A T1W gradient echo image of the same location demonstrates somewhat comparable contrast of the cerebellar tissues. Notice the extensive diamagnetic artifact (*arrows*) in the region of the paranasal sinuses, nasal septum, and complex structures adjacent to the petrous bones. In both cases, the flip angle was 90°, the repetition time was approximately 600 milliseconds, and the echo time was 10 milliseconds.

Those spins in the higher magnetic field strength immediately begin precessing faster than those in the lower magnetic field strength, as illustrated in Fig. 56. Again, the faster spins are represented by the larger circles.

As a consequence of the difference in spin velocity, the individual alignment of spins becomes out of phase. Note that the phase change is uniform along the applied gradient. A given row of spins in the x-direction has an identical phase. The gradient is then shut off, and the spins return to precessing at the same frequency as they were in the same homogeneous magnetic field. The spins retain a "memory" of their relative phase position, however, as shown in Fig. 57.

Unfortunately, it is not possible to extract phase and frequency information simultaneously from a single echo. Data acquisition begins at the same time in each cycle. Suppose that a different strength of phase-encoding gradient is applied on the next cycle. When data collection occurs, the spinning protons are in a slightly different phase than in the preceding cycle. As they spin within the coil, they induce a sinusoidal oscillation of induced current within the coil. If they are in a different phase, the voltage induced is slightly different. Each time this process is repeated, the spins along a given row on the x-axis are given a different phase. When the echo occurs from the 180° pulse, signal is generated from all the spins lying within the excited plane. Each time, however, the process is repeated with a different strength of phase-encoding gradient. The antenna hears a slightly different signal from the protons with a different phase. Later, I show how these data can be combined with frequency encoding to describe the signal of each voxel uniquely.

Changing the phase angle in phase encoding is analogous to different rotational increments of the x-ray beam in computed tomography. The smaller the angle of increment, that is, the greater the number of phase-encoding steps over the 2π radian distance, the more accurate is the representation of the object. If the object is undersampled, the reconstruction is less accurate, giving rise to various artifacts. The price of more accurate information is increased data acquisition time. Each time a new phase-encoding gradient is applied, the entire cycle must be repeated. Thus, if our TR between cycles is 3 seconds and a single average (1 NEX) and 128 phase-encoding steps are obtained, the time of data acquisition is 6.4 minutes. If 256 steps are obtained, the time is doubled to 12.8 minutes.

Echo time

At this point, because of the inhomogeneity in the static magnetic fields, the sample rapidly dephases. Even those in the rows dephase with respect to each other. The FID signal ceases. As

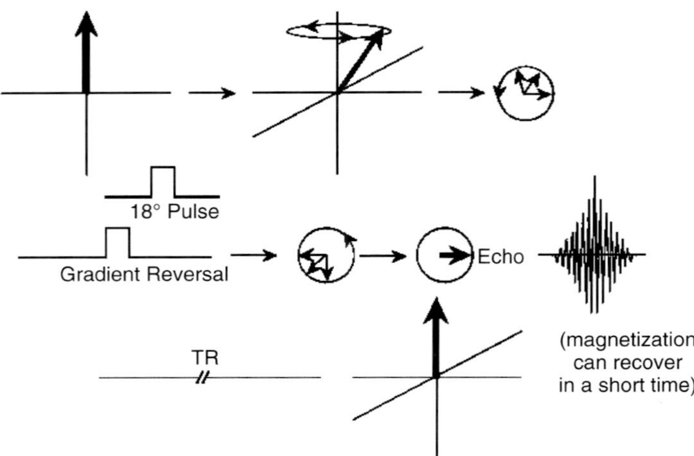

Fig. 51. Limited flip angle. An 18° radiofrequency pulse has been applied to our system. A limited flip angle sequence tips the magnetization vector only a few degrees (less than 90°). By reversing the gradients, the signal lost from gradient effects is recovered and an echo is sampled. Only a small percentage of the available magnetization is sampled for any given pulse. TR, repetition time.

explained previously, a 180° RF pulse is now applied. The time between the 90° pulse and the 180° RF pulse is TE/2, that is, the echo occurs equally spaced from when the 180° pulse occurs. This is one of the important operator-dependent parameters available with SE techniques. The longer we wait before applying the 180° RF pulse, the more "T2W" the sample is. Only those protons with sufficiently long T2 values have signal remaining when the echo is generated. At TE, the vectors in each of the *y*-columns come back into phase; however, they remember the earlier phase change brought about by the phase-encoding gradient as illustrated in Fig. 58.

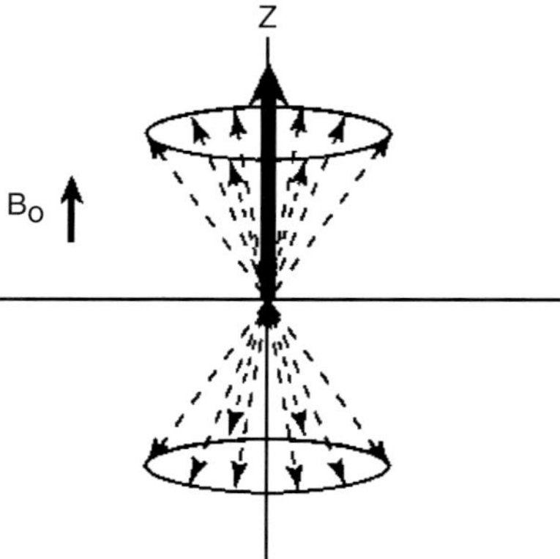

Fig. 52. Precessing vectors for and against the magnetic field, with a net magnetic vector directed toward *z*.

Frequency encoding

The final step in uniquely describing each of the voxels involves the introduction of another gradient that is present while the data are sampled. In this case, it is applied along the *x*-axis. Because the gradient is on during data acquisition, each of the different rows along the *x*-direction is spinning at a different frequency, as illustrated in Fig. 59. If a gradient is applied during data acquisition, do the spins rotate at different frequencies and thus become out of phase again? This is correct. For this reason, a negative lobe is given initially to the frequency gradient to "unwind" the spins, after which the positive gradient is applied, such that at the exact time of the

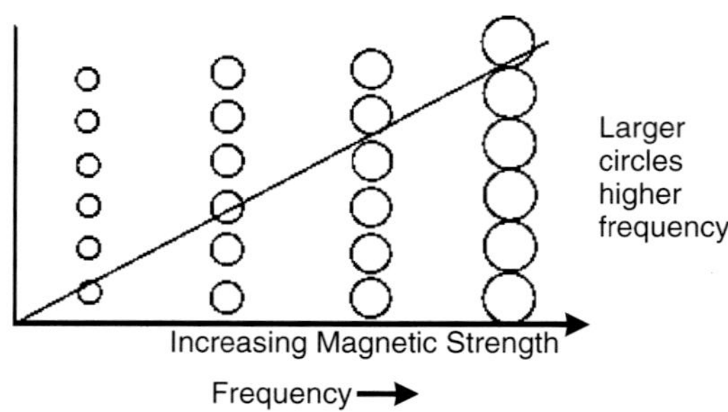

Fig. 53. Magnetic field gradient represented by a sloped line. Increasing precessional frequencies of the protons are indicated by larger circles.

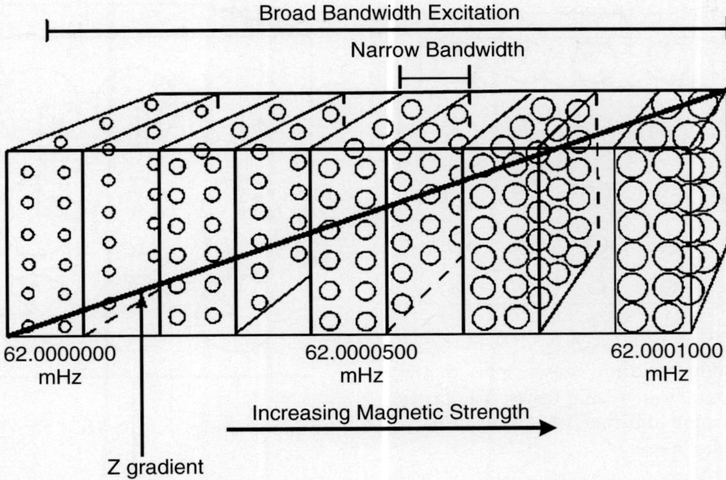

Fig. 54. A gradient across a volume of tissue along the z-axis. With a narrow bandwidth excitation, only the center slab of hydrogen nuclei interacts with the incoming radiofrequency pulse and is thus excited.

maximum echo, all the protons in each voxel are in phase and a coherent signal can be produced. Fig. 59 illustrates that each voxel can be uniquely described in terms of its phase and frequency during data acquisition. In Fig. 60, the entire SE pulse sequence with the appropriate gradients is diagrammatically expressed.

Image reconstruction

The signal detected, amplified, and received by the NMR machine is a group of periodic sine waves of different phases and frequencies. The fact that the signal is already present as sine waves makes the data set ideal for reconstruction by the Fourier transform method. The basis of the Fourier transform is that an object can be represented by an infinite number of sine and cosine waves. The Fourier transform is a mathematic filter that allows conversion of time domain (frequency) to spatial (x, y) coordinates.

Multislice acquisition

To this point, we have discussed the techniques for selective excitation, phase, and frequency encoding for a single slice. The imaging time for a single slice is given by the equation: Time = TR × NEX × Phase-Encoding Steps. Thus, a T2W image with a TR of 3 seconds, 128 matrix, and 1 NEX requires approximately 6 minutes. Were it not possible to acquire multiple images simultaneously, the total imaging time for a 15-slice brain study would be on the order of 90 minutes or longer for a single pulse sequence. An effective method of acquiring multiple slices at once was introduced by Kramer et al [76]. This technique is as follows: an initial slice is excited, the

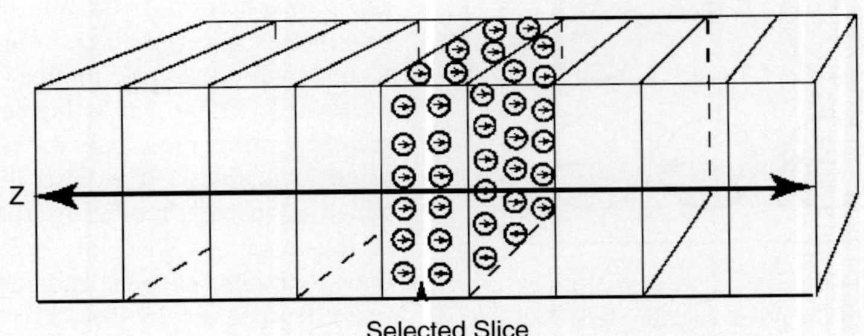

Fig. 55. A slab of selectively excited spins precessing in the x-y plane.

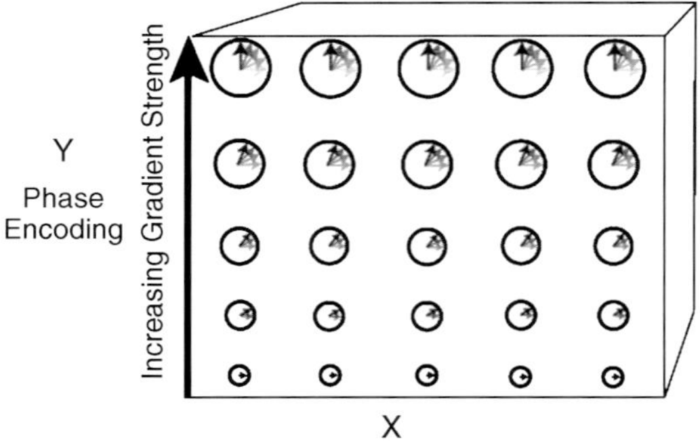

Fig. 56. Phase-encoding gradient causes spins in the stronger part of the gradient to spin faster. The faster spinning protons acquire different phases relative to other lines of precessing nuclei.

appropriate encoding gradients are applied, and the echo is recorded. Note, however, that an additional 2800 milliseconds remain after the echo within the TR before we can re-excite the slice for a different phase-encoding step in the T2W sequence with a TR of 3000 milliseconds as shown in Fig. 61. During this time, the adjacent slice can be excited, encoded, and recorded for a given phase increment, as shown in Fig. 60. After this, there are 2600 milliseconds left during the TR; the process is repeated for the next slice and so on until we have run out of time in our repetition interval and must again return to our initial slice. The first slice is then re-excited, a different strength of phase-encoding gradient is applied, the frequency encoding is performed, and data are

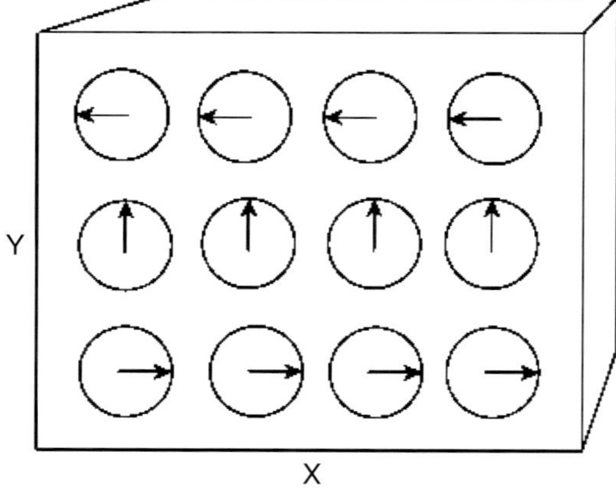

Fig. 57. At the end of the phase-encoding gradient, the phases of the spinning vectors are now uniquely encoded along the *y*-axis.

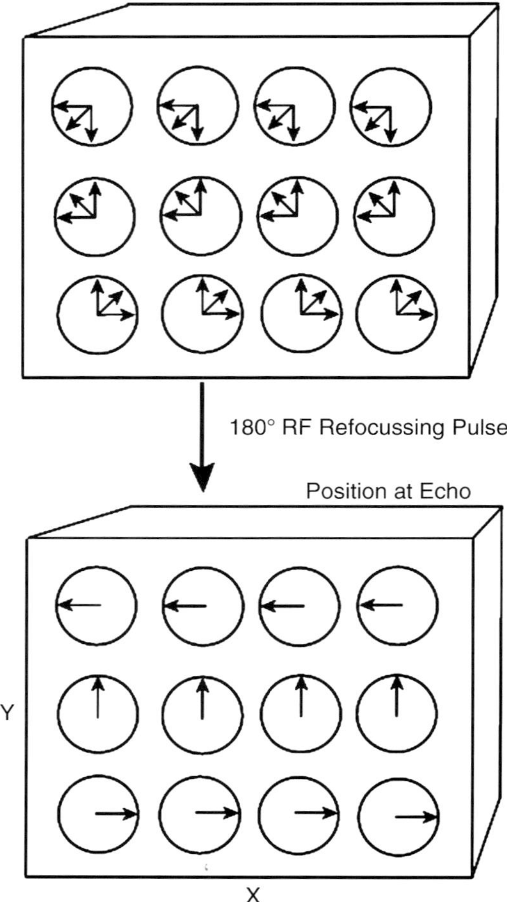

Fig. 58. Rows of spinning protons that begin to dephase are then inverted and resampled by a 180° radiofrequency (RF) pulse. Nevertheless, they "remember" the phase change brought about by the phase-encoding gradient, resulting in a predictable and measurable difference in phase between each of the lines.

sampled again. By the time that we have acquired all the necessary phase-encoding gradients for one slice, information from all the slices has been obtained. From the diagram in Fig. 62, it is easy to understand why the number of slices is limited by the TR. If the TR is increased to 4000 milliseconds, more slices can be sampled during the same acquisition. It is also limited by the TE, which is, in part, limited by the turnaround time of the machine. This duty cycle is the necessary time to excite, encode, and record images selectively from a single slice. For this reason, T1W images that have a short TR are still able to have a relatively similar number of slices compared

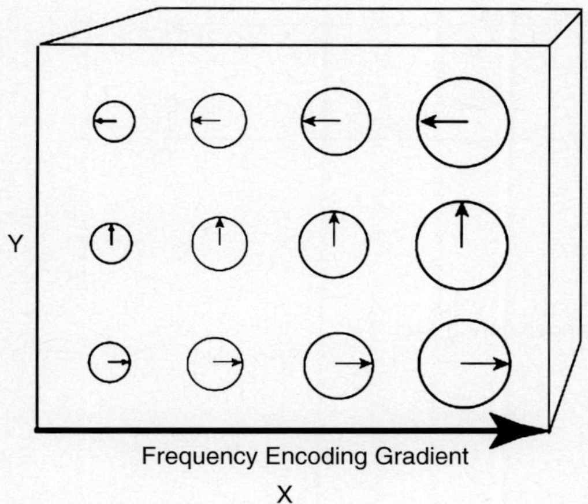

Fig. 59. A frequency-encoding gradient is now applied. The precessing nuclei in the stronger part of the gradient spin at a higher frequency. Each point or voxel within the slice is now defined by a unique phase and frequency.

with T2W sequences (T2W images have a longer TR, but the turnaround time of the machine is also greater as the TE is lengthened).

Single-slice mode

With gradient echo imaging, extremely short TRs and low flip angles may be used. When the TR is so short (on the order of 20–50 milliseconds), only one or two slices can be obtained in a multislice acquisition mode. Therefore, the multislice mode is not time-efficient. Rather, these slices are acquired individually. As shown in Fig. 63, all the phase-encoding steps are acquired for each slice before continuing on to the next slice. The total imaging time for this data acquisition scheme is: Time = TR × NEX × Matrix × Number of Slices.

Gradient echo

The unique feature separating gradient echo pulse schemes from SE is that the 180° RF pulse is omitted. In reality, a gradient echo is performed with each SE pulse sequence; however, data acquisition times and contrast phenomenology are somewhat different. Fig. 64 outlines the timing sequence for gradients and RF pulses for a typical gradient echo data acquisition scheme.

Tissue contrast that can be similar to that in SE imaging is achieved. T1 decay is unchanged. Often, gradient echo acquisition schemes are used in conjunction with low flip angles, which reduces T1 weighting; therefore, the sequence is either proton or T2* weighted. The transverse magnetization rapidly decays with the time constant of T2* as opposed to T2 in SE imaging.

The lack of a 180° refocusing pulse causes several key differences in the appearance of

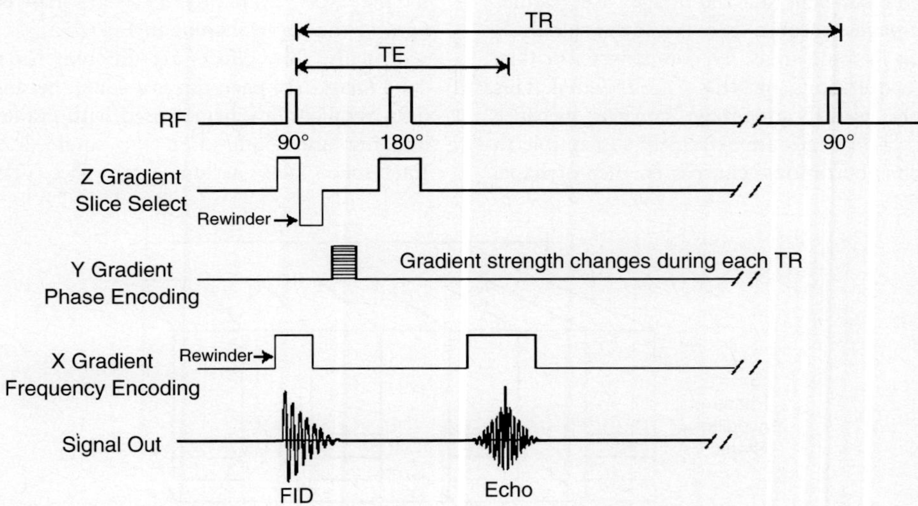

Fig. 60. This spin echo pulse sequence diagram is a bit more complex than the one diagrammed earlier in this article. In this case, the slice-encoding gradients have been added, demonstrating *z*-slice selection with the 90° and 180° pulses. An increasing phase-encoding gradient with each repetition time (TR) and a frequency-encoding gradient that is turned on during the sampling of data at the echo are also present. Rewinder lobes on the slice select and frequency gradients are also present. FID, free induction decay; RF, radiofrequency; TE, echo time.

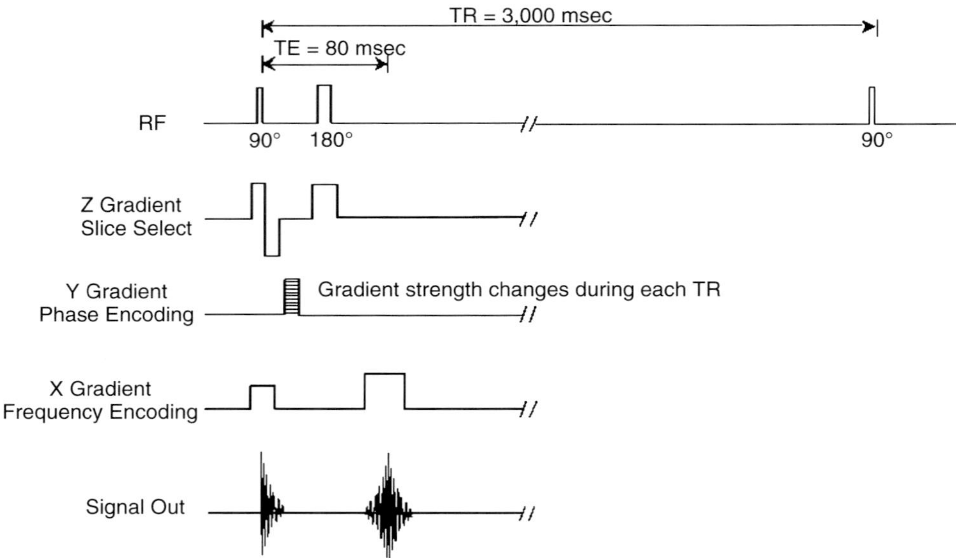

Fig. 61. T2-weighted spin echo pulse diagram with an echo time (TE) of 80 milliseconds. There is a large amount of time still remaining in the repetition cycle (3000 − 80 = 2920 milliseconds) before the next 90° pulse can be applied to that slice of tissue. RF, radiofrequency; TR, repetition time.

gradient echo images as opposed to conventional SE techniques. Phase loss caused by static magnetic field inhomogeneity cannot be recuperated. If a static magnetic field aberration is present, the phase discrepancy induced in these spinning protons is not compensated for by a simple gradient reversal. This means that the images are grainier than SE images, because there is a lower signal-to-noise ratio in some areas. To compensate for this, multiple acquisitions (or NEXs) are required. This can also be used to advantage, however, because gradient echo images are extremely susceptible to local field aberrations caused by hemorrhage, calcification, and paramagnetic or ferromagnetic substances.

A second consequence is that because a 180° RF pulse is not given, there is reduced cross-talk (saturation of the protons of adjacent slices). Serial thin sections can be obtained, as shown by the excellent-quality T1W gradient echo images of the cervical spine in Fig. 65.

Finally, flow effects are different for gradient echo images. In part, this is evident, because many data acquisition schemes used with gradient echo imaging are acquired in the single-slice mode. Each slice acts as an entry slice. Therefore,

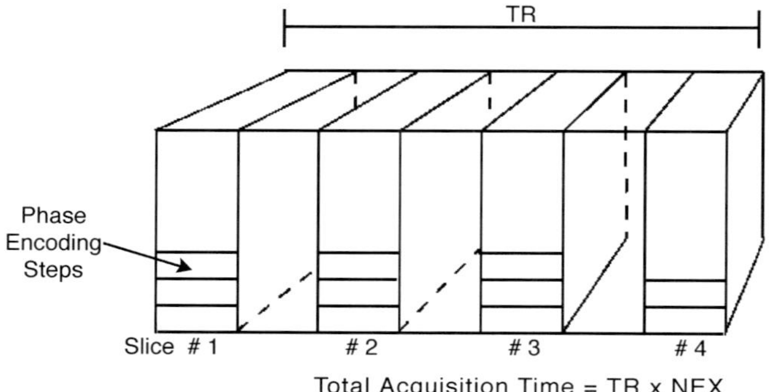

Fig. 62. Multislice acquisition. During each repetition time (TR), phase encoding of multiple slices is performed. Thus, rather than acquiring each slice sequentially, multiple slices are acquired simultaneously using dead time during the TR interval. NEX, number of excitations.

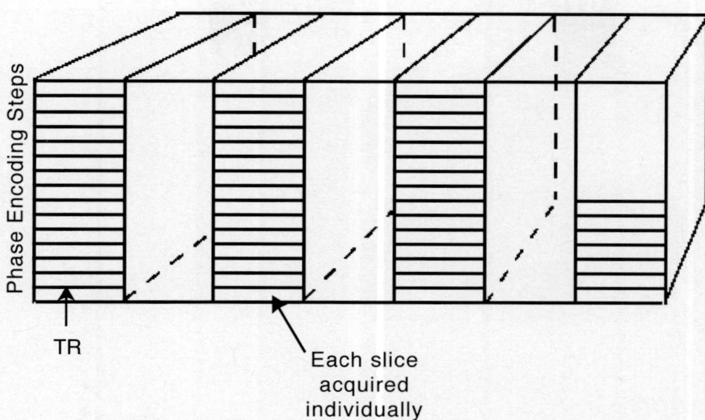

Fig. 63. Single-slice acquisition. If an extremely short repetition time (TR) is used, it is more efficient to acquire each slice individually. In this case, one line of data is acquired during each TR and an entire slice is acquired before moving to the next one. NEX, number of excitations.

flow-related enhancement is more prominent. The second reason why flow effects occur is related to the nonselective nature of gradient refocusing. A selective 90° pulse is given. If the blood flows out of the region of the slice during the time between excitation and data acquisition in SE techniques, this signal is lost. With gradient echo techniques, however, these excited protons are rephased even though they have moved out of the area of interest, and therefore contribute to signal. Gradient echo pulses are often combined with a limited flip angle to achieve extremely short TRs. Imaging time for a slice can be reduced an order of magnitude less than conventional SE.

Gradient echo data acquisition schemes are becoming more popular in clinical use for evaluation of joints, cardiac imaging, and flow studies and are a more sensitive method for detecting

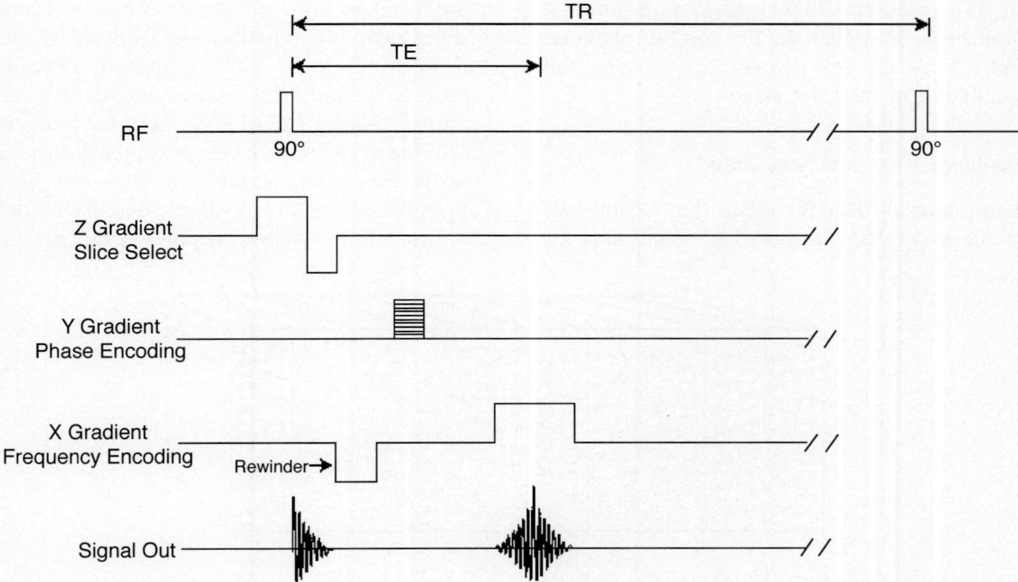

Fig. 64. Gradient echo data acquisition scheme. A simple gradient echo acquisition scheme is presented, where a 90° radiofrequency (RF) pulse is given. The reversal of the slice selection gradients in the *z*-direction and the frequency-encoding gradients in the *x*-direction give an echo as the spins are rephased. TE, echo time; TR, repetition time.

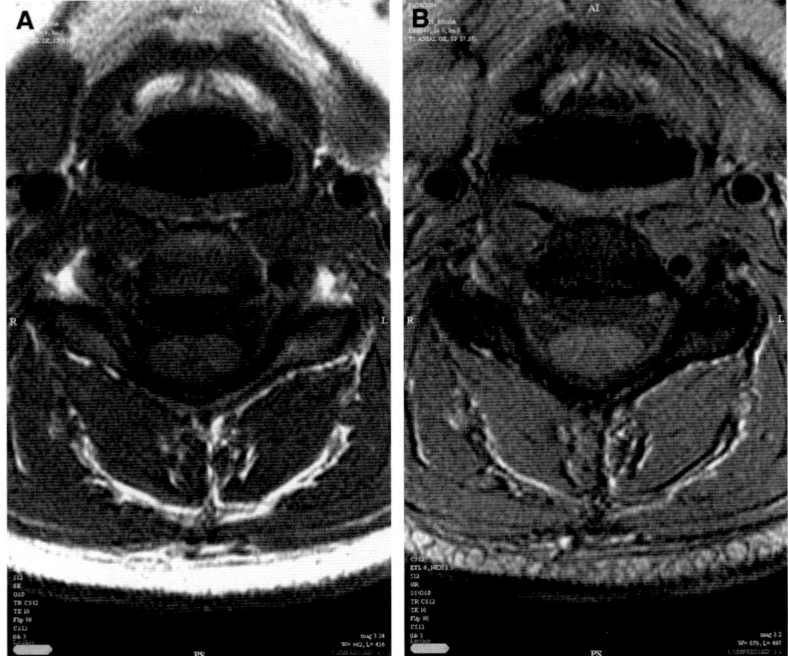

Fig. 65. Thin-section, 3-mm, T1-weighted (T1W), spin echo (SE) versus gradient echo images of cervical spine. (*A*) Thin-section, T1W, SE axial images of cervical spine are fuzzy, and it is difficult to see the nerve roots. (*B*) Same anatomy acquired with the thin-section T1W gradient echo technique. Notice improved contrast and less cross-talk between slices. For thin slices, image quality is visibly better.

hemorrhage and calcification. With extremely short TEs, excellent T1W images with contrast phenomenology similar to SE can be obtained quickly. They are my favorite for imaging the cervical spine in the axial plane.

Three-dimensional data acquisition

Until now, all the data acquisition schemes we have discussed have acquired a single slice at a time. In 3D Fourier transform volume imaging, data from the entire volume of interest is acquired during each TR. Initially, a broadband RF pulse (anywhere from 0°–90°) is applied. Instead of selecting a slice, this excites tissue in a large volume, as shown in Fig. 66. The frequency-encoding gradient can only be applied once, and that is during data acquisition. How can our 3D object be reduced to individual points? The trick is to use two phase-encoding gradients. An

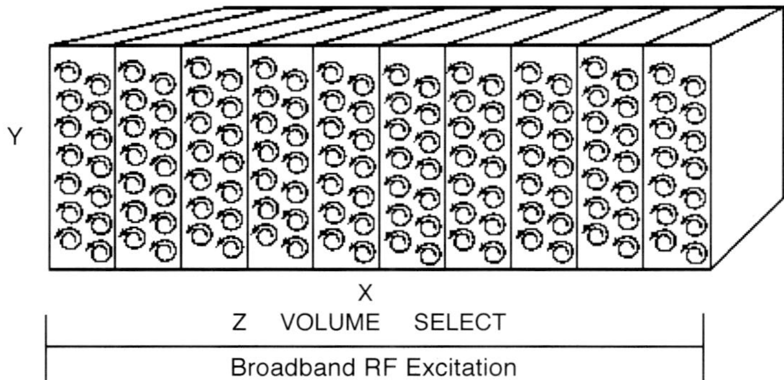

Fig. 66. Three-dimensional imaging. A broadband radiofrequency (RF) excitation excites a large volume of tissue.

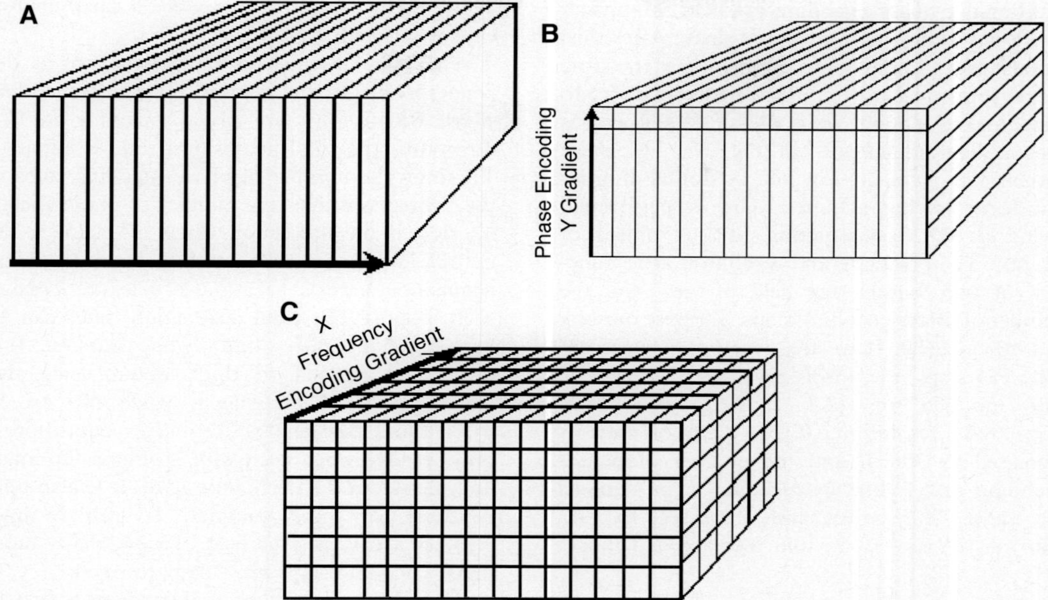

Fig. 67. Three-dimensional (3D) imaging. (*A*) Phase encoding along the *z*-axis establishes uniform phase modulation in our excited box along *z* with unique slabs. (*B*) Phase encoding along the *y*-gradient reduces our 3D object to a series of lines. (*C*) Finally, applying the frequency-encoding gradient during data sampling reduces each individual voxel to unique data.

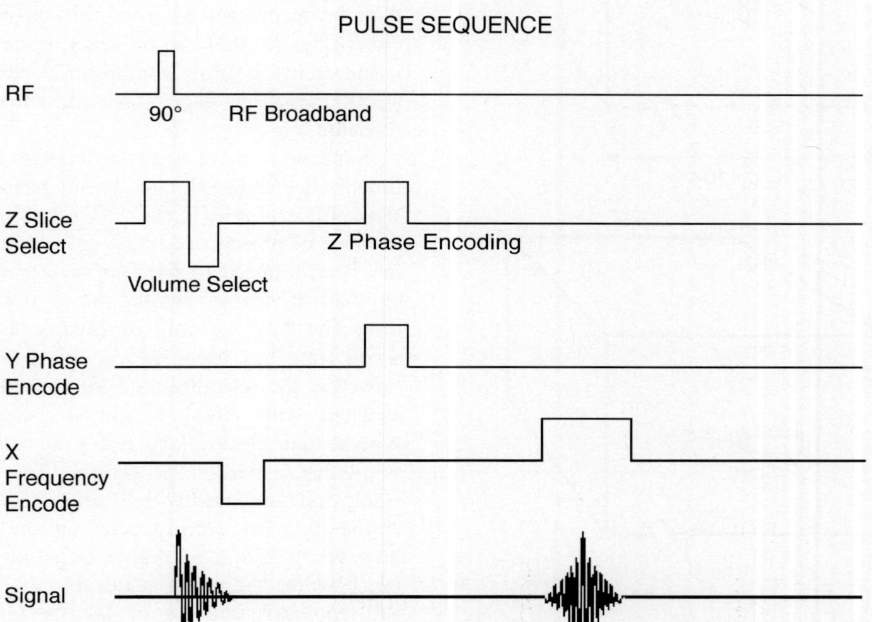

Fig. 68. Pulse sequence diagram for three-dimensional data acquisition incorporating an additional phase-encoding gradient on the *z*-axis.

additional z-phase encoding gradient is applied, which chops our box into small slices. After this, y-phase encoding and then x-frequency encoding are performed taking our 3D object from a slice to a line and to a point, respectively. This process is shown diagrammatically in Fig. 67. The pulse sequence is given in Fig. 68. A double-Fourier transform of the acquired data is performed, giving a 3D reconstruction of our object of interest. The pixel size and resolution are a function of two factors: the field of view and the number of phase-encoding steps. Suppose our box is a 10-cm cube. If we frequency and phase encode 256 steps, the voxel size in our box will be 100 mm/256 or (0.4 mm^3) = 0.064 mm^3 (Fig. 69A) resolution. If our field of view is increased to 30 cm and the number of phase-encoding and frequency-encoding steps remains the same, our voxel size increases to (1.2 mm^3) = 1.7 mm^3, a 27-fold increase in volume.

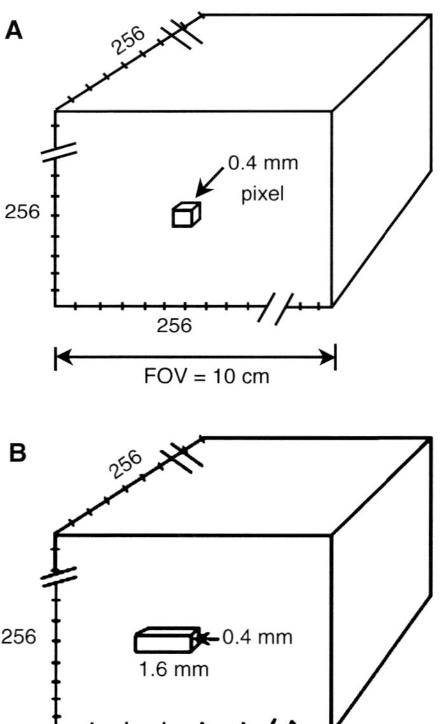

Fig. 69. (*A*) A 10-cm field of view with a 256 matrix on each side yields dimensions of 0.4 mm to each of the pixels or a 0.064 mm^3 voxel size. (*B*) Obtaining a 256 × 256 field of view by 64 yields anisotropic voxels measuring 1.6 mm × 0.4 mm × 0.4 mm, or 0.256 mm^3.

Thus, our resolution is best when a small field of view is selected.

The imaging time in 3D acquisitions is dependent on TR and number of phase-encoding steps. Because we are phase encoding in two directions, the total acquisition time is equal to TR times the number of phase-encoding steps in the z-direction times the number of phase-encoding steps in the y-direction. For a 256 × 256 × 256 matrix and a TR of 50 milliseconds, the total acquisition time is 55 minutes. Clearly, even at such a short TR, total acquisition times can be prohibitive if high-resolution work is desired. It is not even practical to think about using this technique for SE imaging in which TRs are 10 to 50 times this length. 3D image acquisition is only feasible when used with a limited flip angle and ultrashort TR techniques [76]. It is also only practical for small volumes. To achieve high resolution over a large field of view, many more phase-encoding steps must be performed.

One of the advantages of 3D imaging is that all the pixels in the matrix can be made isotropic, that is, of equal size. The data can then be reconstructed in any desired plane, not only in the three orthogonal axes but with the oblique slices reconstructed as well. This is a useful feature, because the data for a given pulse sequence need only be acquired once and any desired plane can then be reconstructed from this information. If one wishes to alter the pulse sequence to change tissue contrast or to administer a paramagnetic agent, however, the pulse sequence must be repeated.

Suppose that we want to decrease acquisition time by decreasing the number of phase-encoding steps, for example, in the z-axis. In Fig. 69B, the number of phase-encoding steps along the z-axis has been reduced to 64. Our pixel size for a 10-cm field of view is then 0.4 mm × 0.4 mm × 1.6 mm. The data are now anisotropic. Data acquisition time has been reduced by a factor of 4; however, the resulting data set cannot be reconstructed with equal resolution in any plane. Notice that the in-plane resolution along x and y still has a 256 × 256 matrix. For this plane, resolution compared with SE imaging is excellent. If the data are reconstructed in the y-z plane, however, a 256 × 64 matrix is present, which is much worse than that achievable with a routine SE sequence. Because of the use of gradient-recalled echo acquisition, these images are T2* weighted and are prone to magnetic susceptibility artifacts.

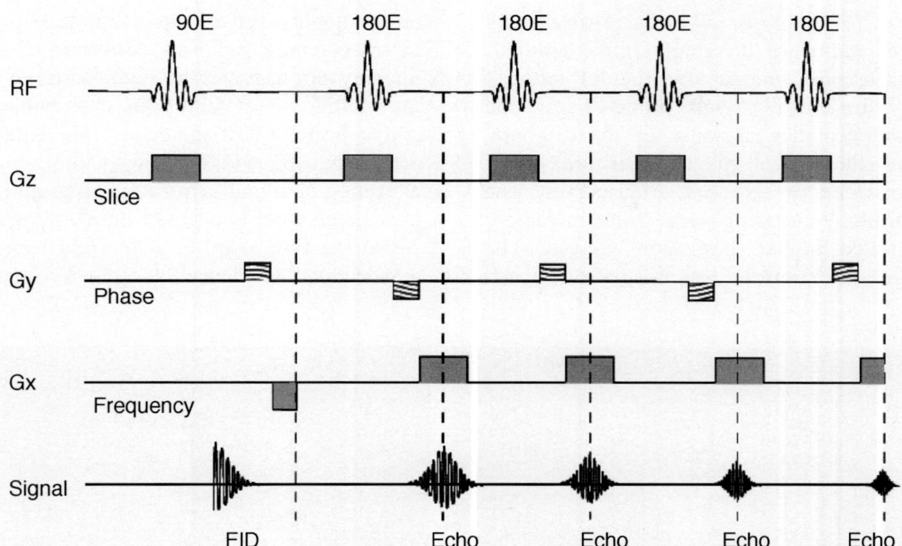

Fig. 70. Fast spin echo pulse sequence diagram. The first part of the sequence is identical to the spin echo sequence. A 90° pulse is given, followed by 180° radiofrequency (RF) refocusing pulse. The difference lies in the fact that multiple 180° RF refocusing pulses are applied, resulting in a stream of echoes after a single excitation pulse. FID, free induction decay.

Because of these limitations, 3D imaging is most suitable in areas in which a small field of view is desirable and multiplanar reconstruction is necessary. These areas include the pituitary gland, the knee and other small joints, and the neuroforamina of the cervical spine.

Fast spin echo technique

Fast spin echo (FSE), or rapid acquisition relaxation enhanced, initially described by Hennig and Friedburg [78] and developed by others [79], is probably the single most important advance in faster imaging within the past decade. FSE is really a hybrid of the multislice SE and echoplanar techniques. Any long TR or long TE pulse sequence (especially with newer and faster gradient technology) has substantial dead time. Rather than acquire one line at a time in a multislice mode, multiple 180° pulses with incremental phase encoding are performed during a single TE (Fig. 70). Instead of acquiring one line of k-space during an echo, four or more lines are acquired. This is shown diagrammatically in Fig. 71. Eight lines of k-space are acquired per single echo within a given repetition cycle, and data from many slices can be obtained during each TR. This makes FSE one of the most efficient available methods for acquiring MRI data. This is especially true for T2W images. Because the TRs are long, many slices can be obtained. The TEs are also long, allowing multiple lines of k-space to be sampled during one TE, more than 100 (ie, single-shot FSE) with some machines. FSE imaging adds another dimension to MRI parameters that can affect image quality and speed (ie, echo train length). In a study by Tien et al [80] of FSE imaging parameters using a 16-kHz bandwidth, an echo train length of 8 and TRs between 3000 and 4000 milliseconds were determined to be optimal.

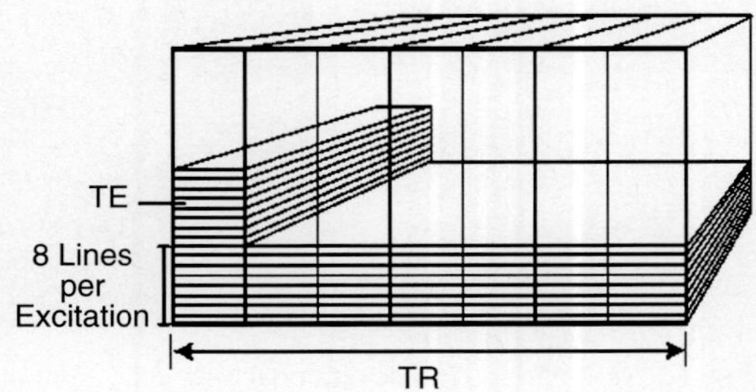

Fig. 71. Fast spin echo multislice acquisition. In this case, multiple lines are obtained using multiple echoes from a single excitation. This vastly increases the acquisition efficiency, particularly on long repetition time (TR) sequences. The k-space can be filled much faster. In this case, eight lines are obtained during each echo. TE, echo time.

FSE can be compared with the revolutionary advance of multislice imaging. Unlike gradient echo images, FSE images are true RF-induced echoes and are much less susceptible to magnetic field inhomogeneities. Because of the dramatic increase in efficiency of image acquisition, multiple averages can be acquired. Alternatively, the number of phase-encoding steps can be increased, yielding much higher resolution images. The bottom line is extremely fast images or superb image quality for an equal amount of time investment compared with conventional SE. FSE imaging can improve the signal-to-noise ratio per unit time by a factor of 8 compared with conventional SE if an echo train length of 16 echoes is used [81]. Looked at another way, the efficiency of signal acquisition is proportional to how much time is devoted purely to reading the signal. In FSE with an echo train length of 33, a calculated efficiency of 50% is obtained. By

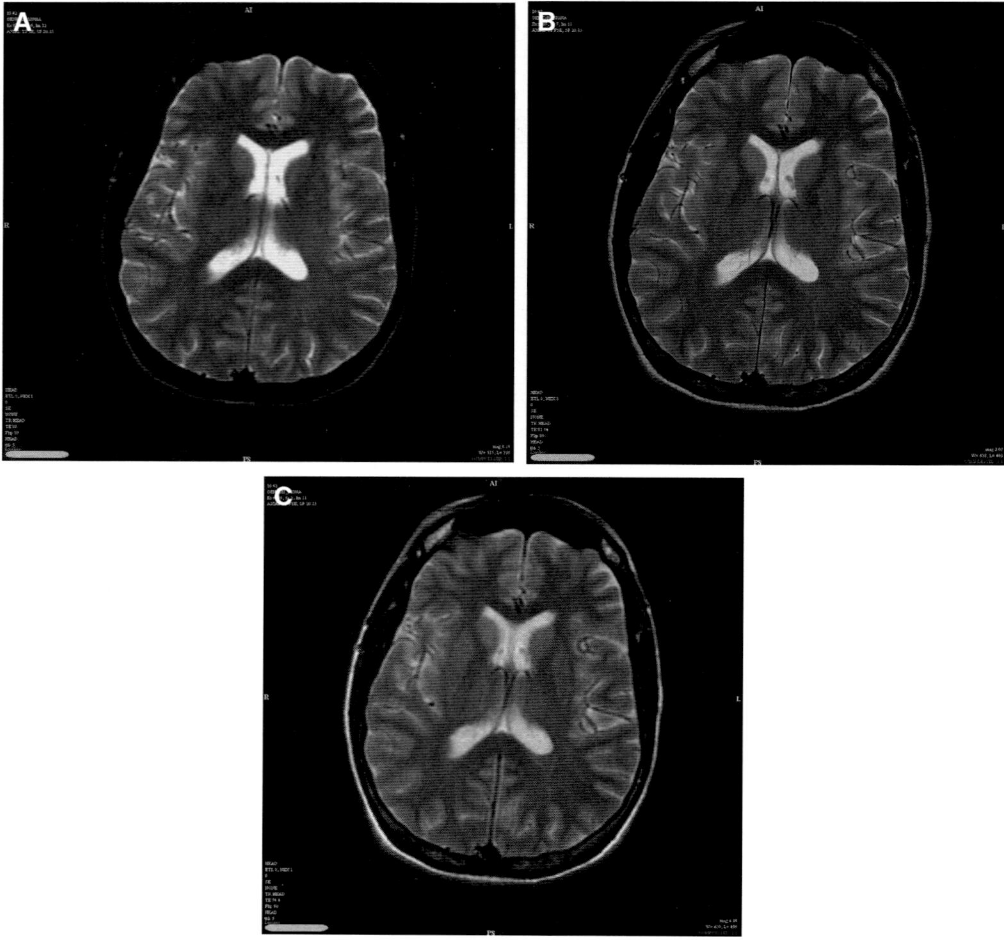

Fig. 72. Comparison of conventional spin echo (SE) and fast spin echo (FSE). (*A*) SE (repetition time [TR] = 3000 milliseconds, echo time [TE] = 80 milliseconds, 5-mm thick slices, 18 images in 7 minutes and 48 seconds, 256 × 192 matrix, number of excitations [NEX] = 1). (*B*) FSE (TR = 3000 milliseconds, effective TE = 84 milliseconds, 5-mm slice thickness, echo train length = 8, 12 images in 7 minutes and 18 seconds, 512 × 512 matrix, NEX = 3). In this case, the imaging time is comparable to that of Fig. 72A. With FSE, however, there is a dramatic improvement in the signal-to-noise ratio and resolution. (*C*) Alternatively, one can use the benefits of FSE to decrease the acquisition time. In this case (TR = 3000 milliseconds, TE = 80 milliseconds, echo train length = 8 milliseconds, 5-mm slice thickness, 256 × 192 matrix, NEX = 1), FSE yielded 18 images in 1 minute. The image quality is comparable to that of the conventional SE image, which required nearly 8 minutes, representing an eight-fold improvement in efficiency.

comparison, SE imaging has approximately 20% efficiency [82]. Thus, FSE imaging not only acquires images faster but acquires more signal per unit time. A series of images comparing a conventional SE sequence and a FSE sequence is shown in Fig. 72. From this series of images, we can see that with FSE images, tradeoffs can be made between image quality and speed [83].

Image contrast in fast spin echo imaging

The central region of k-space corresponding to low frequencies (low gradient strength) is primarily responsible for image contrast. The more peripheral high-frequency components are responsible for edge detail [84]. FSE requires strong gradients, because phase encoding must be performed quickly. Strong gradients dephase signal. The central part of k-space, near the gradient isocenter, receives the least dephasing. Therefore, measurable signal differences between tissues are greatest and produce most of the contrast in the image for echoes sampled near the center of k-space. Whether the center of k-space is sampled early or late determines in part whether an image is T1W or T2W. If the periphery of k-space is sampled first, followed by the central echoes, it is T2W.

T1-weighted fast spin echo

For T1W imaging, the first echoes (ie, those at the beginning of the phase encoding) are used to sample the central k-space to achieve T1W contrast. This has the undesirable effect of

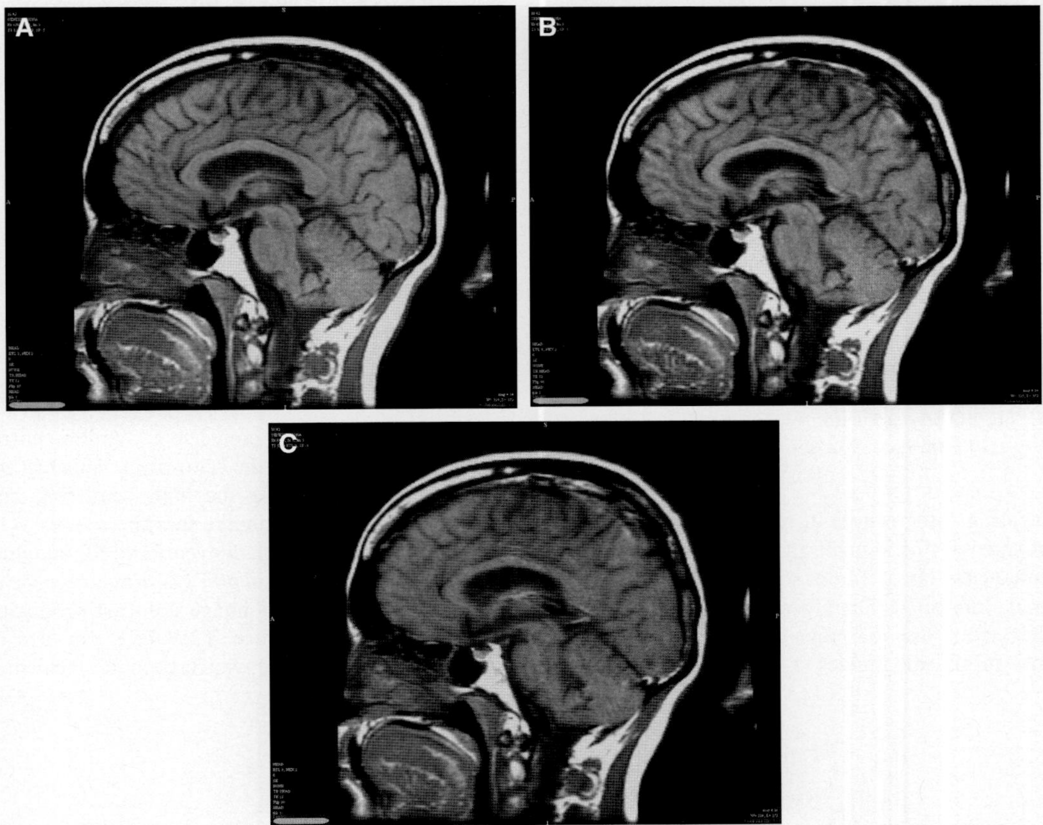

Fig. 73. This is a comparison of T1-weighted fast spin echo (FSE) images showing loss of edge detail with increasing echo train length. A series of FSE (TR = 600 milliseconds, TE = 15eff milliseconds, 5-mm slice thickness, 2.5-mm spacing, 256 × 192 matrix, NEX = 2, 22-cm field of view images). (*A*) Echo train length of 2. (*B*) Echo train length of 4. (*C*) Echo train length of 8. Notice how the gyral detail is obscured with increasing echo train length. The corpus callosum and adjacent cerebrospinal fluid are not as sharply defined. The pons appears fuzzy. The cerebellar folia are not as well delineated.

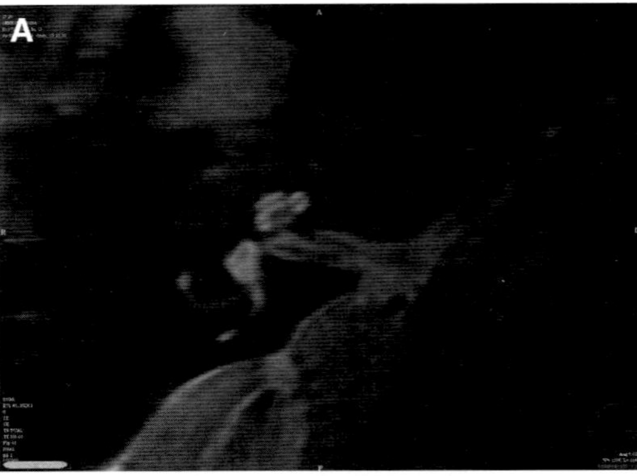

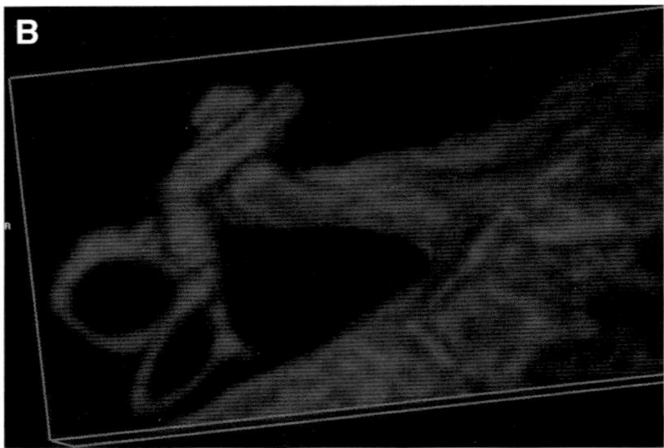

Fig. 74. Axial fast spin echo images through the internal auditory canals and petrous bones (TR = 4400 milliseconds, TE = 109 milliseconds, echo train length = 48 milliseconds, 512 × 256 matrix, three-dimensional [3D] axial 0.8-mm slice thickness). The individual seventh and eighth nerves can be identified in the internal auditory canal. (*A*) Collapsed region reconstruction of the 3D data. (*B*) 3D reconstruction of the 3D FSE data set on a Novarad (American Fork, Utah) workstation.

relegating later echoes to acquire the more peripheral lines of k-space that correspond to high frequencies. These echoes show progressive loss of signal intensity. Therefore, T1W FSE images suffer from loss of edge detail compared with conventional SE images (Fig. 73). Increasing the echo train length causes progressive loss of image sharpness. Furthermore, because the TR of T1W images is relatively short (500–1000 milliseconds), the introduction of multiple additional echo trains prolongs the acquisition time and drastically reduces the number of slices available. For example, an eight–echo train, T1W, FSE pulse sequence requires approximately 160 milliseconds. Only 4 slices can be acquired compared with a conventional SE sequence, in which 35 slices can be acquired. Therefore, FSE imaging is not highly efficient for T1W imaging.

When sampling a longer echo train, there is progressive T2 decay of all tissues in an exponential fashion. Those echoes sampling high-frequency data are performed last and have the lowest intensity and the highest noise. Furthermore, those tissues that have the shortest T2 suffer the most in loss of spatial information. Therefore, areas such as bone interfaces show poor edge detail with adjacent tissues as CSF. The longer the echo train length, the greater signal intensity difference there is between the first and last echoes.

FSE imaging can be acquired in a 3D mode. As such, the edge blurring found on T1W images can be directed out of the image plane and into the *z*-slice select direction by reordering the *x*- and *y*-directions of phase encoding. This technique was used by Weinberger et al [85] to acquire 3D T1W images of the pediatric spine, acquiring 28 images at 1-mm thickness in a period of 8.5 minutes.

T2-weighted fast spin echo

FSE T2W images, conversely, acquire central k-space much later in the echo train. This has the advantage of acquiring the high-frequency data first. Edge clarity and image sharpness seem to be slightly better than with conventional SE imaging. There is an accentuation of T2 contrast because of the late acquisition of image contrast-producing echoes in central k-space. T2W FSE can also be obtained in a 3D mode, which becomes efficient if

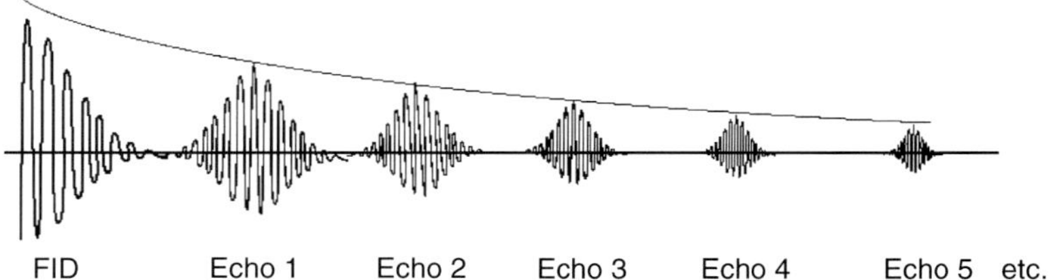

Fig. 75. With each echo, the signal intensity drops. Thus, lines of data acquired at echo 8 suffer degradation and distortion compared with those acquired at echo 1. FID, free induction decay.

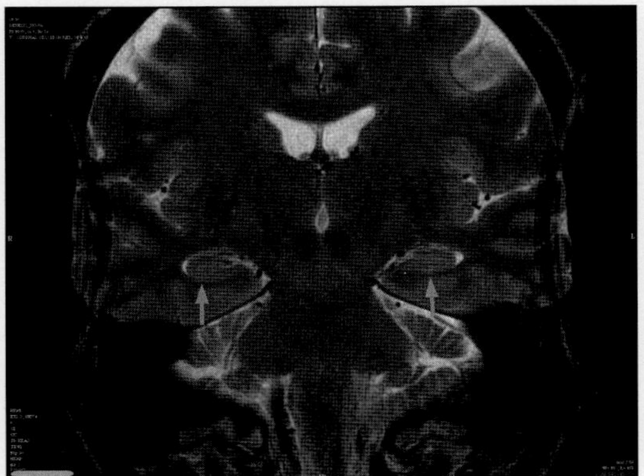

Fig. 76. Fast spin echo (TR = 4000 milliseconds, TE = 92 milliseconds, echo train length = 8, 18-cm × 14-cm field of view, 3-mm slice thickness, 512 × 384 matrix, NEX = 4) images through the temporal lobe allow excellent delineation of the hippocampal formations (*arrows*). This technique is useful for screening of mesiotemporal sclerosis.

a long echo train length is used. Such a sequence is useful for high-resolution images of structures that have long T2, such as the semicircular canals of the inner ear (Fig. 74) [86].

Disadvantages

Nothing is completely free. FSE has a few disadvantages. It is not particularly well suited for T1W images because of the short TEs required for T1 weighting. Traditional T2 contrast as seen on brain imaging is a little different from FSE imaging. To begin with, each of the echoes is not identical. There is gradual loss of signal with the refocusing of each echo (Fig. 75). The more echoes that are attempted for each TE, the more distortion there is between each line. FSE also suffers from a number of artifacts, which include blurring of images with T1W images (see Fig. 71) and edge enhancement artifacts found with T2W images [87]. Furthermore, because more echoes are sampled for each TE, the gradients are driven harder. This, in turn, induces more eddy currents and magnetic field inhomogeneities. With the large number of 180° RF pulses (some of which are off-resonant) and because multislice imaging is being performed, a significant amount of magnetization transfer occurs. Magnetization transfer is the most important reason for signal loss in comparison with SE [88]. FSE imaging can acquire single- or double-echo sequences [89]. The TE is really a false TE time; the TE is determined by when the central phase-encoding data are obtained. Most systems describe this as the TEeff.

Clinical applications

Early results predicted (and these have largely been borne out in practice) that FSE imaging would replace conventional SE imaging for most

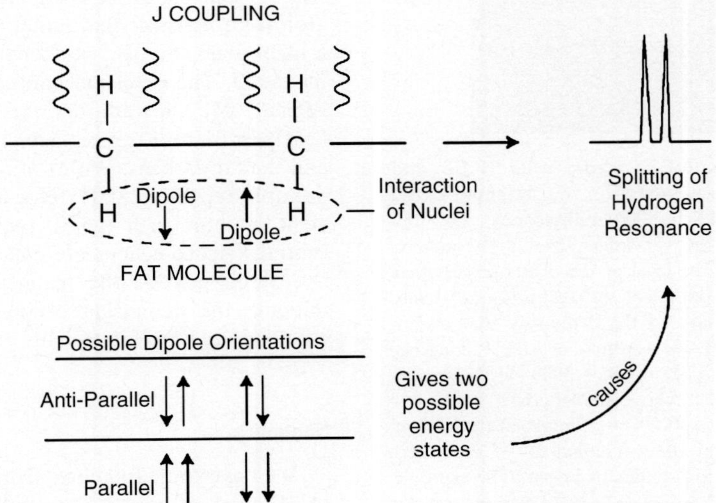

Fig. 77. J coupling. Hydrogen nuclei on adjacent carbon atoms have their own small magnetic field, which interacts with adjacent atoms. As a result of this interaction, the spectrum of the hydrogen nuclei is altered—a phenomenon known as splitting. The dipoles can exist in one of two orientations, parallel or antiparallel. When the dipoles are parallel, they tend to repel each other, altering the magnetic field, and thus altering the resonant frequency of the hydrogen nuclei.

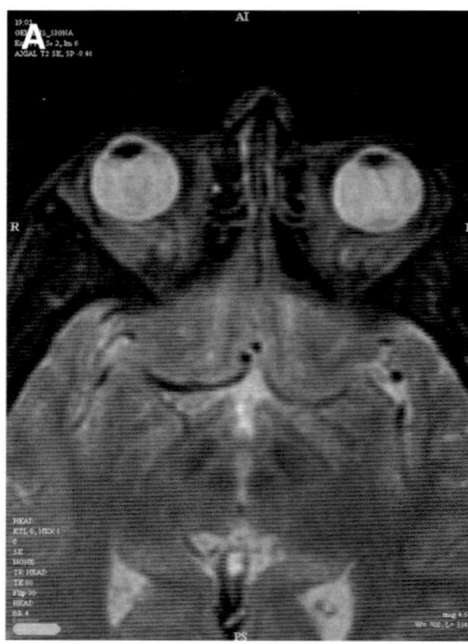

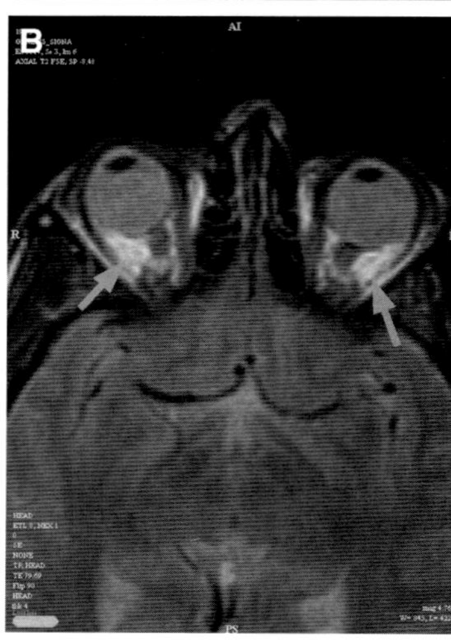

Fig. 78. Comparison of fast spin echo (FSE) and conventional spin echo (SE) for fat brightness. (*A*) Conventional SE (TR = 3000 milliseconds, TE = 80 milliseconds, 5-mm slice thickness, 256 × 192 matrix, NEX = 1) image at the level of the orbits reveals that the intraorbital fat is dark. The scalp fat is also relatively dark. This is secondary to the dephasing that occurs within fat molecules as a result of the J coupling phenomenon. (*B*) FSE (TR = 3000 milliseconds, TE = 80 milliseconds, echo train length = 8 milliseconds, 256 × 192 matrix, NEX = 1) image at the level of the orbits reveals that the intraconal fat of the orbits (*arrows*) and the scalp fat remain bright. The multiple echo train of the FSE sequence helps to average out the micromolecular magnetic perturbations within the fat molecule.

brain [90] and spine imaging [91] for intradural [92] and extradural disease [93] of the spine. Heavily T2W images can be sampled, creating myelographic-like visualization of the spine. Numerous clinical studies comparing the efficacy of FSE with conventional SE have demonstrated it to be comparable or superior in the detection of multiple sclerosis lesions [94], in the evaluation of infarcts [95], for the pelvis [96], and for the evaluation of intracranial neoplasms [97]. The improved resolution is also helpful for evaluation of the temporal lobes (Fig. 76).

Hemorrhagic lesions do not show quite as much susceptibility effect, although lesion conspicuity is similar in actual practice [98]. Additionally, FSE imaging is less sensitive for the diagnosis of meniscal tears compared with conventional SE imaging at comparable image resolution [99]. Susceptibility effects decrease with increasing echo train length, which may account for its lowered sensitivity in these conditions [100].

J coupling

Fat signal also tends to have different characteristics on T2W FSE images from conventional SE images [101–103]. This has been attributed to a phenomenon known as J coupling (Fig. 77). J coupling is commonly found in NMR spectra in which hydrogen nuclei interact with one another across a carbon-carbon or other bond. The net effect is splitting of the resonance of the hydrogen atoms. In essence, this might be thought of as a micromagnetic field perturbation at the molecular level. The exact mechanism remains controversial [104]. On traditional SE images, this local field perturbation causes dephasing of the nuclei and the fat darkens. With FSE imaging, there are multiple repetitive 180° refocusing pulses, often eight or more in a typical sequence, before the central k-space echoes are collected. This repetitive refocusing of the magnetic field tends to mitigate the dephasing ordinarily caused by J coupling, and the fat remains bright (Fig. 78).

Summary

We have come full circle from spinning quarks to 3D medical images. The bulk of MRI is now performed using slice-selective gradients, during which RF energy is applied to excite the hydrogen nuclei. By stepping a phase-encoding gradient during each TR and using a frequency-encoding gradient as the data are sampled, the 3D human object can be reduced to many individual points or voxels. By acquiring multiple slices at once, the time efficiency of imaging can be vastly improved. Many newer strategies use variations of this technique to acquire multiple lines of data during a single echo, enshrining spin warp imaging as the most important method of signal acquisition for MRI.

References

[1] Purcell EM, Torrey HC, Pound RV. Nuclear induction experiment. Phys Rev 1946;70:474–85.

[2] Bloch F, Hansen WW, Packard M. Resonance absorption by nuclear magnetic moment in a solid. Phys Rev 1946;69:37–8.

[3] Williams WSC. Nuclear and particle physics. Oxford (NY): Oxford University Press; 1991.

[4] Fullerton GD. Basic concepts for nuclear magnetic resonance imaging. Magn Reson Imaging 1982; 1(1):39–53.

[5] Levin I. Nuclear-magnetic-resonance spectroscopy. Phys Chemistry 1978;671–80.

[6] Gordon RE. Magnets, molecules and medicine. Phys Med Biol 1985;30:741–69.

[7] Lerski RA. Principles of nuclear magnetic resonance (NMR)—current state-of-the art. J Med Eng Technol 1985;9(3):112–6.

[8] Pykett SL, Newhouse JH, Buonanno BS, Brady TJ, et al. Principles of nuclear magnetic resonance imaging. Radiology 1982;143:157–68.

[9] Pykett IL. NMR imaging in medicine. Sci Am 1982;246:78–88.

[10] Gore JC, Emery EW, Orr JS, Doyle FH. Medical nuclear magnetic resonance imaging: I. Physical principles. Invest Radiol 1981;18(4):269–74.

[11] Hennel JW, Klinowski J. Fundamentals of nuclear magnetic resonance. Essex: Longman Sci Tech; 1993. p. 61–7.

[12] Dwek RA. Nuclear magnetic resonance (NMR) in biochemistry: applications to enzyme systems. Oxford: Clarendon Press; 1973. p. 15.

[13] Hallick D, Resnick R, et al. Fundamentals of physics. New York: John Wiley & Sons; 1974.

[14] Dwek RA. Relaxation, chemical shifts, spin-spin coupling constants and chemical exchange. NMR Biochem 1973;11–47.

[15] Koenig SH, Brown RD, Spiller M, Lundbom N. Relaxometry of brain: why white matter appears bright in MRI. Magn Reson Med 1990;14:482–95.

[16] Mitchell DG, Burk DL, Vinitski S, Rifkin MD. The biophysical basis of tissue contrast in extracranial MR imaging. AJR Am J Roentgenol 1987;149: 831–7.

[17] Boyko OB, Burger PC, Shelburne D, Ingram P. Non-heme mechanisms for T1 shortening: pathologic, CT and MR elucidation. AJNR Am J Neuroradiol 1992;13(5):1439–45.

[18] Fullerton GD, Cameron IL, Ord VA. Frequency dependence of magnetic resonance spin-lattice relaxation of protons in biological materials. Radiology 1984;151(1):135–8.

[19] Koenig SH, Brown RD, Adams D, Emerson D, Harrison CG. Magnetic field dependence of $1/T_1$ of protons in tissue. Invest Radiol 1984;19:76–81.

[20] Wehrli FW, MacFall JR, Shutts D, Breger R, Herfkens RJ. Mechanisms of contrast in NMR imaging. J Comput Assist Tomogr 1984;8(3):369–80.

[21] Kj?r L, Henriksen O. Comparison of different pulse sequences for in vivo determination of T1 relaxation times in the human brain. Acta Radiol 1988; 29(Fasc 2):231–6.

[22] Young IR. Considerations affecting signal and contrast in NMR imaging. Br Med Bull 1984;40(2): 139–47.

[23] Breger RK, Rimm AA, Fischer ME, Papke RA, Haughton VM. T1 and T2 measurements on a 1.5-T commercial MR imager. Radiology 1989; 171:263–76.

[24] Damadian R. Tumor detection by nuclear magnetic resonance. Science 1971;171:1151–3.

[25] Cameron IL, Ord VA, Fullerton GD. Characterization of proton NMR relaxation times in normal and pathological tissues by correlation with other tissue parameters. Magn Reson Imaging 1984; 2(2):97–106.

[26] LeBas JF, Benabid AL, et al. NMR of brain tumors. J Comput Assist Tomogr 1984;8(6):1048–57.

[27] Jackson JA, Schneiders NJ, Ford JJ, Bryan RN. Improvements in the clinical utility of calculated T_2 images of the human brain. Magn Reson Imaging 1985;3(2):131–43.

[28] Just M, Thelan M. Tissue characterization with T1, T2 and proton density values: results in 160 patients with brain tumors. Radiology 1988;169:779–85.

[29] Hoehn-Berlage M, Tolxdorff T, Bockhorst K, Okada Y, Ernestus R-I. In vivo NMR T_2 relaxation of experimental brain tumors in the cat: a multiparameter tissue characterization. Magn Reson Imaging 1992;10:935–47.

[30] Jackson EF, Ginsberg LE, Schomer DF, Leeds NE. A review of MRI pulse sequences and techniques in neuroimaging. Surg Neurol 1997;47:185–99.

[31] Zimmerman R, Gibby WA, Carmody RF. Neuroimaging, clinical and physical principles. New York (NY): Springer-Verlag; 2000.

[32] Hahn EL. Spin-echoes. Phys Rev 1955;80:580–94.

[33] Wehrli FW, MacFall JR, Glover GH, Grigsby N, et al. The dependence of nuclear magnetic resonance (NMR) image contrast on intrinsic and pulse sequence timing parameters. Magn Reson Imaging 1984;2(1):3–16.

[34] Perman WH, Hilar SK, Simon HE, Maudsley AA. Contrast manipulation in NMR imaging. Magn Reson Imaging 1984;2(1):23–32.

[35] Plewes DB. The AAPM/RSNA physics tutorial for residents: contrast mechanisms in spin-echo MR imaging. Radiographics 1994;14(6):1389–404.

[36] Wehrli FW, Breger RK, MacFall JR, Daniels DL, et al. Quantification of contrast in clinical MR brain imaging at high magnetic field: original investigations. Invest Radiol 1985;20(4):360–9.

[37] Nelson TR, Hendrick RE, Hendee WR. Selection of pulse sequences producing maximum tissue contrast in magnetic resonance imaging. Magn Reson Imaging 1984;2(4):285–94.

[38] Carr HY, Purcell EM. Effects of diffusion on free precession in nuclear magnetic resonance experiments. Phys Rev 1954;94:630–8.

[39] Meiboom S, Gill D. Carr-Purcell-Meiboom-Gill sequence (CPMG). Rev Sci Instrum 1959;29:688–91.

[40] Bydder GM, Young IR. MR imaging: clinical use of the inversion recovery sequence. J Comput Assist Tomogr 1985;9(4):659–75.

[41] Wehrli FW, MacFall JR, Shutts D, et al. Mechanisms of contrast in NMR imaging. J Comput Assist Tomogr 1984;8(3):369–80.

[42] Edelstein WA, Bottomley PA, Hart HR, Smith LS. Signal, noise and contrast in nuclear magnetic resonance (NMR) imaging. J Comput Assist Tomogr 1983;7(3):391–401.

[43] Moran PR, Kumar NG, Karstaedt N, Jackels SC. Tissue contrast enhancement: image reconstruction algorithm and selection of TI in inversion recovery MRI. Magn Reson Imaging 1986;4:229–35.

[44] Huk W, Heindel W, Deimling M, Stetter E. Nuclear magnetic resonance (NMR) tomography of the central nervous system: comparison of two imaging sequences. J Comput Assist Tomogr 1983;7(3): 468–75.

[45] Atlas SW, Grossman RI, Hackney DB, Goldberg HI, Bilaniuk LT, Zimmerman RA. STIR MR imaging of the orbit. AJNR Am J Neuroradiol 1988;9:969–74.

[46] Takehara S, Tanaka T, Uemura K, Shinora Y, et al. Optic nerve injury demonstrated by MRI with STIR sequences. Neuroradiology 1994;36: 512–4.

[47] Johnson G, Miller DH, MacManus D, Tofts PS, et al. STIR sequences in NMR imaging of the optic nerve. Neuroradiology 1987;29(13):238–45.

[48] Tien RD. Fat suppression MR imaging and neuroradiology: techniques and clinical application. AJR Am J Roentgenol 1992;158(2):369–79.

[49] Krinsky G, Rofsky NM, Weinreb JC. Non-specificity of short inversion time inversion recovery (STIR) as a technique of fat suppression: pitfalls in image interpretation. AJR Am J Roentgenol 1996;166:523–6.

[50] Hittmair K, Mallek R, Prayer D, Schindler EG, Kollegger H. Spinal cord lesions in patients with multiple sclerosis: comparison of MR pulse sequences. AJNR Am J Neuroradiol 1996;17:1555–65.

[51] Rydberg JN. Fast FLAIR. Radiology 1993;193: 173–80.

[52] Rydberg JN. FLAIR. Magn Reson Med 1995;34: 868–77.

[53] Alexander JA, Sheppard S, Davis PC, Salverda P. Adult cerebrovascular disease: role of modified rapid fluid-attenuated inversion-recovery sequences. AJNR Am J Neuroradiol 1996;17:1507–13.

[54] Filippi M, Yousry T, Baratti C, Hounsfield HA, et al. Quantitative assessment of MRI lesion load in multiple sclerosis: a comparison of conventional spin-echo with fast fluid-attenuated inversion recovery. Brain 1996;119:1349–55.

[55] Hajnal JV, Bryant DJ, Kasuboski L, Pattany PM, et al. Use of fluid attenuated inversion recovery (FLAIR) pulse sequences in MRI of the brain. J Comput Assist Tomogr 1992;16(6):841–4.

[56] Murata T, Itoh S, Koshino Y, Sakamoto K, et al. Serial cerebral MRI with FLAIR sequences in acute carbon monoxide poisoning. J Comput Assist Tomogr 1995;19(4):631–4.

[57] DeCoene B. MR of brain FLAIR. AJNR Am J Neuroradiol 1992;13:1555–64.

[58] Araki Y, Ashikaga R, Takahashi S, Ueda J, Ishida O. High signal intensity of the infundibular stalk on fluid-attenuated inversion recovery MR. AJNR Am J Neuroradiol 1997;18:89–93.

[59] Brant-Zawadzki M, Atkinson D, Detrick M, Bradley WG, Scidmore G. Fluid-attenuated inversion recovery (FLAIR) for assessment of cerebral infarction: initial clinical experience in 50 patients. Stroke 1996;27(7):1187–91.

[60] Rosen BR, Wedeen VJ, Brady TJ. Selective saturation NMR. J Comput Assist Tomogr 1984;8(5): 813–8.

[61] Simon JH, Szumowski J. Proton (fat/water) chemical shift imaging in medical magnetic resonance imaging. Current status. Invest Radiol 1992; 27(10):865–73.

[62] Mills TC, Ortendahl DA, Hylton NM, Crooks LE, Carlson JW, Kaufman L. Partial flip angle MR imaging. Radiology 1987;162:531–9.

[63] Lauterbur PC. Image formation by induced local interactions; examples employing nuclear magnetic resonance. Nature 1973;242:190–1.

[64] Hinshaw WS, Andre ER, Bottomley PA, et al. NMR images by the multiple sensitive point method; application to larger biological systems. Phys Med Biol 1977;22(5):971–4.

[65] Damadian R, Minkoff I, Goldsmith M. NMR in cancer XXI. FONAR scan of the live human abdomen. Physiol Chem Phys 1978;10(6):561–3.

[66] Pykett IL. NMR imaging in medicine. Sci Am 1982;246(5):78–88.

[67] Hinshaw WS, Bottomley PA, Holland GN. A demonstration of the resolution of NMR imaging in biological systems. Experentia 1979;35(a): 1268–76.

[68] Crooks L, Hoenninger J, Arakawa M, et al. Tomography of hydrogen with nuclear magnetic resonance. Radiology 1980;136:701–6.

[69] Mansfield P, Maudsley AA. Medical imaging by NMR. Br J Radiol 1977;50(591):188–94.

[70] Kumar A, Welti D, Ernst RR. NMR Fourier zeugmatography. J Magn Reson Imaging 1975;18: 69–83.

[71] Lauterbur PC, Lai C-M. IEEE Trans Nucl Sci 1980;27:1227–31.

[72] den Boef JH, van Uijen CMJ, Holzcherer CD. Multiple-slice NMR imaging by three-dimensional Fourier zeugmatography. Phys Med Biol 1984; 29(7):857–67.

[73] Edelstein WA, Hutchison JMS, Johnson G, Redpath T. Spin warp NMR imaging and applications to human whole-body imaging [letter to the editor]. Phys Med Biol 1980;25:751–6.

[74] Hinshaw WS, Andrew ER, Bottomley PA, Holland GN, et al. An in vivo study of the forearm and hand by thin section NMR imaging. Br J Radiol 1979;52:36–43.

[75] Bottomley PA, Andrew ER. RF magnetic field penetration, phase shift and power dissipation in biological tissue: implications of NMR imaging. Phys Med Biol 1978;23(4):630–43.

[76] Kramer DM, Guzman RJ, Carlson JW, Crooks LE, Kaufman L. Physics of thin-section MR imaging at low field strength. Radiology 1989; 173(2):541–4.

[77] Jezzard P, Duewell S, Balaban RA. MR relaxation times in human brain: measurement at 4 T1. Radiology 1996;199:773–9.

[78] Hennig J, Friedburg H. RARE imaging: a fast imaging method for clinical MR. Magn Reson Med 1986;3(6):823–33.

[79] Jolesz FA. Fast spin-echo technique extends versatility of MR. Diagn Imaging 1992;14:78–86.

[80] Tien RD, Felsberg GJ, MacFall J. Practical choices of fast spin-echo pulse sequence parameters: clinically useful proton density and T2-weighted contrasts. Neuroradiology 1992;35:38–41.

[81] Constable RT, Smith RC, Gore JC. Signal-to-noise and contrast in fast spin-echo (FSE) and inversion recovery FSE imaging. J Comput Assist Tomogr 1992;16(1):41–7.

[82] Feinberg DA, Keifer B, Litt AW. High resolution GRASE MRI of the brain and spine: 512 and 1024 matrix imaging. J Comput Assist Tomogr 1995;19(1):1–7.

[83] Melki PS, Mulkern RV, Panych LP, Joesz FA. Comparing the FAISE method with conventional dual-echo sequences. J Magn Reson Imaging 1991; 1(3):319–26.

[84] Choen MS, Weisskoff RM. Ultra-fast imaging. Magn Reson Imaging 1991;9(1):1–37.

[85] Weinberger E, Murakami JW, Shaw DW, et al. Three dimensional fast spin-echo T1 weighted imaging of the pediatric spine. J Comput Assist Tomogr 1995;19(5):721–5.

[86] Tien RD, Felsberg GJ, MacFall J. Fast spin-echo high resolution MR imaging of the inner ear. AJR Am J Roentgenol 1992;159:395–8.

[87] Melki PS, Jolesz FA, Mulkern RV. Partial RF echo-planar imaging with the FAISE method. I. Experimental and theoretical assessment of artifact. Magn Reson Med 1992;26:328–41.

[88] Constable RT, Anderson AW, Zhong J, Gore JC. Factors influencing contrast and fast spin echo MR imaging. Magn Reson Imaging 1992;10: 497–511.

[89] Noll DC. Variable averaging RARe. Magn Reson Med 1994;31:323–7.

[90] Norbash AM, Glover GH, Enzmann DR. Intracerebral legion contrast with spin echo and fast spin-echo pulse sequences. Radiology 1992;185(3): 661–5.

[91] Jones KM, Mulkern RV, Schwartz RB, et al. Fast spin-echo MR imaging of the brain and spine: current concepts. AJR Am J Roentgenol 1992;158: 1313–20.

[92] Sze G, Merriam M, Oshio K, Jolesz FA. Fast spin-echo imaging in the evaluation of intradural disease of the spine. AJNR Am J Neuroradiol 1992;13: 1383–92.

[93] Chappell PM, Glover GH, Enzmann DR. Contrast on T2-weighted images of the lumbar spine using fast spin-echo and gated conventional spin-echo sequences. Neuroradiology 1995;37:183–6.

[94] Thorpe JW, Halpin SF, MacManus DG, et al. A comparison between fast and conventional spin-echo in the detection of multiple sclerosis lesions. Neurology 1994;36(5):388–92.

[95] Susuki T, Kakiuchi H, Sugiki S, et al. Detection of cortical infarcts in brain MR imaging; feasibility of short-TR-T2-weighted imaging using a fast spin-echo sequence. Nippon Igaku Hoshasen Gakkai Zasshi 1995;55(4):260–2.

[96] Smith RC, Reinhold C, Lange RC, et al. Fast spin-echo MR imaging of the female pelvis. Part I. Use of a whole volume coil. Radiology 1992; 184:665–9.

[97] Tice HM, Jones KM, Mulkern RV, et al. Fast spin-echo imaging of intracranial neoplasms. J Comput Assist Tomogr 1993;17(3):425–31.

[98] Jones KM, Mulkern RV, Mantello MT, et al. Brain hemorrhage: evaluation with fast spin-echo images. Radiology 1992;182(1):53–8.

[99] Rubin DA, Kneeland JB, Listerud, et al. MR diagnosis of meniscal tears of the knee: value of fat spin-echo vs. conventional spin-echo pulse sequences. AJR Am J Roentgenol 1994;162:1131–5.

[100] Reimer P, Allkemper T, Schuierer G, Peters PE. Brain imaging: reduced sensitivity of RARE-derived techniques to susceptibility effects. J Comput Assist Tomogr 1996;20(2):201–5.

[101] Nghiem HV, Herfkens RJ, Franscis IR, et al. The pelvis: T2-weighted fast spin-echo MR imaging. Radiology 1992;185(1):213–7.

[102] Wright G.A. Lipid signal enhancement in spin echo trains. In: Proceedings of the Mtg Soc Magn Reson. 1992. p. 437.

[103] Henkelman RM, Hardy PA, Bishop JE, et al. Why fat is bright in RARE and fast spin-echo imaging. J Magn Reson Imaging 1992;2:533–40.

[104] Williamson DS, Mulkern RV, Jakab PD, Josesz FA. Coherence transfer by isotropic mixing in Carr-Purcell-Meiboom-Gill imaging: implications for the bright fat phenomenon in fast spin-echo imaging. Magn Reson Med 1996;35:506–13.

[105] Ling CR, Foster MA, Hutchison JMS. Comparison of NMR water proton T1 relaxation times of rabbit tissues at 24 mHZ and 2.5 mHZ. Phys Med Biol 1980;25:748–51.

[106] Bottomley PA, Foster TH, Argersinger RE, Pfeifer LM. A review of normal tissue hydrogen NMR relaxation times and relaxation mechanisms from 1–100 MHz: dependence on tissue type, NMR frequency, temperature, species, excision and age. Med Physic 1984;11(4):425–48.

[107] Hopkins AL, Yeung HN, Barton CB. Multiple field strength in vivo T1 and T2 for cerebrospinal fluid protons. Magn Reson Med 1986;3: 303–11.

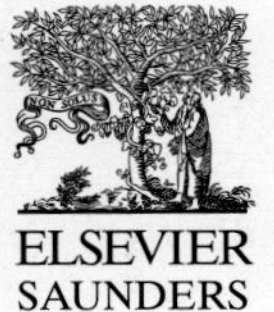

ELSEVIER
SAUNDERS

Neurosurg Clin N Am 16 (2005) 65–75

NEUROSURGERY
CLINICS
OF NORTH AMERICA

Quasi–real-time neurosurgery support by MRI processing via grid computing

Heiko Lippmann, PD*, Frithjof Kruggel, MD

Max-Planck-Institute for Human Cognitive and Brain Sciences, Stephanstraße 1, D-04103 Leipzig, Germany

Motivation

In neurosurgery, the resection of brain tumors may be planned on the basis of high-resolution preoperative anatomic MRI scans of the patient's head. To gain more information about the function of regions adjacent to the tumor, a functional MRI (fMRI) scan may also be acquired. This information is useful in assisting the surgeon's navigation during the intervention and in minimizing the risk of potential functional damage.

After the skull is opened, several effects take place that lead to nonlinear distortions of the brain, which are collectively called the brain shift phenomenon. Thus, functional information acquired before surgery cannot be easily mapped onto anatomic images acquired during surgery. This is the major shortcoming of image-guided surgical planning based on fMRI data acquired before surgery, because the occurrence of surgically induced deformations invalidates positional information about functionally relevant areas.

Referring to observations in the article by Nabavi et al [1] and a survey by Ferrant et al [2], brain shift is understood as a nonrigid and relatively slow process. The deformation of the brain during surgery mainly occurs because of physical manipulation of the tissue: dura opening, retraction and resection, and draining and leakage of cerebrospinal fluid (CSF). Further impact on brain shift occurs from physiologic reactions of the brain to anesthetics and osmotic agents as a result of the properties of living tissue as well as conditions that are different from a normal state. The opening of the dura and the leakage of CSF cause a gravitational shift because of the disappearance of tension and pressure forces at the brain and ventricular boundaries. Further on, retraction and resection of brain tissue always affects neighboring brain tissue. The change in blood pressure as well as hydration or dehydration of the brain caused by medication administered during surgery causes the patient's brain to swell or shrink. All these factors lead to deformation of the brain during surgery.

This problem has been addressed previously in many publications. For example, Nimsky et al [3] report a manual brain shift correction procedure using intraoperative MRI. This technique is reported to be quite effective and can be done in 15 minutes. Unfortunately, it is limited to anatomic data only and is also costly.

Hastreiter et al [4] try to visualize brain shift using a deformable surface model, which they apply to pre- and intraoperative data sets to show the movement of the brain's surface. To take into account the shift of structures that lie below the brain surface, a voxel-based approach is used, which allows calculation of volume deformation. They use mutual information to perform a nonlinear registration of three-dimensional (3D) piecewise linear patches gained from the transformed data set. Although no quantitative statements referring to accuracy are made, neither of the presented techniques seems to model the brain shift extremely accurately.

Other approaches [2,5–9] try to model the brain shift using a biomechanical finite element model (FEM). These models operate with a limited

This work was supported by the European Union under the IST Programme Framework V, Project IST-2001-37153.

* Corresponding author.
E-mail address: lippmann@cbs.mpg.de
(H. Lippmann).

1042-3680/05/$ - see front matter
doi:10.1016/j.nec.2004.07.009

number of nodes; the number of nodes is usually lower than the resolution of the volumetric image from which the FEM was extracted. Thus, not all the brain's fine structure can be modeled. These models use forces that are estimated from the movement of the brain surface using stereo cameras or intraoperative MRI scans to deform the biomechanical brain model. This deformation can be applied to almost any type of preoperative data for correction with respect to brain shift. Most approaches model the brain as a homogeneous tissue that only deforms elastically, however. Correct matching of the brain surface during surgery is quite difficult, and interaction between deformed brain tissue and skull is always a problem in these models. Another problem occurs if tissue (eg, tumor) is resected. Here, the surface matching is much harder; in addition, the FEM needs to be updated to reflect the changes in topology. As far as we know, when using the FEM, the only method that is capable of modeling brain shift if tissue has been resected is the one by Ferrant et al [2]. If cameras are used to track the surface's deformation as in the study by Skrinjar et al [6], problems with specularities on the wet brain surface occur, which complicates the stereo reconstruction. Despite all these problems, the accuracy of these techniques is described to be sufficient if no tissue has been resected, and computation time (caused by the use of parallel computers in some cases) is reported to be acceptable in clinical use.

A similar technique using a physics-based approach is used by Hagemann et al [10]. These investigators use a biomechanical model of the human head comprising different materials, such as bone and brain tissue, with different elasticities. Requiring manual interaction, such as tumor and resection area outlining, the method achieves good registration results using synthetic and real patient data. The disadvantage is that the method has only been tested in two-dimensional (2D) imaging and an extension to 3D imaging may be computationally expensive.

Hata et al [11] tried to measure volumetric brain deformation using intraoperative MRI with a volumetric optical flow method. Because of vulnerabilities to contrast variations in intraoperative data, they observed that the best results were achieved if the skin was segmented out. They reported an average error of 3.5 mm, determined from landmarks on a phantom test model. Unfortunately, they also applied their method only to anatomic data sets before and after the opening of the dura mater, so no discontinuities caused by tissue resection are reported.

In this article, the problem is addressed by nonrigid image registration using a viscous fluid model proposed by Christensen et al [12] with respect to intraoperative MRI. The core idea is the nonlinear registration of preoperative fMRI to intraoperative MRI acquired by an open MRI scanner. Whenever an intraoperative data set is acquired, an image processing chain must be executed, which includes correction of intensity nonuniformities in the scan data; linear registration with a preoperative data set, followed by nonlinear registration to obtain a 3D deformation field; application of the deformation; overlaying of preoperative fMRI data to the intraoperative data; and, finally, transfer to a presentation device.

This chain also has a high computation cost that scales with the resolution of the processed MRI scans. To decrease computation time, parallel computers are used. We present a parallel image processing chain that is able to fulfill these requirements.

The chain is currently under development in the European grid-enabled medical simulation services (GEMSS) project [13], which examines the possibilities of the use of grid computing for medical applications. With the utilization of distributed computing over the Internet, which tries to make the power of large computation centers available to simple Internet-connected terminals, we try to achieve an execution time for this chain within 10 minutes.

Grid computing

The idea of providing the computation power of large computation centers to simple terminals over the Internet is understood as grid computing. The aim is to develop a transparent service that abstracts from the Net infrastructure. The user of such a service should not have to care about the availability of certain servers or computation centers somewhere in the Net. He simply requests a service from the grid, and the grid provides the necessary resources using software agents. Those agents are able to determine the computation centers that are capable of providing the requested service with respect to the special conditions specified by the user. Such conditions may include special requests referring to execution time, cost of the service, or security issues.

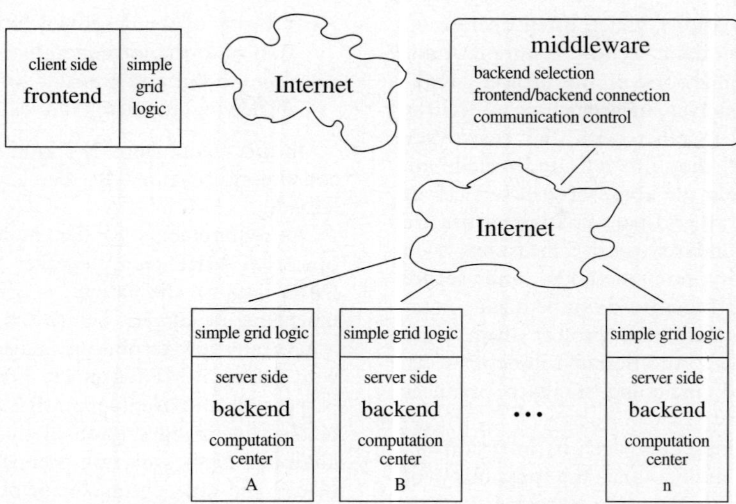

Fig. 1. Grid infrastructure within the grid-enabled medical simulation services (GEMSS) project.

Various projects such as the National Aeronautics and Space Administration's Information Power Grid or European Centre for Nuclear Research DataGrid have been launched to explore the possibilities of the realization of grid environments and to develop the necessary infrastructure. Current grid technologies (eg, Globus Toolkit, Globus Alliance, http://www.globus.org) have evolved principally to meet the needs of high-performance computing resource sharing in the academic community. Those technologies are designed for scientific purposes. When considering their use to support outsourcing of medical applications on a commercial and quasi–real-time basis, it is clear that they do not support the necessary business models, quality of service, and tightly controlled access to applications and data. The GEMSS project was initiated to meet those requirements.

Within the GEMSS project, the grid is realized in a three-tier environment consisting of the client side, middleware, and application back end. To grid-enable an application, it must be split up into two parts. The first part is usually the application front end, which is computationally insensitive, together with simple grid communication logic. On this side, all the input parameters and service requirements are defined by the user. The second part is the often parallel, computational expensive back end, which must also be able to communicate with the grid to obtain its input data and to transmit its output data. The connection between these two parts of an application forms the middleware component, which acts as a service broker. The middleware is contacted by the front end, and the service request is transmitted. Examining this request, the broker chooses and contacts an appropriate back end. Once the link between the front end and the back end has been established, all the applications communication is controlled by the middleware via a simple interface. The client simply loads up input data and waits for the job to start. If the job has been started, it can be monitored or, if necessary, canceled. If the data have been transferred, the application on the back end is invoked with the information as to where it can find its input data and where to place its output data and status information. After the completion of the back end's task, the status is set to "finished." The client detects that through the grid interface and initiates the download of the back end's output data and presents it to the user. Note that all the communication that takes place flows through the middleware over encrypted channels. Fig. 1 shows the described infrastructure schematically.

A scenario similar to the one described here is applied to the image processing chain described in this article. The vision is that the information the user has to provide to run the application is reduced to a minimum. The relevant data here are the location of the patient data and the requested maximum run time. Irrelevant information for surgery, such as where the job is run, how much memory is needed, or how many processors are used, is determined automatically.

Because of the fact that the grid infrastructure developed within GEMSS project should be used for medical applications, which often operate on the basis of patient data, security is an important aspect. In the framework of the project, weaknesses of the used Net infrastructure as well as possible attacks, together with the costs they would produce if they are left undetected, are examined. To avoid the abuse of grid services or confidential data, all grid-participating parties are equipped with standard security measures, such as firewalls, encryption methods, and secure communication protocols to authenticate communications and data and protect them from unauthorized access. Additionally, in-depth security is maintained, including standard practices like logging.

Beyond that, measures, such as intrusion detection, security audits, and the possibility of installing security updates, are examined. It is also planned to apply software security, such as virus scanners on systems, for example, on machines running clients of certain medical services, where this will be useful. On each grid site, a trust model will be created for each specific security infrastructure to determine security weaknesses. It can then be seen how weak links in a security infrastructure affect the stronger links, and action can be taken to reduce the dependency on the weak links or to improve the security strength of the weak links.

The overall goal is to enable GEMSS project participants to use the grid without excessive cost while maintaining acceptable security.

Description of the image processing chain

In this section, a detailed description of the exact application flow of the image processing chain is given. The required steps of the chain include the following:

1. Transfer of anatomic images from the scanner
2. Correction of intensity nonuniformities in the scan data caused by magnetic field inhomogeneities of the scanner
3. Linear registration of the usually low-resolution intraoperative scan with a high-resolution preoperative scan
4. Intensity adjustment between both scans to improve the results of nonlinear registration
5. Nonlinear registration of both scans to yield a 3D deformation field
6. Application of the deformation field to the preoperative fMRI data set
7. Overlay of the deformed functional information onto the intraoperative data
8. Conversion and transfer to the presentation device (eg, monitor, surgical microscope)

In this chain, steps 2, 3, and 5 are quite time-consuming. Fortunately, these steps can be parallelized.

As requirements for the chain to work, a preoperative MRI scan, together with its aligned fMRI data on the patient, is needed. During the first stage of surgery before the skull is opened, a generally low-resolution image (A) is acquired with the open MRI scanner. After the correction of possible radiofrequency (RF) field inhomogeneities, linear registration of this image with the anatomic high-resolution preoperative data takes place. The nine optimal registration parameters, which include three translation, three rotation, and three scaling parameters, are stored as a starting position for further linear registration steps. The registered image is the reference for further steps of the chain.

After the skull is opened, a sequence of intraoperative images (B) is acquired. These images are also corrected with respect to possible intensity nonuniformities and are registered with the first intraoperative data set A using the stored parameter set P as the initial position. Before the nonlinear registration step is executed, a linear intensity adjustment is performed to obtain the same intensity distribution in both input images A and B. The resulting displacement field of the nonlinear registration process is applied to the preoperative fMRI data. In the final step, the deformed fMRI scan is overlaid on the linearly registered open-skull data set B and later sent to a presentation device.

The nonlinear registration method that is based on fluid dynamics produces the best results if its input images are acquired by the same scanner. That is the reason why the first (closed skull) intraoperative image, A, is acquired and used as a reference image for further processing and not the preoperative high-resolution data, which are usually not acquired with an open MRI scanner. Fig. 2 shows the chain schematically (Fig. 3).

Elements of the image processing chain

A brief overview of the theory behind the individual steps of the image processing chain, together with their limitations and problems, is given in this section.

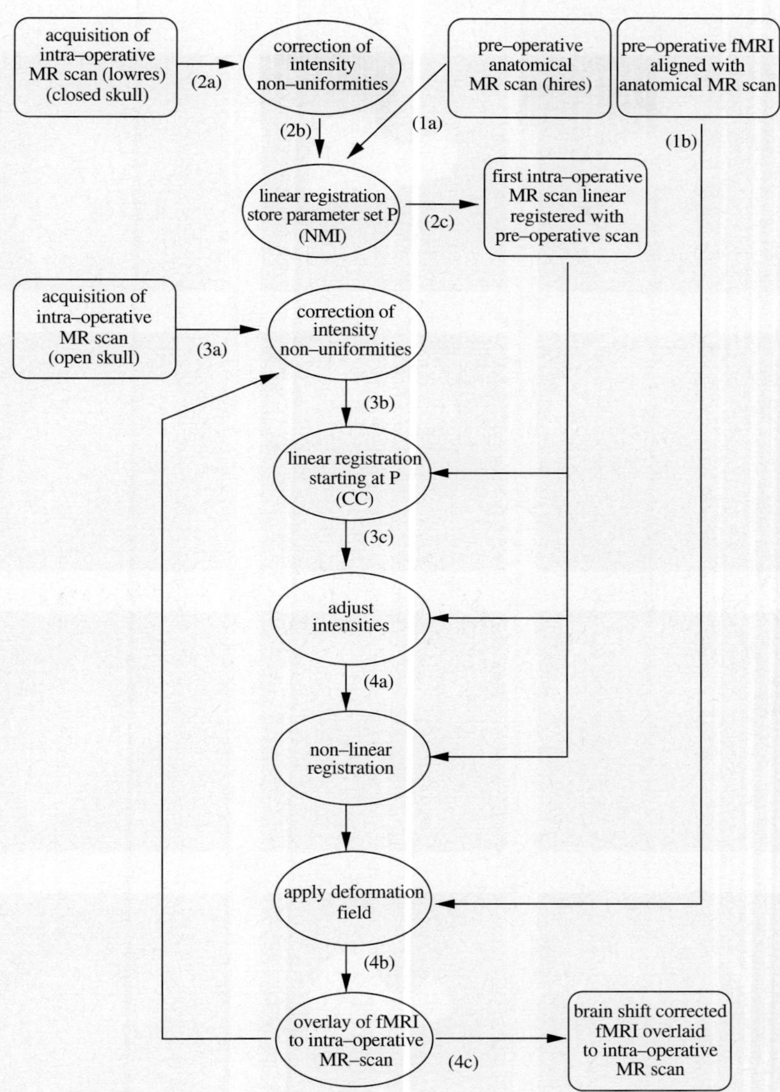

Fig. 2. Image processing chain. The result of each step written in brackets is shown in the corresponding subfigure of Fig. 3.

Data transfer and conversion

Currently, an implementation of this step does not exist. Instead, input data are expected to be in files in a machine-independent format. Later, a direct transfer from the open MRI scanner to the application for intraoperative data is planned.

Correction of intensity nonuniformities

With today's MRI techniques, acquired data often contain inhomogeneities that may be caused by nonuniformities in the RF field of the scanner during acquisition. These inhomogeneities can cause serious misregistration during later processing steps. To address this problem, an adaptive fuzzy C-means (AFCM) algorithm [14,15] is used. Although this algorithm was originally a segmentation method, it can be applied to obtain intensity-corrected MRI scans, because it has been shown [16] that correction of inhomogeneities is strongly coupled with segmentation. The AFCM algorithm segments an MRI scan while estimating a multiplicative bias field that can be used to correct image intensities.

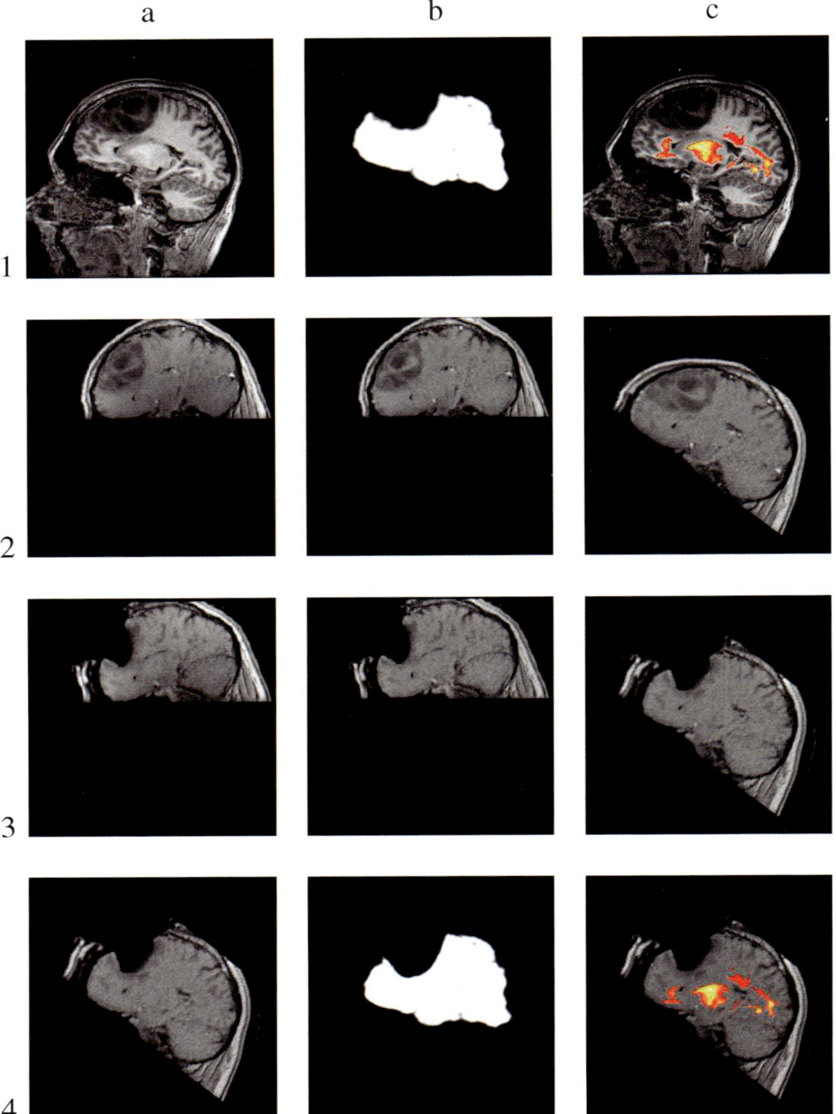

Fig. 3. Single steps of the image processing chain. Subfigures correspond to the results of the step written in brackets in Fig. 2. Subfigure 1*C* shows overlaid preoperative anatomic MRI and functional MRI data. Because of the lack of corresponding fMRI data, a synthetically generated data set was used.

Application of the AFCM algorithm is time-consuming because of the solution of a huge linear system. To improve speed, the linear system is only coarsely solved within a multiresolution framework, which is sufficient to estimate a proper bias field. Further speed improvement is obtained by restricting the analysis to a head mask extracted from the data set. The greatest improvement in performance is obtained by computing the solution of the linear system in parallel. The algorithm was enhanced to work in a multiprocessor shared memory environment with nearly linear speed-up. This was realized by an overlap of iterations. Thus, the next iteration is starting as soon as all necessary data have been computed, although the current iteration is not yet finished. This is the reason why the maximum number of usable processors is limited by the number of slices in the MRI scan.

A different strategy is applied in a distributed memory environment. Here, the data set is partitioned into blocks, and each block is solved independently of the others. If the volume is split up into n blocks, n−1 additional blocks are processed, which are centered over the borders of two neighboring blocks. If the algorithm converged for each block, the n blocks are put together again; on the borders of those blocks, where the convergence is usually worse than near the center of a block, slices from the additional n−1 blocks are filled in. Finally, the last iteration of the algorithm runs serially on the full volume to correct remains of the artifacts in the data caused by the partitioning.

Linear registration

The registration of the low-resolution intraoperative data set to a high-resolution preoperative image is realized by maximizing the normalized mutual information (NMI) [17] or the cross-correlation (CC), respectively. NMI is used when data from different scanners are registered, and CC is used for data sets originating from the same scanner. Fourier-Mellin transform-based methods [18,19] cannot be applied, because the Fourier spectra of intraoperative and preoperative images can vary dramatically because of their possibly different structures (eg, a few intraoperative slices should be registered with a full preoperative image of the head).

Linear registration has to embrace translation, rotation, and scaling that define a nine-dimensional search space in 3D space. To achieve a fast convergence, the downhill simplex optimization algorithm is used, which performs well [20] and does not require any gradient information. Computation time of the gradient of the NMI cost function, for example, would be nine times greater than the evaluation time of the cost function itself. To improve the speed of the registration, a parallel evaluated speculative downhill simplex that converges exactly like the original method but twice as fast was developed. Further nearly linear speed-up was gained by evaluating the cost function (NMI and CC) in parallel by partitioning the data into blocks and assigning each block to a single processor. The results of the processed subvolumes are totalled to obtain the cost function value. All these parallel computed parts of the linear registration can be used in a shared and distributed memory environment.

Currently, the success of linear registration depends on the initial orientation of both images, because it cannot be assumed that the global optimum is found during optimization. A strategy needs to be developed to increase the probability of convergence to the global optimum.

Intensity adjustment of two scans

The result of the nonlinear registration step of the processing chain depends, among other things, on the similarity of the intensities of both images. To achieve this, a codomain of tissue voxels in both images is computed. The mean and standard deviation of voxel intensities of the source image are then adjusted to match those of the reference.

This step is optional because it is often not necessary. Because it is not time-consuming, it can be performed serially.

Nonlinear registration

To obtain a deformation field that can be applied to an fMRI scan, nonlinear registration is required. In this chain, a method based on fluid mechanics [12,21] is applied. The time-consuming part here is, once again, the solution of a huge linear system. To speed this up and to avoid local minima, the system is solved using a multiresolution approach. Further speed-up is achieved by solving the system in parallel in a shared memory environment. Here, each processor operates on a single "slice" of the system.

If there is only a distributed memory environment available, all multiresolution steps except the last one, which needs more computation time than all the other steps before combined, are computed serially. For the last resolution level, the data are again partitioned into blocks, and each block is processed by its own processor in parallel. The blocks are computed independently of each other. To avoid partitioning artifacts, the blocks have an overlap of two slices on each border.

In Fig. 4, the brain's surface within the intraoperative data set with the opened skull, together with the deformation field obtained from the nonrigid registration with the intraoperative data set with the closed skull, is visualized. Regions colored in red mean a contraction, and regions colored in blue mean an expansion of the brain tissue. Additionally, small arrows indicate the direction of the shift of the tissue.

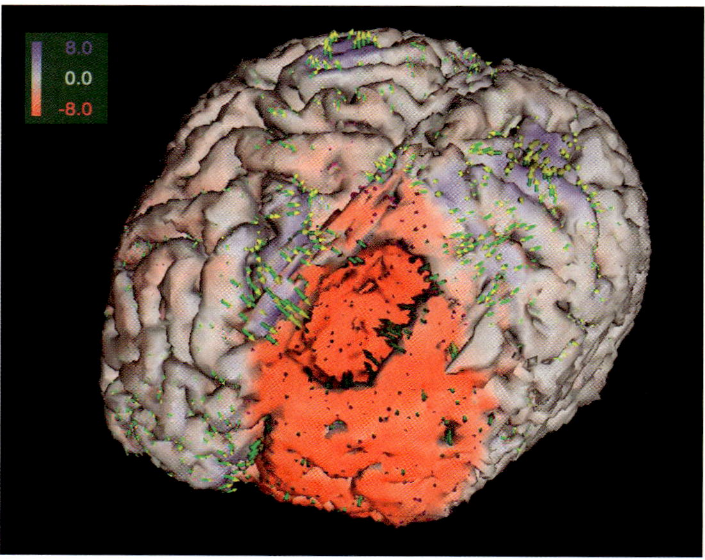

Fig. 4. Surface of the brain within the intraoperative data set with an opened skull, together with the deformation field obtained by nonrigid registration. Red means contraction, and blue means expansion of the brain volume. Arrows indicate the direction of the tissue shift.

Application of a deformation field to functional MRI data

The deformation field obtained by nonlinear registration is applied to an fMRI data set by shifting each voxel of the data set by its corresponding vector from the displacement field. This step is not time-consuming and can be performed serially.

Overlay of the deformed functional MRI data with intraoperative data

In this step, which is again performed serially, the deformed preoperative functional data set that was initially aligned with the preoperative anatomic MRI scan is overlaid to the rigidly registered intraoperative image to show regions of activation with respect to the brain shift.

Conversion and transfer to presentation device

This step has also not been implemented yet. Data are converted into a format that can be viewed with a visualization tool. As in step 1, automatic transfer of the data to a chosen presentation device is imaginable.

Executing the chain over the grid

To decrease the computation time of an unoptimized serial processing chain, which needed approximately 4 hours on a Pentium III single processor with 500 MHz, to a clinically acceptable 10 minutes, the software experienced a lot of optimization. In addition, we will probably need a parallel machine with 10 to 12 processors at a clock rate of 1.6 GHz to achieve this goal. This would mean that a personal computer (PC) cluster has to be available not far away from the MRI scanner to compute a usable result within 10 minutes.

Because of the fact that parallel computers are expensive, need maintenance, and are often underloaded, the idea of using external computation centers on demand is attractive. This is the main idea behind grid computing. The presented image processing chain will be implemented to work within the grid infrastructure provided by GEMSS project.

A common use for our application could be that before an operation begins, an available computation center is determined by the GEMSS project middleware. After automatically negotiating terms of necessary resources, payment, and security issues, the preoperative as well as closed-skull intraoperative anonymous patient data are transferred to the target computation center. Right after that, the preprocessing can start. After the acquisition of another intraoperative MRI scan, now with the skull opened, the new data are transferred to the center and the main part of the image processing chain is executed remotely. After the computation has finished, the result is transferred to the operating room. There, the data can be displayed in a surgical microscope or monitor. Now, further intraoperative data sets can be uploaded, and the main part of the chain can be restarted.

The only computation hardware that is required in the operating room is an inexpensive terminal connected to the MRI scanner, the Internet, and a presentation device. Of course, the grid service is not free of charge, but compared with the setup and maintenance of a local PC cluster, which will probably need a special room with a controlled climate, this may be an interesting alternative.

Quality of service

The middleware that is under development within the GEMSS project provides access to computation centers using common Web transport protocols like hypertext transfer protocol (HTTP). For security reasons, the secure socket layer-encrypted version of HTTPs is used. The client side does not require a special network environment; specifically, network ports do not need to be opened, which always entails a potential security risk. If a Web browser operates correctly, communication with the middleware is ensured. This framework also does not need any modification of current firewall configurations. The only requirement is a fast Internet connection to have low transfer times for the MRI data sets. The size of one data set can vary from 4 to 12 MB for an anatomic data setup to 50 MB for an fMRI data set.

Before any transfer over the Internet is initiated, patient data can be made anonymous, if necessary, to protect the identity of the patient.

The server side of the application, which can be installed in all the computation centers that plan to provide this special service, contains the described image processing chain controlled by the middleware. In its final version, the middleware estimates resource requirements of the current application using abstract performance models. Such a performance model may, for example, predict the application's memory use and its execution time, depending on the current input parameters and the current load of the computation center. These parameters as well as the price for the requested service are compared with the requirements stated by the client. Based on this negotiation, a suitable computation center is chosen.

Performance

Currently, the performance and the quality of the results of the chain are examined on a local PC cluster. The cluster contains four nodes with two Advanced Micro Devices AthlonMP (Advanced Micro Devices, Sunnyvale, California) 1800+ processors at a clock rate of 1.6 GHz. Nodes are equipped with 1 GByte of random-access memory and connected via a 100-MBit/s Ethernet network. Each component of the chain uses a message passing interface framework to communicate with other processes in this distributed memory environment. Table 1 shows the execution times of the chain for a different number of used processors compared with the serial execution of the chain on one processor compared with the run time in a two-processor shared memory environment (SHR) provided by a single node of the cluster and compared with a large PC cluster used over the grid. The last column of the table lists transfer times for the data sets, including data packing and unpacking, but does not include any overhead introduced by communication over the grid middleware. The values are gained for the processing of only one real data set because of the lack of further patient data. The preoperative MRI scans have a resolution of 256 × 192 × 256 voxels, and the intraoperative data sets have a resolution of 256 × 256 × 60 voxels.

The poor speed-up gained by using 10 processors instead of 1 is caused by the high communication overhead and because of the fact that each parallel component contains serial parts that cannot be parallelized. In a distributed memory environment, data must be transferred multiply between the nodes. This overhead grows with an increasing number of processors. In a SHR, which is used seldom because of its high price, all processors can directly access the data, and this problem does not appear.

Varying the number of processors always produces a different partitioning of the data. This can result in the effect that with one partitioning, the finding of the optimum requires more iterations than with another partitioning. Thus, it can occur that although there are more processors used now than before, a special step of the chain requires more computation time, although there are more processors used as seen in the

Table 1
Performance of the chain

	SER (1)	SHR (2)	MPI (4)	MPI (6)	MPI (8)	GRD (10)
Preprocessing						
Upload	0 min 0 s	0 min 0 s	0 min 0 s	0 min 0 s	0 min 0 s	0 min 44 s
Inhom	2 min 51 s	2 min 15 s	2 min 36 s	2 min 39 s	2 min 29 s	2 min 16 s
Linreg	4 min 21 s	3 min 4 s	2 min 14 s	2 min 13 s	2 min 5 s	1 min 47 s
Σ	6 min 12 s	5 min 19 s	4 min 50 s	4 min 52 s	4 min 34 s	4 min 47 s
Processing						
Upload	0 min 0 s	0 min 0 s	0 min 0 s	0 min 0 s	0 min 0 s	0 min 8 s
Inhom	2 min 58 s	2 min 20 s	2 min 44 s	2 min 28 s	2 min 19 s	2 min 1 s
Linreg	8 min 16 s	5 min 13 s	3 min 42 s	2 min 33 s	2 min 31 s	1 min 50 s
Intens	0 min 4 s	0 min 4 s	0 min 4 s	0 min 4 s	0 min 4 s	0 min 3 s
Fluidreg	6 min 56 s	4 min 31 s	3 min 57 s	4 min 2 s	2 min 39 s	2 min 34 s
Shift	0 min 21 s	0 min 16 s	0 min 12 s	0 min 16 s	0 min 16 s	0 min 20 s
Overlay	0 min 4 s	0 min 4 s	0 min 4 s	0 min 4 s	0 min 4 s	0 min 3 s
Download	0 min 0 s	0 min 0 s	0 min 0 s	0 min 0 s	0 min 0 s	0 min 9 s
Σ	18 min 39 s	12 min 28 s	10 min 43 s	9 min 27 s	7 min 53 s	7 min 8 s
Overall Σ	24 min 51 s	17 min 47 s	15 min 33 s	14 min 19 s	12 min 27 s	11 min 55 s

Abbreviations: Fluidreg, nonlinear registration; GRD, grid; Inhom, correction of inhomogeneities; Intens, intensity adjustment; Linreg, linear registration; min, minutes; Overlay, overlay of fMRI to anatomic MRI data; s, seconds; SER, serial execution; Shift, apply deformation field; SHR, shared memory environment.

The number of processors is shown in brackets. The values for GRD have been obtained on a different cluster.

preprocessing section of Table 1 between the columns showing the results for four and six processors as well as in the processing section for fluid registration.

As already mentioned, the required number of processors is approximately 10 to 12 to complete the chain in 10 minutes in a grid scenario, including transfer times and input/output times of every single software component. In praxis it has to be taken into account that on a grid site, input/output times can vary significantly, depending on the current load of the cluster that might be produced by other tasks.

Summary

One problem of providing time-critical medical services over the grid is always its dependency on the Internet. It cannot be assumed that transfer of a certain amount of data over the Internet is always achieved during a specified period. Such a requirement cannot be fulfilled by the infrastructure of the Web. There is always the risk of a network delay or even an overload. Because of this, another goal of this project is the evaluation of grid services versus the use of local services.

A further point for future research related to the chain has to deal with the optimization approach for the linear registration step. Because the optimization uses the downhill simplex algorithm in a nine-dimensional search space, the number of iterations needed to find the optimum can vary dramatically. This makes linear registration the most unpredictable step of the chain in terms of execution time. It cannot be assured that the global optimum is found.

Additional work has to be done in validating the registration accuracy, including the examination of the influence of intensity variations between intraoperative images as well as the influence of tumor resection and the presence of the opened skull versus the closed skull in the fluid-based registration.

References

[1] Nabavi A, Black PM, Gering DT, Westin CF, Mehta V, Pergolizzi PS, et al. Serial intraoperative MR imaging of brain shift. Neurosurgery 2001;48:787–98.

[2] Ferrant M, Nabavi A, Macq B, Black PM, Jolesz FA, Kikinis R, et al. Serial registration of intraoperative MR images of the brain. Med Image Anal 2002;6:337–59.

[3] Nimsky C, Ganslandt O, Hastreiter P, Fahlbusch R. Intraoperative compensation for brain shift. Surg Neurol 2001;56:357–65.

[4] Hastreiter P, Rezk-Salama C, Nimsky C, Lürig C, Greiner G, Ertl T. Registration techniques for the

analysis of the brain shift in neurosurgery. Comput Graph 2002;24:385–9.

[5] Ferrant M, Warfield SK, Nabavi A, Jolesz FA, Kikinis R. Registration of 3D intraoperative MR images of the brain using a finite element biomechanical model. Delp SL, DiGioia AM, Jaramaz B, editors. In: Medical image computing and computer-assisted intervention—MICCAI 2000. Berlin: Springer; 2000. p. 19–28.

[6] Skrinjar O, Nabavi A, Duncan J. Model-driven brain shift compensation. Med Image Anal 2002;6:361–74.

[7] Warfield SK, Ferrant M, Gallez X, Nabavi A, Jolesz FA, Kikinis R. Real-time biomechanical simulation of volumetric brain deformation for image guided neurosurgery. In: High performance networking and computing conference—SC 2000. IEEE Computer Society: Washington, DC; 2000. p. 1–16.

[8] Paulsen K, Miga M, Kennedy F, Hoopes P, Hartov A, Roberts D. A computational model for tracking subsurface tissue deformation during stereotactic neurosurgery. IEEE Trans Biomech Eng 1999;46:213–25.

[9] Clatz O, Delingette H, Bardinet E, Dormont D, Ayache N. Patient specific biomechanical model of the brain: application to Parkinson's disease procedure. In: International symposium on surgery simulation and soft tissue modeling (IS4TM) 2003, vol. 2673. Lecture Notes in Computer Science, Institut National de Recherche en Informatique et en Automatique Sophia Antipolis. Springer: Heidelburg; 2003. p. 321–31.

[10] Hagemann A, Rohr K, Stiel HS, Spetzger U, Gilsbach JM. Non-rigid matching of tomographic images based on a biomechanical model of the human head. In: Hanson E, editor. SPIE medical imaging 1999. Proceedings of the SPIE International Symposium. Society of Photo-optical Instrumentation Engineers: Bellingham, Washington; 1999. p. 583–92.

[11] Hata N, Nabavi A, Wells WM, Warfield SK, Kikinis R, Black PM, et al. Three-dimensional optical flow method for measurement of volumetric brain deformation from intraoperative MR images. J Comput Assist Tomogr 2000;24:531–8.

[12] Christensen G, Joshi S, Miller M. Volumetric transformation of brain anatomy. IEEE Trans Med Imaging 1997;16:864–77.

[13] GEMSS project. Grid-enabled medical simulation services. Available at: http://www.gemss.de. Accessed September 8, 2004.

[14] Pham DL, Prince JL. An adaptive fuzzy c-means algorithm for image segmentation in the presence of intensity inhomogeneities. Patt Recog Lett 1999; 20:57–68.

[15] Pham DL, Prince JL. An adaptive fuzzy segmentation algorithm for three-dimensional magnetic resonance images. Information Processing in Medical Imaging. Lecture Notes in Computer Science 1999; 1613:140–53.

[16] Styner M, Brechbühler C, Szekely G, Gerig G. Parametric estimate of intensity inhomogeneities applied to MRI. IEEE Trans Med Imaging 2000; 19:153–65.

[17] Pluim JPW, Maintz JBA, Viergever MA. Mutual information based registration of medical images: a survey. IEEE Trans Med Imaging 2003;22: 986–1004.

[18] Chen Q, Defrise M, Deconinck F. Symmetric phase-only matched filtering of Fourier-Mellin transforms for image registration and recognition. Transactions on Pattern Analysis and Machine Intelligence 1994; 16:1156–68.

[19] Reddy BS, Chatterji BN. An FFT-based technique for translation, rotation, and scale-invariant image registration. IEEE Trans Image Process 1996;5: 1266–71.

[20] Maes F, Vandermeulen D, Suetens P. Comparative evaluation of multiresolution optimization strategies for multimodality image registration by maximization of mutual information. Med Image Anal 1999;3:373–86.

[21] Wollny G, Kruggel F. Computational cost of non-rigid registration algorithms based on fluid dynamics. IEEE Trans Med Imaging 2002;11:946–52.

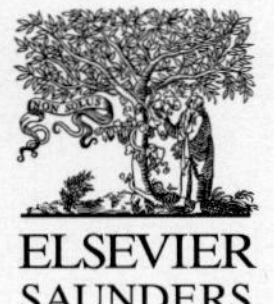

ELSEVIER
SAUNDERS

Neurosurg Clin N Am 16 (2005) 77–99

NEUROSURGERY
CLINICS
OF NORTH AMERICA

Functional MRI localizing in the cerebellum

Wolfgang Grodd, MD[a,*], Ernst Hülsmann, MD[a], Hermann Ackermann, MD, MA[b]

[a]*Section on Experimental Magnetic Resonance of Central Nervous System, Department of Neuroradiology, University of Tüebingen, Hoppe-Seyler Straße 3, D72076, Tübingen, Germany*

[b]*Department of Neurology, University of Tüebingen, Hoppe-Seyler Straß 3, 72076, Tübingen, Germany*

The cerebellum contains approximately half of the brain's neurons, but its particular nerve cells are so small that the cerebellum constitutes only 10% to 15% of the entire brain weight, approximately 140 g in human beings. It is composed of a highly convoluted cerebellar cortex and a core of white matter with three nuclei are embedded on each side (Fig. 1). It is located dorsal to the brain stem in the posterior fossa, inferior to the tentorium cerebelli, and internal to the occipital bone. It overlies the pons and medulla, connecting with these structures and with the mesencephalon through three peduncles on each side. The cerebellum has a superior surface apposed to the tentorium and a convex inferior surface that abuts the inner surface of the occipital bone.

There are three major lobes, the anterior, posterior, and flocculonodular, and these can be further subdivided into a series of lobules. The lobules have been given proper names, but this nomenclature has largely been replaced by the numbering system introduced by Larsell [1], which consists of a Roman numeral applied to each of the folia of the vermis (Fig. 2). On the basis of phylogenetic and embryologic studies, the lobules have been grouped into three components: the archicerebellum, paleocerebellum, and neocerebellum. The archicerebellum consists of the flocculonodular lobe, and the paleocerebellum comprises the vermis of the anterior lobe (culmen and lobulus centralis) plus the lower vermis with the pyramis, uvula, and paraflocculus. The neocerebellum comprises both hemispheres and has developed together with the telencephalon as the latest phylogenetic structure and is thus most prominent in mammals, especially in hominids [2].

All inputs to the cerebellar cortex are mediated by two sorts of afferents: mossy fibers and climbing fibers. It is now well established that all climbing fibers emerge from the inferior olivary nucleus, whereas all other afferent fiber systems originate from the spinal cord, the vestibular nuclei, and the pons terminate as mossy fibers with synapse on dendrites of granule cells [3]. With respect to their origin, the three cerebellar components are also called the vestibulocerebellum, spinocerebellum, and ponto- or cerebrocerebellum. The archicerebellum receives its major input from the vestibular system (Fig. 3). Fibers from the spinal cord ascend within the spinocerebellar tract and terminate in the paleocerebellum, mainly in the anterior lobe. The human neocerebellum receives its major input from large masses of cells in the pons and from the inferior olivary nucleus in the medulla. All output fibers leave the cerebellar cortex via Purkinje cells and project to a set of deep cerebellar nuclei. The fastigial nucleus receives fibers from the midline vermal zone and projects to the lateral vestibular nucleus. The interposed nuclei comprising the nucleus globosus and emboliformis receive fibers from the paravermal zone and project via the superior cerebellar peduncle to the contralateral red nucleus. The dentate nucleus is by far the largest nucleus; it receives output fibers of the cerebellar hemisphere and projects contralateral to the ventrolateral nucleus of the thalamus.

* Corresponding author.

E-mail address: wolfgang.grodd@med.uni-tuebingen.de (W. Grodd).

1042-3680/05/$ - see front matter
doi:10.1016/j.nec.2004.07.008

neurosurgery.theclinics.com

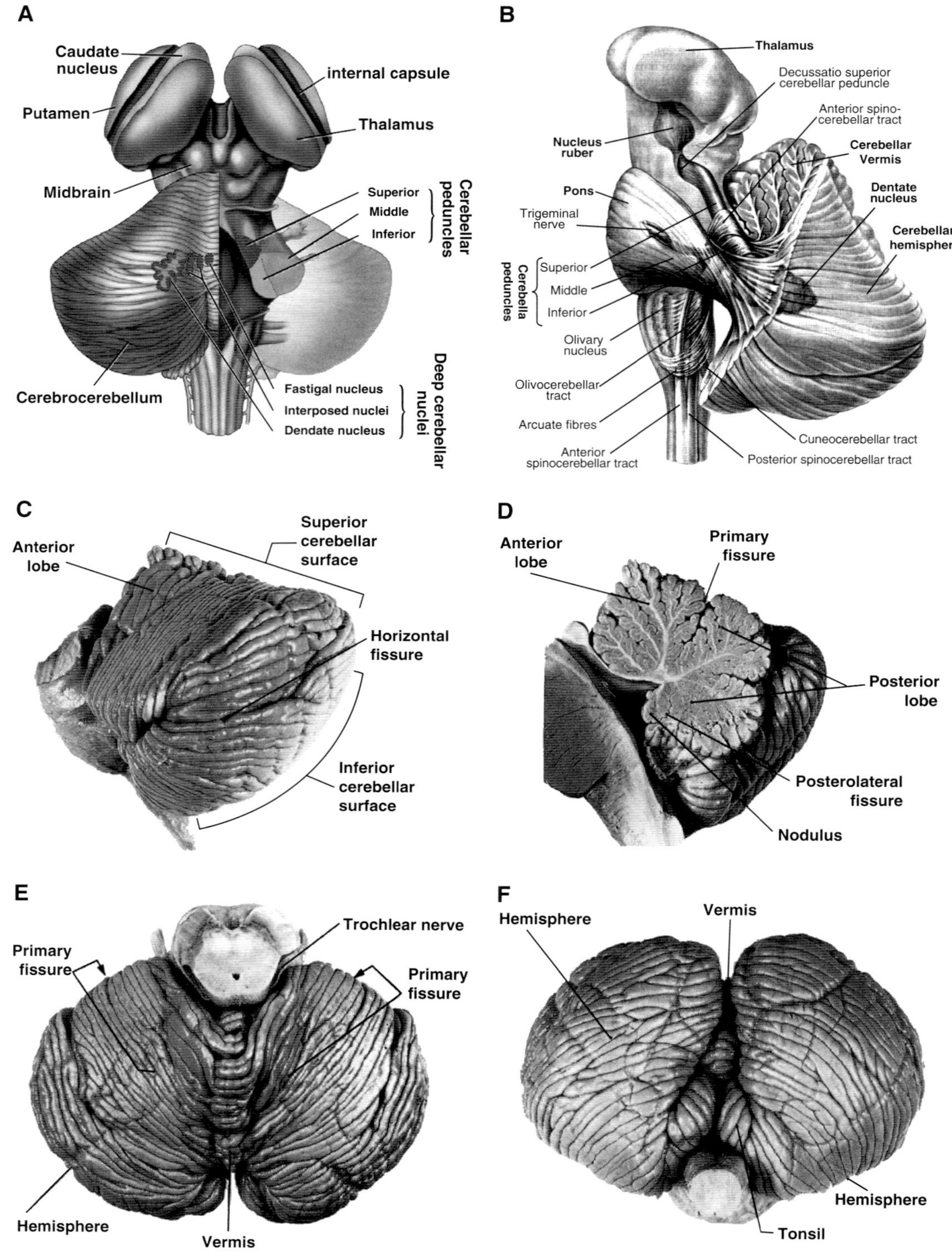

Grodd: fMRI of the cerebellum

Brief history of functional assignment in the cerebellum

The existence of functional assignment within the cerebellum was first recognized almost two centuries ago by comparative anatomic and physiologic studies. Careful analyses of the motor disturbances led Flourens [4] to conclude in 1824 that the cerebellum is neither an initiator nor an actuator but instead serves as a coordinator of movements. An animal with a damaged cerebellum still initiates and executes movements but only in a clumsy manner. From that time on, most investigators recognized the specifically motor role of the cerebellum. In 1991, more than 60 years later, Luciani [5] observed that cerebellar lesions did not impair coordinated movement as such but were caused by more elemental deficits, which he called atonia, asthenia, and astasia. Atonia is the loss of muscle tone, asthenia is weakness of muscles, and astasia is a deficit in the regularity and stability of muscle contraction. He also recognized that motor disturbances caused in an animal by a partial lesion of the cerebellum were gradually compensated for because of the functional plasticity of cerebellar tissues.

In 1904, Bolk [6] introduced his scheme of functional organization after he had examined the cerebella of more than 60 different mammalian species. He reasoned that the cerebellum is probably made up of a number of centers, each of which controls the actions of a different group of muscles. He suggested that movements can be subdivided into two basic types: one group of movements that require a muscular collaboration across the midline of the body and being represented in an unpaired structure of the cerebellum like the vermis and a second group of unilateral movements which can perform independently and are controlled by lateral structures. He concluded that the midline vermis controls bilaterally synchronized movements, whereas the cerebellar hemispheres direct unilateral movements. He also proposed sagittal continuity of the cerebellar cortex across the folia of the vermis and hemispheres and transverse continuity between the vermis and hemispheres. According to his subdivision, the sulcus primarius anterior or fissura prima splits the cerebellum into an anterior lobe and a posterior lobe (Fig. 4).

In 1910, Comolli [7] introduced the concept of paleo- and neocerebellum to differentiate the oldest and youngest cerebellar regions, respectively. According to this concept, the vermis and the flocculus represent the paleocerebellum and the hemispheres represent the neocerebellum. The cerebellar hemispheres are prominent in mammals but are barely discernible in birds [8]. Furthermore, in the superior mammals, most strikingly in hominids, the vermis is progressively reduced in size, whereas the cerebellar hemispheres are markedly enlarged, [2]. Because the hemispheres are widely connected with the cerebral cortex through the pontine nuclei, their progressive development is related to the concurrent development of the pons.

In 1934, Larsell [1] proposed a further subdivision of the cerebellar areas. His research extending over more than 30 years was posthumously was published in 1971 in a book by Larsell and Jansen [9]. His work provided a comparative anatomic basis of cerebellar localization and served as the basis for our present concepts of cerebellar morphology. He started from the observation that the fissure that appears most precociously in ontogeny as well as in phylogeny is the posterolateral fissure. This fissure splits the cerebellum into two lobes, the flocculonodular lobe and the corpus cerebelli, which encompass the whole remaining cerebellum. The corpus cerebelli is further subdivided into two lobes, anterior and posterior, by the fissura prima. According to Larsell [1], the craniocaudal course from the lingula to the nodulus is divided into 10 lobuli (vermis: I–X, hemisphere: HI–X). These are subdivided into up to six lamellae (a–f; see Fig. 2). Larsell's subdivision constituted the final step in a series of the classifications of cerebellum anatomy.

At the beginning of the 1940s, new functional assignments emerged from electrophysiologic investigations. Adrian [10] recorded cerebellar unitary discharges during joint displacements, muscle stretching, or tactile stimulation in anesthetized cats and monkeys as well as in decerebrate cats. He demonstrated that proprioceptive and exteroceptive information is somatotopically arranged

◄

Fig. 1. Anatomy of the cerebellum. Dorsal (*A*) and lateral (*B*) views of the cerebellum with depiction of the cerebellar nuclei and peduncles and the course of the cerebellar peduncles as well as the other major input tract. (*Adapted from* Nieuwenhuys R, Voogd J, Huijzen C. The human central nervous system. 3rd edition. New York: Springer; 1988.) Depiction of cerebellar lateral (*C*), midsagittal (*D*), superior (*E*), and inferior (*F*) surfaces. (*Adapted from* Haines DE. Fundamental neuroscience. New York, Churchill Livingstone; 1997.)

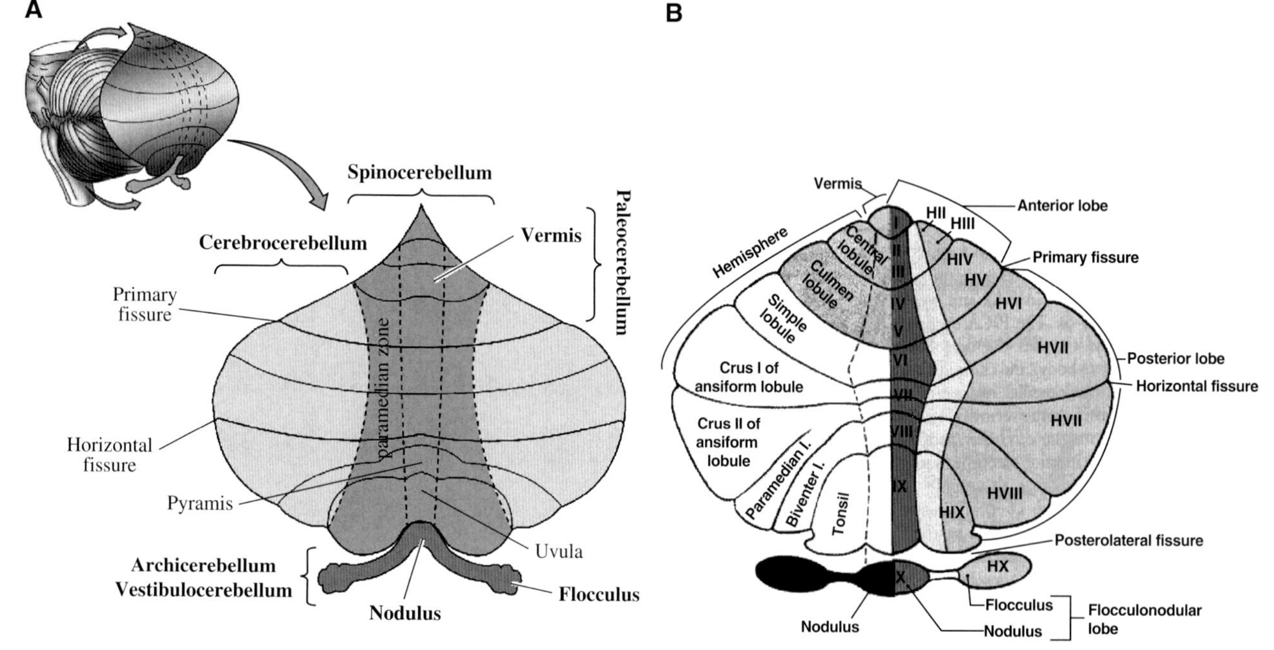

Grodd: fMRI of the cerebellum

Fig. 2. Anatomic assignments of the cerebellum. (*A*) Unfolded cerebellar surface with display of major compartments and anatomic nomenclature. (*B*) Assignment of major lobules according to Larsell [1].

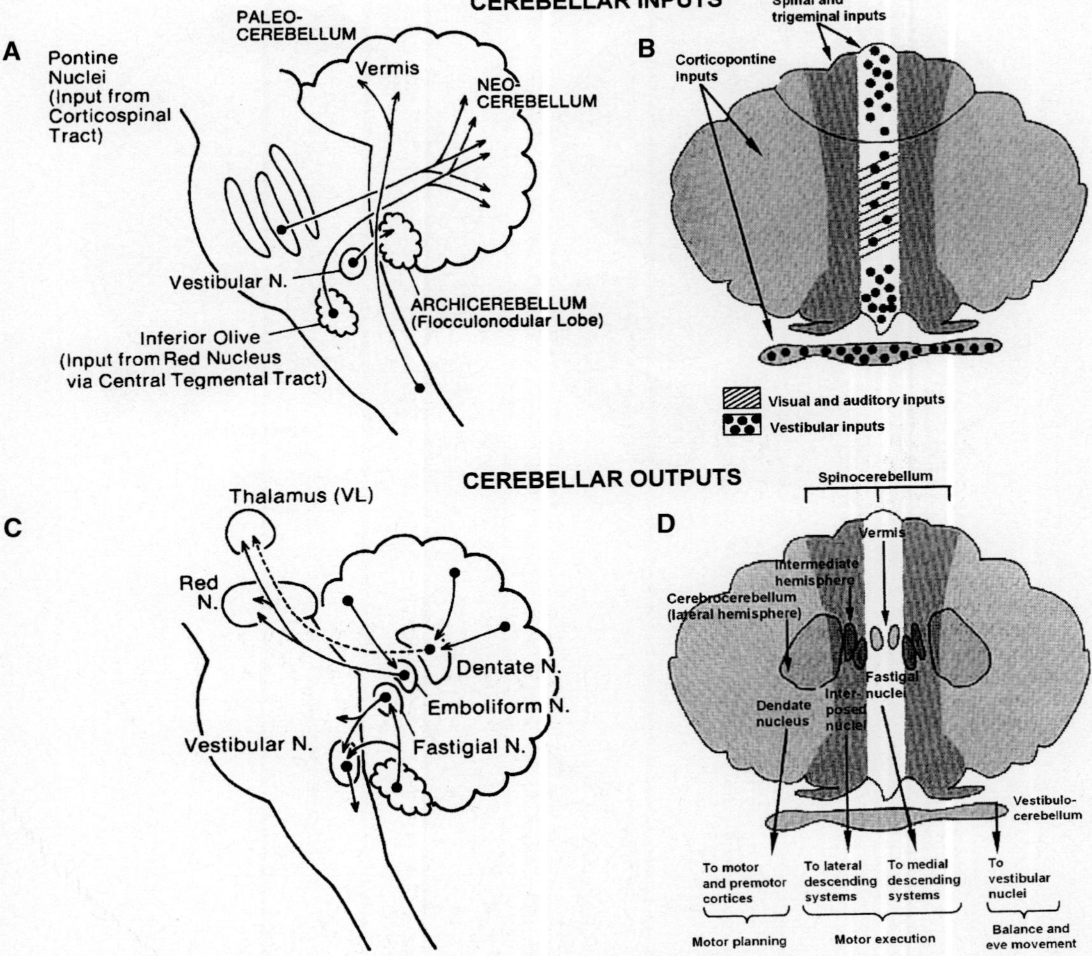

Fig. 3. Cerebellar input and output channels. Overview of the major cerebellar input (*A*, *B*) and output (*C*, *D*) pathways with their corresponding cerebellar compartments (*B*, *D*).

in the anterior lobe. Specifically, hind limb afferents project to vermian and hemispheric regions of the lobulus centralis (Larsell's lobules III and HIII), forelimb afferents project to the culmen (lobules IV, V, HIV, and HV), and face afferents project to the lobulus simplex (lobules VI and HVI).

Similarly, in 1944, Snider and Stowell [11] revealed two inverted somatotopic maps in the anterior lobe and paramedian lobule in anesthetized cats and monkeys, where exteroceptive information from hair or vibrissae is projected (see Fig. 4). Their mapping was based on recordings of surface potentials, which reflect the predominant cerebellar input. The body map in the anterior lobe has the hind limbs oriented forward, whereas the face extends backward into the first lobule of the posterior lobe. The map in the paramedian lobule has the head forward and the limbs represented on either side of the midline. Arms and legs are represented adjacent to the vermis over the intermediate cortex of the hemispheres. The projections to the anterior lobe are strictly ipsilateral, whereas the afferents to the paramedian lobule are bilateral, although with a slight bias toward the ipsilateral projection. In addition, these investigators described slightly overlapping auditory and visual inputs to the vermis (lobulus simplex, folium, and tuber vermis), probably reaching the cerebellum through the colliculi and the tectocerebellar tract. The somatotopic representation demonstrated for exteroceptive and proprioceptive

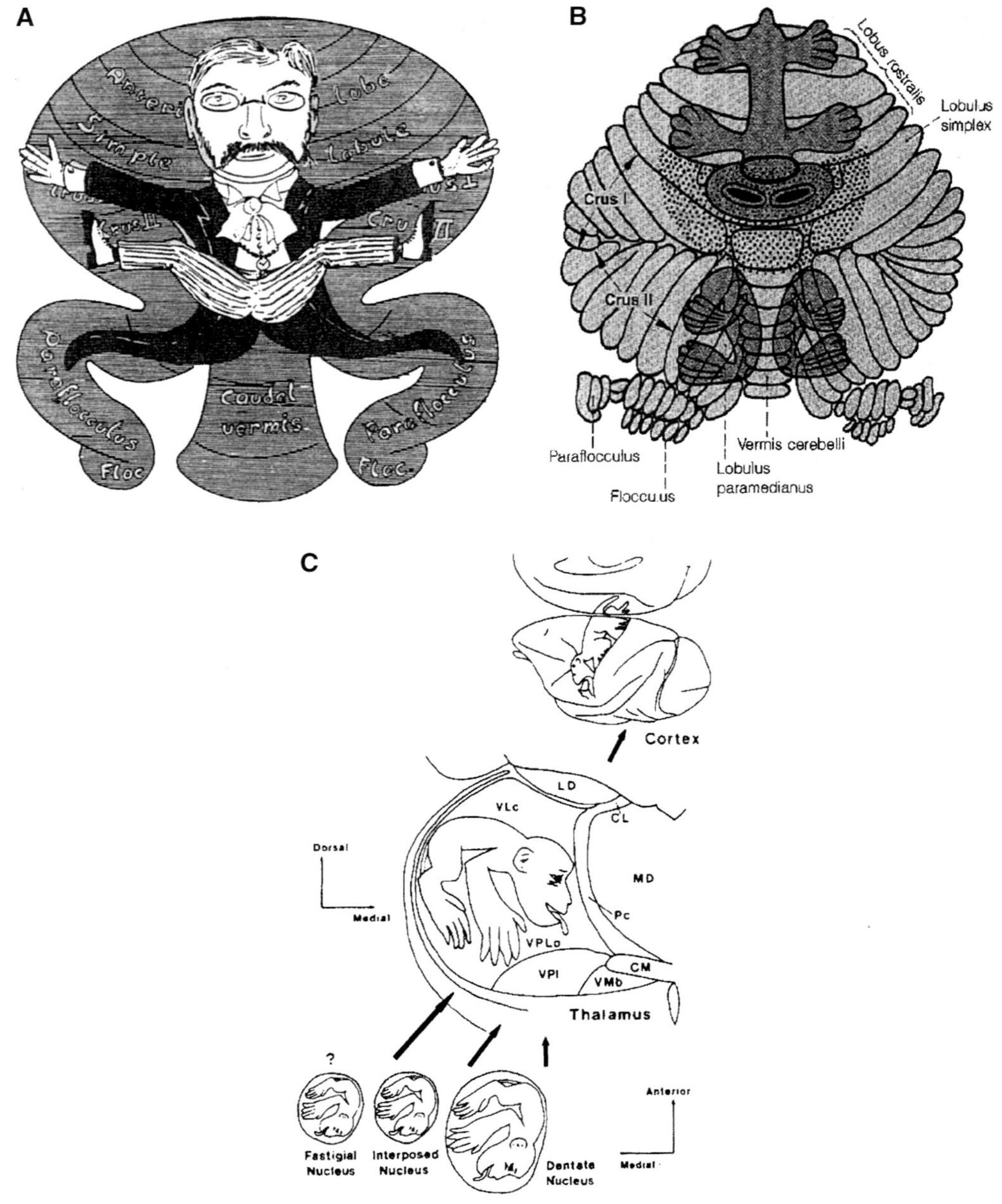

Fig. 4. Cerebellar somatotopy. Cortical arrangement of body parts as seen by Bolk (*A*) and Snider and Eldred (*B*) and somatotopic organization of the deep cerebellar nuclei as predicted by Asanuma (*C*). (*A: From* Glickstein M, Yeo C. The cerebellum and motor learning. J Cogn Neurosci 1990;2:69–80; with permission. *B: From* Snider R, Stowell A. Receiving areas of the tactile, auditory and visual systems in the cerebellum. J Neurophysiol 1944;7:331–57; with permission. *C: Adapted from* Asanuma C, Thach WT, Jones EG. Brain stem and spinal projections of the deep cerebellar nuclei in the monkey, with observations on the brain stem projections of the dorsal column nuclei. Brain Res Rev 1983;5:299–322.)

inputs mediated by spinocerebellar pathways was also valid for neocortical afferents, which reach cerebellar regions via the pontine nuclei. Subdivisions of the primary motor cortex (M1) that represent the face, arms, and legs project within the cerebellum into the same areas as the spinocerebellar projections from the face, arms, and legs, respectively, demonstrating an elegant somatotopic arrangement of inputs, regardless of the site of origin.

Soon after the discovery of the somatotopic organization of cerebellar afferents, experiments were performed to elucidate the efferent projections of the cerebellum. In the absence of anesthesia, stimulation of the cerebellar cortex evokes localized movements. As for the anterior lobe, stimulation of the lobule simplex evokes head movements of the face and jaw, stimulation of the culmen evokes forelimb movements, stimulation of the centralis evokes hind limb movements, and stimulation of the lingula evokes tail movements. Trunk muscles are represented medially, whereas limb muscles are represented laterally. This scheme, which was first disclosed in the decerebrate animal, was confirmed in intact animals by means of chronically implanted electrodes. Hampson et al [12] reported that in the decerebrate cat, dog, and monkey, electrical stimulation of the anterior lobe provoked inhibition of hypertonus in the ipsilateral limbs and increased hypertonus in the contralateral limbs.

More recent studies have revealed that in the mammalian cerebellum, the main afferent and efferent projections have a parasagittal band-like topographic organization [13,14]. This somatotopic organization was demonstrated for climbing and mossy fiber afferents as well as for efferent Purkinje cell projections to cerebellar and lateral vestibular nuclei. In the pars intermedia of the anterior lobe, as far as the climbing fibers are concerned, the hind limb is represented in the lobus centralis and the forelimb is represented in the culmen. Similarly, in the vermian portion of the anterior lobe, a sagittal organization was found, with the forelimb and hind limb represented medially and laterally, respectively [15,16]. Electrophysiologic studies in primates show that deep cerebellar nuclei are also somatotopically organized (see Fig. 4). They are arranged to receive projections from the two maps on the dorsal and ventral surfaces of the intermediate and lateral zones of the cerebellar cortex and project contralateral to the red nucleus and M1 through the thalamus [17].

At a finer level of resolution, experimental studies based on single-cell recordings in mammals have shown that body parts are not represented continuously over larger areas of the cerebellar cortex but are broken down into smaller discontinuous patches. A small area that receives sensory input from the arm (by way of mossy fiber–granule cell connections) might be located adjacent to an area that receives input from a noncontiguous region of the same upper extremity. In addition, each body part is represented in several locations. This spatial pattern of representation is referred as fractured somatotopy [18].

On the basis of numerous experimental findings, similar somatotopic maps have been hypothesized in human beings, but a relative uncertainty exists as to what extent the spino- and neocerebellum serve sensorimotor functions and which part serves other brain functions, especially sensory and cognitive processing [19]. The existing clinical topodiagnostic scheme in human beings still attributes motor deficits only to the lateral, intermediate, and vermal zones. In general, this notion is consistent with the experimental findings [11] in that (1) lateral cerebellar damage predominantly results in a delay of movement initiation and decomposition of multijoint movements, which are invariably more pronounced in the arm; (2) paramedian lesions often cause dysarthria; and (3) lesions to the vermis yield ataxia of stance and gait [20].

Functional imaging of the cerebellum

Detailed functional mapping of the human cerebellum first became possible with the advent of positron emission tomography (PET) and functional MRI (fMRI) in the 1980s. Although both neuroimaging techniques are of an indirect nature because they are coupled via a hemodynamic response function to the underlying neuronal events, they have nevertheless opened a wide range of cerebellar investigations. As a result, a steadily increasing number of imaging studies have been published regarding functional localization in the cerebellum. In this article, we summarize some of the major results in assigning sensorimotor, language, and other sensory and cognition functions to the cerebellum.

Spatial normalization of the cerebellum

Because functional mapping shows considerable differences in individual brain anatomy, PET and fMRI of the cerebrum are usually subjected to a group statistic. The latter is accomplished within a normalization procedure using a defined reference space to achieve probabilistic mapping. The most applied normalization procedure refers to the Talairach space, originally developed for stereotactic procedures to the thalamus, which thus does not include the cerebellum [21]. Nevertheless, this normalization approach is still commonly applied in human neuroimaging studies and implemented in a number of evaluation programs [22,23]. Meanwhile, a three-dimensional MRI atlas of the human cerebellum in a proportional stereotaxic space has been introduced by Schmahmann et al [24], in which the Talairach space is simply modified by extending the coordinate system caudally. In addition, on the basis of this extended reference frame, a first MRI atlas with detailed coordinates of the cerebellar nuclei has been published [25].

Nevertheless, better reduction of variance caused by differences in individual anatomy is achieved by applying a transformation procedure specific for the cerebellum, because this approach accounts for variations in the medullopontine angulation. Such a transformation can easily be realized analogous to the Talairach normalization by introducing an appropriate reference frame and specific anatomic landmarks for the cerebellum. By defining three orthogonal planes centered on the floor of the fourth ventricle and introducing seven predefined landmarks, one can achieve spatial normalization by adjusting the individual landmarks to the determined values by means of linear expansion or compression along these three axes [26]. The superiority of this approach compared with Talairach normalization is especially pronounced for the inferior cerebellar surface (Fig. 5).

Sensorimotor functions

Cortical topography

By applying such cerebellar-centered normalization procedure, Grodd et al [26] have recently determined the areas of activation in the cerebellar cortex in 46 human subjects during a series of motor tasks with fMRI (Fig. 6). The representation areas for movements of the lips, tongue, hands, and feet were found to be sharply confined to lobules, sublobules, and the sagittal zones in the rostral and caudal spinocerebellar cortex. There was a mirror-like symmetry aligned to the midline. The activation maps separate into two distinct homunculoid representations: one, a more extended representation, was located upside down in the superior cerebellum, and a second one, doubled and smaller, was located in the inferior cerebellum. The two representations were remarkably similar to those proposed by Snider and Eldred [27] five decades ago (Fig. 7). In the upper representation, intralimb somatotopy for the right elbow, wrist, and fingers was likewise revealed. The maps seem to confirm earlier electrophysiologic findings of sagittal zones in animals. They differed, however, from micromapping reports on fractured somatotopy in the cerebellar cortex and most likely reflect the input integration of afferent peripheral and central information in the cerebellar cortex.

Active versus passive movement

The former study was restricted to active movements and did not investigate the patterns of activation during passive limb excursions, and it is still unknown whether a similar dual representation for afferent inputs to the cerebellum exists, as reported in the cat and monkey. If this would be the case, the question arises whether the two areas have comparable roles in motor and sensory processing or whether there are differences in these areas during voluntary movement and passive kinesthetic sensory stimulation. The aim of the cerebellar fMRI study by Thickbroom et al [28] was thus to determine whether a dual representation can also be demonstrated with passive movement and to compare the patterns and degree of cerebellar activation with kinematically comparable active and passive limb movement. They compared differences between active and passive index finger movement and detected activation ipsilateral in the anterior and posterior lobes during both tasks (Fig. 8). During passive movement, dual activation was detected in the ipsilateral cerebellum, in the anterior lobe, and in the posterior lobe. A similar pattern of activation was observed during voluntary movement; however, the overall magnitude was approximately doubled in both areas. They conclude that the rostral representation is the dominant one but that both areas may be involved in kinesthetic sensory and motor processing.

Executed versus imagined movement

The question as to what extent imagery and perception share the same neuronal substrates or whether they are based on completely different neuronal mechanisms, such as abstract

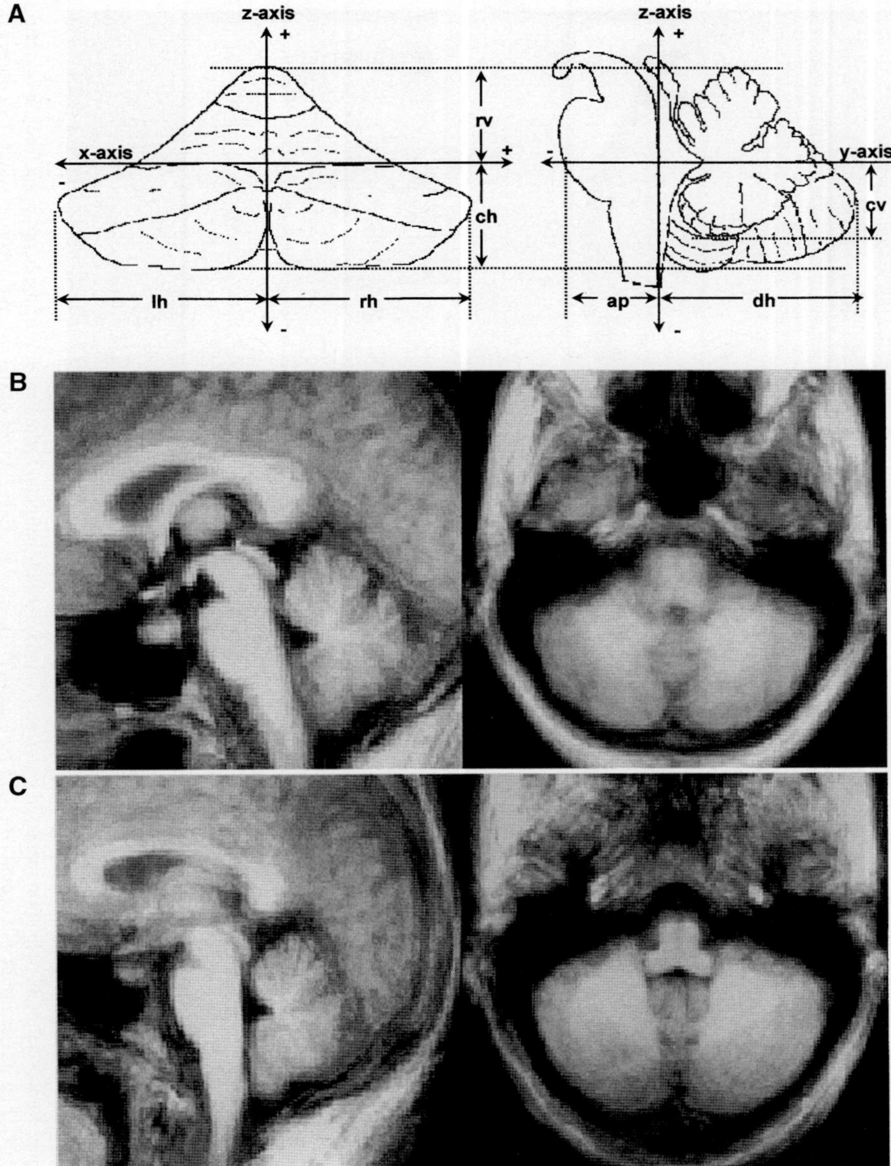

Fig. 5. Cerebellar transformation. (*A*) Linear transformation of the cerebellum. Three perpendicular planes (midsagittal x-plane, y-plane along the floor of the fourth ventricle, and z-plane through the apex of the fourth ventricle) centered at the dorsal pons with definition of seven anatomic landmarks (ap, anterior pons; ch, caudal hemisphere; cv, caudal vermis; dh, dorsal hemisphere; lh, left hemisphere; rh, right hemisphere; rv, rostral vermis) used for cerebellar transformation. (*B, C*) Results of two transformation procedures on the averaged cerebellar anatomy of 10 subjects in a midsagittal view (*left*) and axial view (*right*) on the inferior cerebellar surface. Talairach transformation (*B*) and cerebellum-centered transformation (*C*) according to Grodd et al [26]. Note the superior outline of the spinal cord and cerebellar tonsils in *C*.

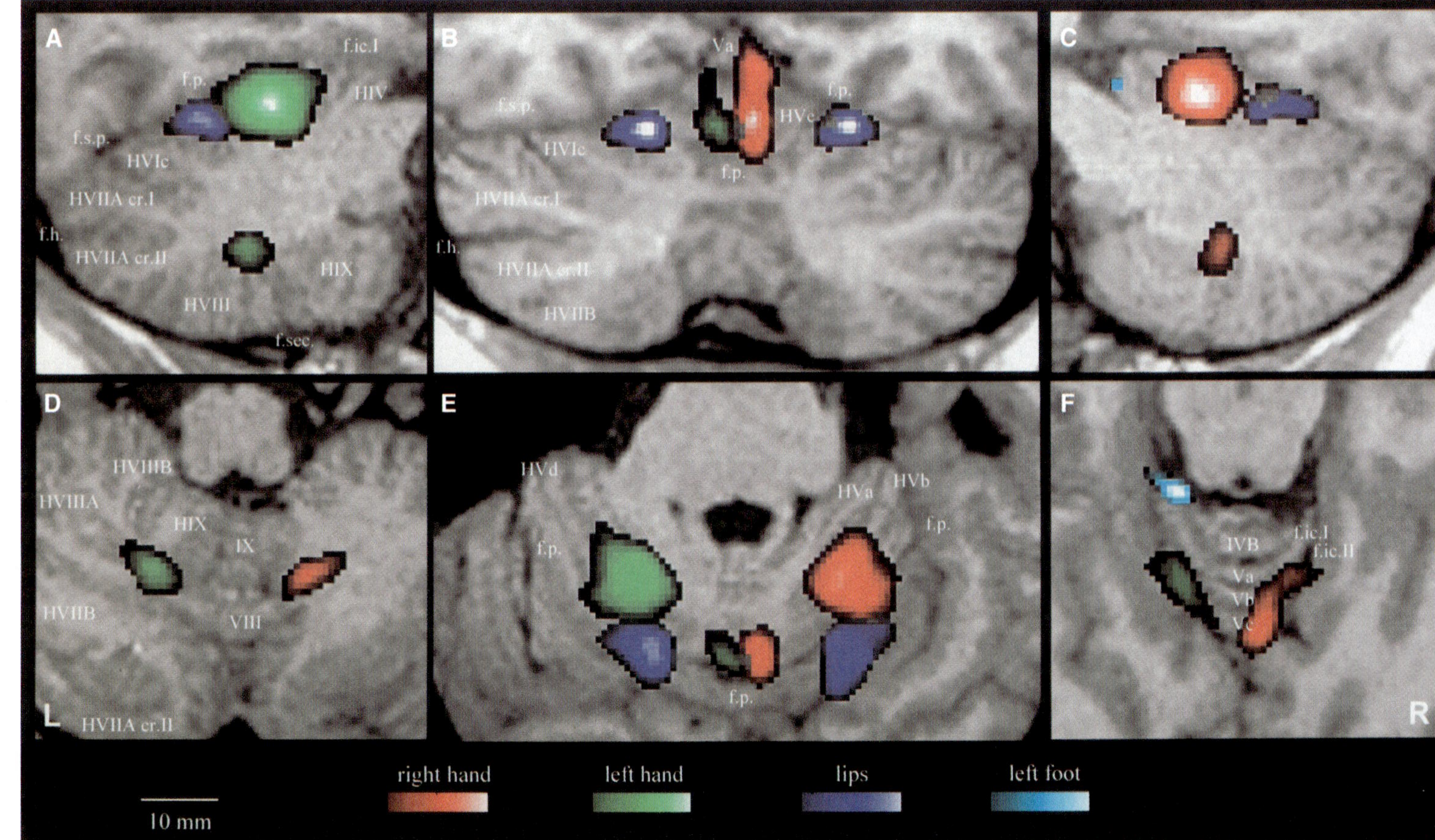

Fig. 6. Topography of cerebellar activation. Functional MRI activation displayed on an individual cerebellar template for movements of the hands (*right* [red], *left* [green]), the lips (blue), and the feet (cyan) ($P < 0.01$). Left parasagittal (*A*), coronal (*B*), right parasagittal (*C*), inferior axial (*D*), medioaxial (*E*), and superior axial (*F*) sections. f.h., fissura horizontalis; f.p., fissura prima; f.sec., fissura secunda; f.s.p., fissura superior posterior; L, left; R, right. (*From* Grodd W, Hülsmann E, Lotze M, Wildgruber D, Erb M. Sensorimotor mapping of the human cerebellum: fMRI evidence of somatotopic organization. Hum Brain Mapp 2001;13:55–73; with permission.)

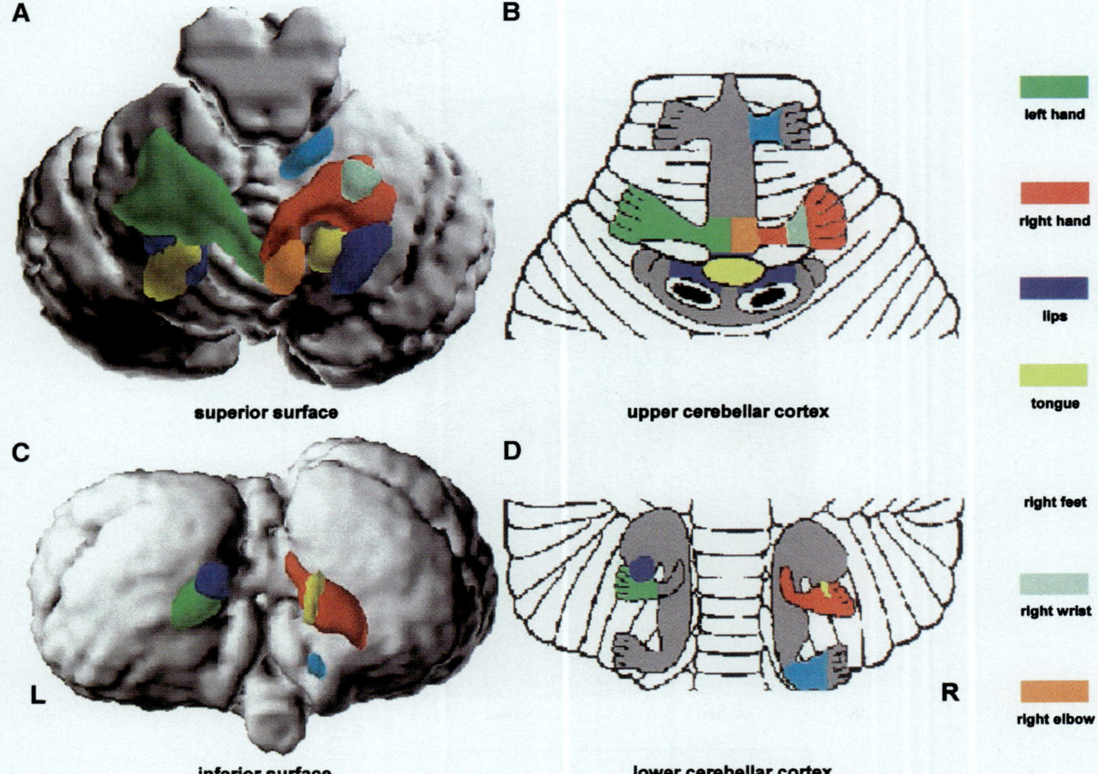

Fig. 7. Functional somatotopy of the cerebellum. Display of cerebellar surface with superimposed color-coded functional MRI activation volumes on the superior (*A*) and inferior (*C*) cerebellar surface with corresponding display of the cerebellar homunculi (*B, D*) as represented by Snider and Eldred. (*Data from* Brain Innovation B.V. Web site. http://www.brainvoyager.com. Accessed September 27, 2004.)

postperceptual representations, is an ongoing debate in the neurosciences. The discussion has mainly focused on visual imagery; evidence from neuroimaging and neuropsychologic testing suggests that imagery and perception use the same brain areas. Motor imagery may have different characteristics, in which it is not the virtual environment that is imagined but introspective kinesthetic feelings of moving the limb [29]. Movement imagery as an internal process may be compared with movement preparation, two processes that might be functionally equivalent. Lotze et al [30] have studied fMRI brain activation during executed movement (EM) and imagined movement (IM) of both hands. In conjunction with electromyographic control of the musculi flexor digitorum superficialis and training of high vividness of IM before image acquisition, they determined regional cerebral activation for EM and IM compared with rest in selected regions. In all subjects, the supplementary motor area (SMA), premotor cortex, and primary motor cortex M1 showed significant activation during both conditions, but only the somatosensory cortex (S1) was significantly more highly activated during EM. The prefrontal and parietal regions revealed no significant changes during both conditions, but in the cerebellum, ipsilateral activation was decreased during IM compared with EM (Fig. 9). In addition, the foci of maximal cerebellar activation between IM and EM differed significantly. High ipsilateral activation was observed in the anterior lobe (lobule HIV-HV) during EM, whereas during IM, a smaller activation area was found distant approximately 2 cm dorsolateral in lobule HVII. Although the cortical results support the hypothesis that motor imagery and motor performance possess similar neural substrates, the activation in the cerebellum during EM and IM may be in accordance with the assumption that the posterior cerebellum is involved in the inhibition of movement execution during imagination.

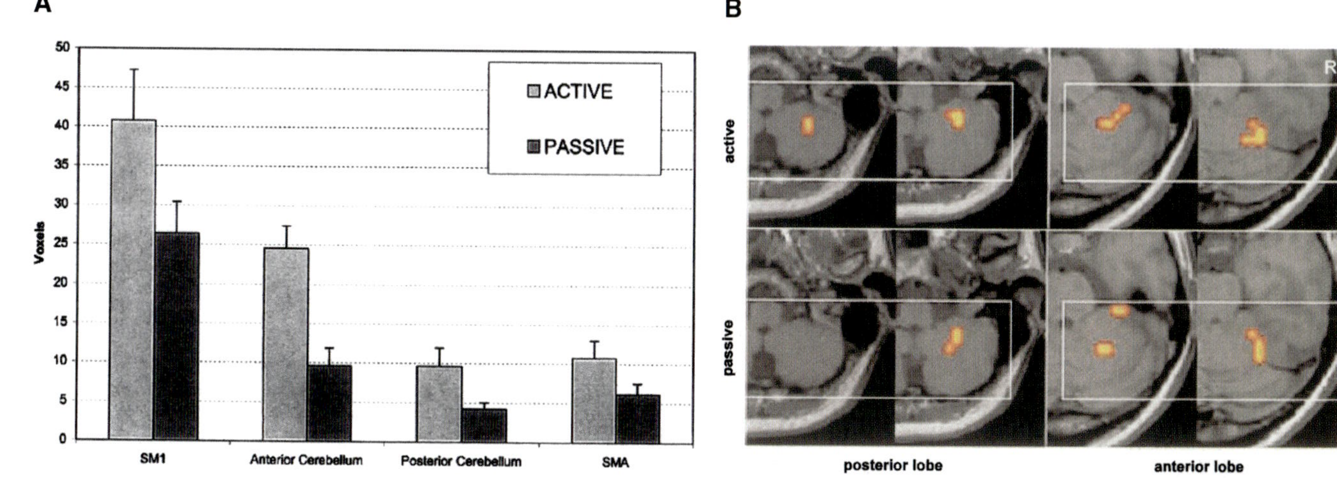

Fig. 8. Comparison of active and passive movement. (*A*) Group data comparing the number of activated voxels in the contralateral sensorimotor cortex (SM1), supplementary motor area (SMA), and anterior and posterior ipsilateral cerebellar hemispheres during voluntary and passive movement (mean and standard error). (*B*) Cerebellar activation during voluntary right index finger movement of one subject in axial planes of two contiguous slices in the anterior (*left*) and posterior (*right*) lobes for active (*top*) and passive movement (*bottom*). (*From* Thickbroom GW, Byrnes ML, Mastaglia FL. Dual representation of the hand in the cerebellum: activation with voluntary and passive finger movement. Neuroimage 2003;18:670–4; with permission.)

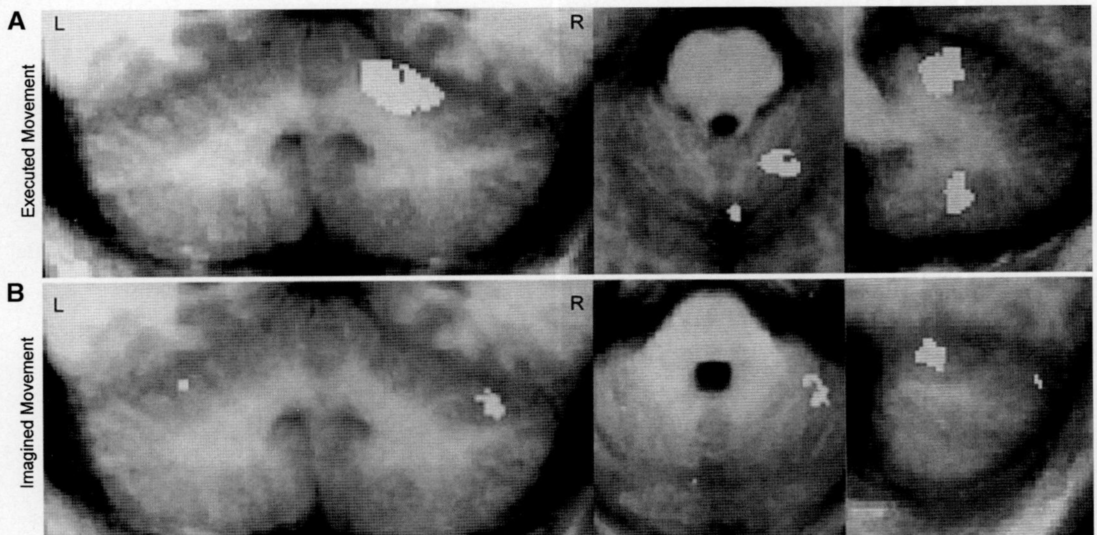

Fig. 9. Comparison of executed movement (EM) and imagined movement (IM). Cerebellar activation during EM (A) and IM (B) of the hand projected on normalized cerebellum of 10 subjects in coronal (*left*), axial (*middle*), and parasagittal views (*right*). Note that the activation maximum for EM is ipsilateral in the anterior hemisphere (lobule HIV-V) and that the activated maximum for IM is smaller and in the posterior hemisphere (lobule HVII) located 2.2 cm lateral and 1 cm dorsal to EM. (*Adapted from* Lotze M, Montoya P, Erb M, Hülsmann E, Flor H, Klose U, et al. Activation of cortical and cerebellar motor areas during executed and imagined hand movements: an fMRI study. J Cogn Neurosci 1999;11:491–501.)

Frequency of voluntary movements

For voluntary movements, a number of functional imaging studies have indicated a mass activation effect within the hand representation area of the sensorimotor cortex during finger-tapping or finger-to-thumb opposition tasks in terms of a stepwise or linear function between movement rate and hemodynamic response. With respect to subcortical structures of the sensorimotor system, there is, by contrast, only preliminary evidence for nonlinear rate/response functions within the basal ganglia and cerebellum. Therefore, Riecker et al [31] performed an fMRI study with externally paced finger tapping of six frequencies: 2, 2.5, 3, 4, 5, and 6 Hz. Parametric analysis revealed the expected increase of the hemodynamic response within the left mesiofrontal cortex and sensorimotor cortex in parallel to the movement rate (with the plateau phase at the sensorimotor cortex for frequencies greater than 4 Hz) (Fig. 10). By contrast, the left caudate nucleus, putamen, and external pallidum showed a negative linear rate/response relation.

Interestingly, two hemodynamic responses emerged ipsilateral in the anterior and posterior lobes of the cerebellum, which both exhibited a stepwise rate/response function. In accordance with clinical findings, these data indicate that the cerebellum responds different to movement frequencies less than or greater than approximately 3 Hz, respectively.

Timing of voluntary movements

Timing is essential for the execution of skilled movement, but our knowledge of the neuronal systems underlying timekeeping operations is limited. A number of studies suggested that the internal generation of precisely timed movement is dependent on at least three interrelated neural systems: one that is involved in explicit timing (basal ganglia and SMA) [32], one that mediates sensory memory, and one that is involved in sensorimotor processing (sensorimotor cortex and cerebellum) [33]. In an intriguing experiment, Hülsmann et al [34] monitored the time scale of corticocerebellar interaction during a delayed motor response by event-related fMRI. They assumed that the cerebellum has to be consulted within a limited window of time prior to a planned action and that cerebellar activation should thus occur in a time-dependent manner with respect to the corresponding telencephalic areas.

They evaluated the activation for simple thumb movement with a time-shifted

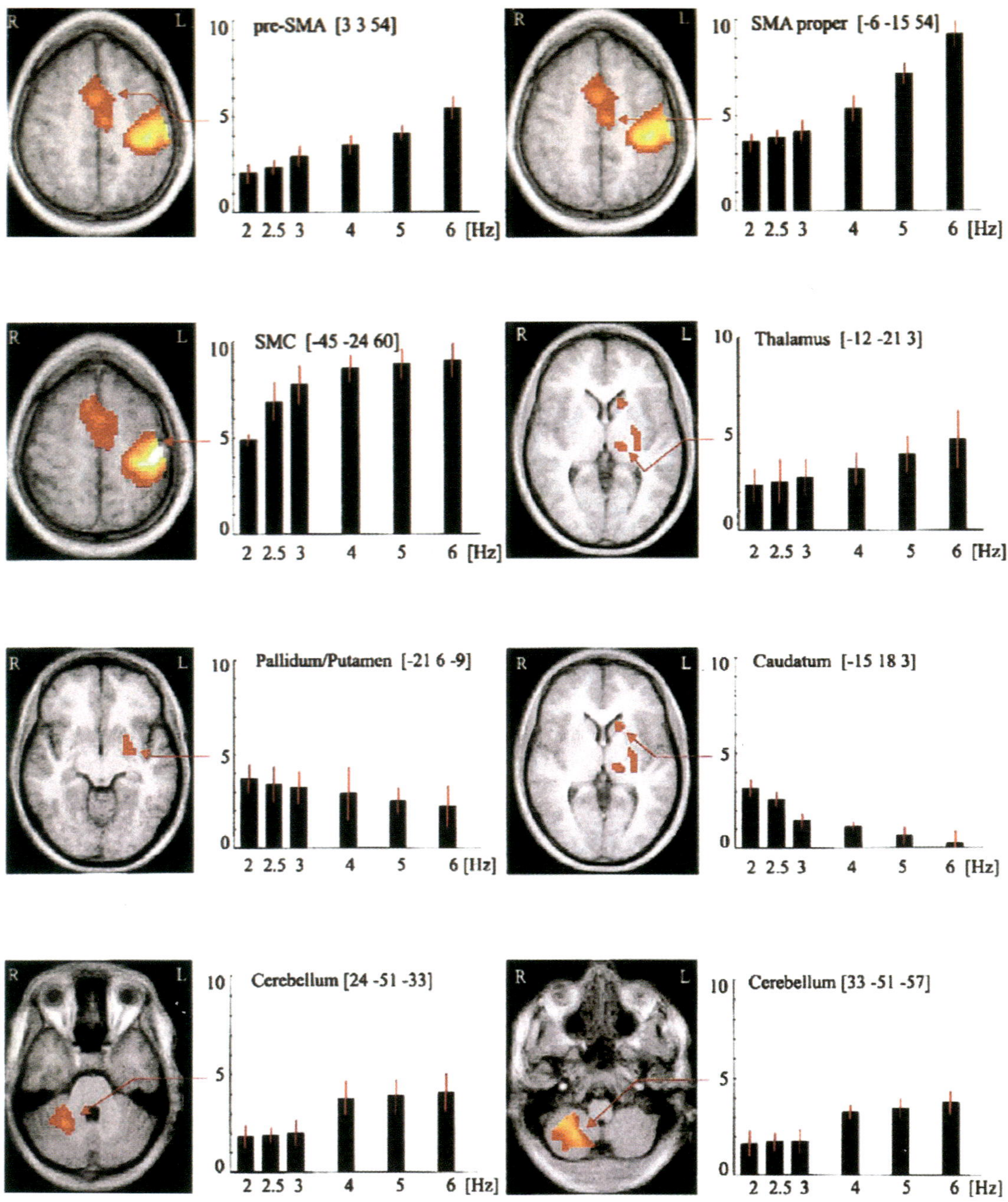

Fig. 10. Frequency dependence of voluntary movement. Parametric analysis of hemodynamic activation of group data (n = 8). The different rate/response functions (size of effect and variance of signal intensity calculated in arbitrary units by Statistical Parameter Mapping [SPM]) within the respective activated clusters (displayed on transverse sections of the averaged anatomic reference images) across all six different rates. SPM coordinates are given in square brackets. L, left; R, right; SMA, supplementary motor area; SMC, sensorimotor cortex. (*From* Riecker A, Wildgruber D, Mathiak K, Grodd W, Ackermann H. Parametric analysis of rate dependent hemodynamic response functions of cortical and subcortical brain structures during auditorily cued finger tapping: an fMRI study. Neuroimage 2003;18:731–9; with permission.)

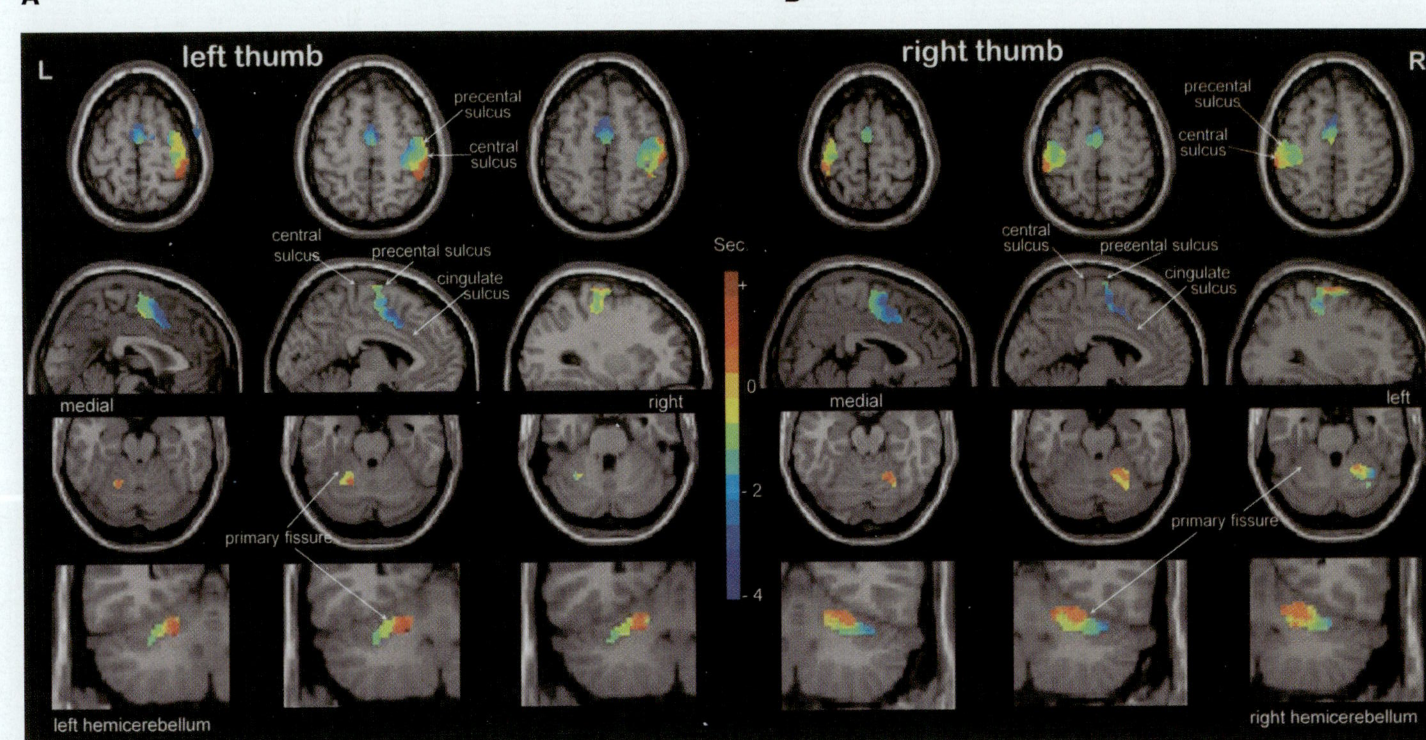

Fig. 11. Time course of cortical and cerebellar activation for thumb movement. Color-coded delay map depicting the time points of maximal t values of single voxels in the contralateral medial prefrontal cortex, the sensorimotor cortex, and the ipsilateral hemicerebellum superimposed on anatomic axial (running from top to bottom), sagittal (running from medial to outside), and coronal (running from posterior to anterior) slices of a single subject brain (MNI) for left (*A*) and right (*B*) thumb movement. Cingulate motor areas on both sides of the cingulate sulcus showed the earliest activation, followed by the presupplementary motor area and supplementary motor area (SMA) proper. The premotor activation occurred 2 seconds before movement onset, and anterior to the precentral sulcus in the sensorimotor cortex, it occurred 0.5 to 1 second before movement onset and proceeded toward the central sulcus. In the cerebellum, early activation located in lobule HVI, caudal to the primary fissure, was in time with the late anterior cingulate and SMA, whereas late cerebellar activation was located in spinocerebellar lobule HV, rostral to the primary fissure, in time with the sensorimotor cortex. (*From* Hülsmann E, Erb M, Grodd W. From will to action: sequential cerebellar contribution to voluntary movements. Neuroimage 2003;20:1485–92; with permission.)

hemodynamic response and found spatially and temporally separated cerebral and cerebellar activations, which accompanied the entire process, from conscious planning to final motor output, within a time frame of 6 seconds (Fig. 11). The cerebral activations spread from the anterior cingulate cortex through the SMA and premotor area to the primary motor and sensory cortices. This cascade was temporally in parallel with cerebellar activations propagating from the neocerebellum to the spinocerebellum. An early lateral cerebellar recruitment of 3 seconds prior to movement onset confirms its involvement in early motor planning (Fig. 12). A later medial activation occurring close to movement onset most probably reflects spinocerebellar kinesthetic feedback. Between these two points, a striking lateromedial succession was found, which is in line with the hypothesis of the existence of multiple internal models residing in the cerebellum, with each communicating with its own corresponding telencephalic region.

Somatosensory cancellation

In an elegant fMRI study, Blakemore et al [35] investigated how the cerebellum uses a signaled efference copy for the prediction of central motor commands. They compared the responses when subjects experienced a tactile stimulus that was self-produced or externally applied. More activity was found in S1 when the stimulus was externally produced. In the cerebellum, less activation was associated with a movement that generated a tactile stimulus than with a movement that did not (Fig. 13). The reduction in S1 to self-produced tactile stimuli is likely to be the physiologic correlate of the reduced perception associated with this type of stimulation, whereas the selective deactivation in the right anterior lobe by self-produced tactile stimulus suggests that the cerebellum differentiates between movements depending on their specific sensory consequences. This reasoning is consistent with the theory that the cerebellum is a component of a system that provides (via an internal forward model [36]) precise prediction of the sensory consequences of motor commands, which, when congruent with the actual sensory consequences, are used to cancel the perception of a tactile stimulus.

Language and cognitive processing

PET and fMRI studies have consistently reported on cerebellar activation associated with mental operations, such as memory retrieval, verbal fluency, language comprehension, and control of attention [37,38]. Neuropsychologic studies have shown that patients with focal or diffuse cerebellar pathologic findings are impaired on a wide range of cognitive tasks, especially those associated with higher executive control [39].

Speech production

Although the cortical areas like the left inferior frontal lobe (Broca's area), left superior temporal lobe (Wernicke's area), and M1 bilaterally are well known to be involved in language production and comprehension, the localization and extent of cerebellum participation are less secure. fMRI investigations of speech production and singing [40] have revealed that the superior cerebellum is activated reciprocally to the concomitant cortical areas of the dominant hemisphere (ie, right-sided activation for speech and left-sided activation for singing) (Fig. 14).

Because a variety of data indicate that the cerebellum participates in speech tasks that require precise representation of temporal information, Wildgruber et al [41] have determined whether the cerebellum is prone to differences in syllable speed. Therefore, fMRI was performed during silent repetitions of the syllable "ta" at three different rates (2.5, 4.0, and 5.5 Hz). Again, as for finger tapping [31], the spatial extent and magnitude of hemodynamic responses at the level of the motor cortex showed a positive correlation to production frequencies, whereas the lower rates (2.5 and 4.0 Hz) gave rise to higher magnitudes of activation within the left putamen as compared with the 5.5-Hz condition (Fig. 15). In contrast, cerebellar responses were rather restricted to fast performance (4.0 and 5.5 Hz) and exhibited a shift in a caudal direction during 5.5 Hz as compared with 4.0 Hz. These findings corroborate the suggestion of a differential role of various cortical and subcortical areas depending on speech motor speed, and the data are closely parallel to clinical findings: extensive acoustic analyses of syllable repetition tasks in cerebellar patients found slowed maximum repetition rates that do not seem to fall below 3 Hz [42]. Presumably, these effects must be considered a characteristic sign of cerebellar dysfunction.

Language perception and temporal discrimination

Access to the word form of a lexical item requires, among other functions, the processing of durational parameters of verbal utterances. Assuming the cerebellum to participate in explicit

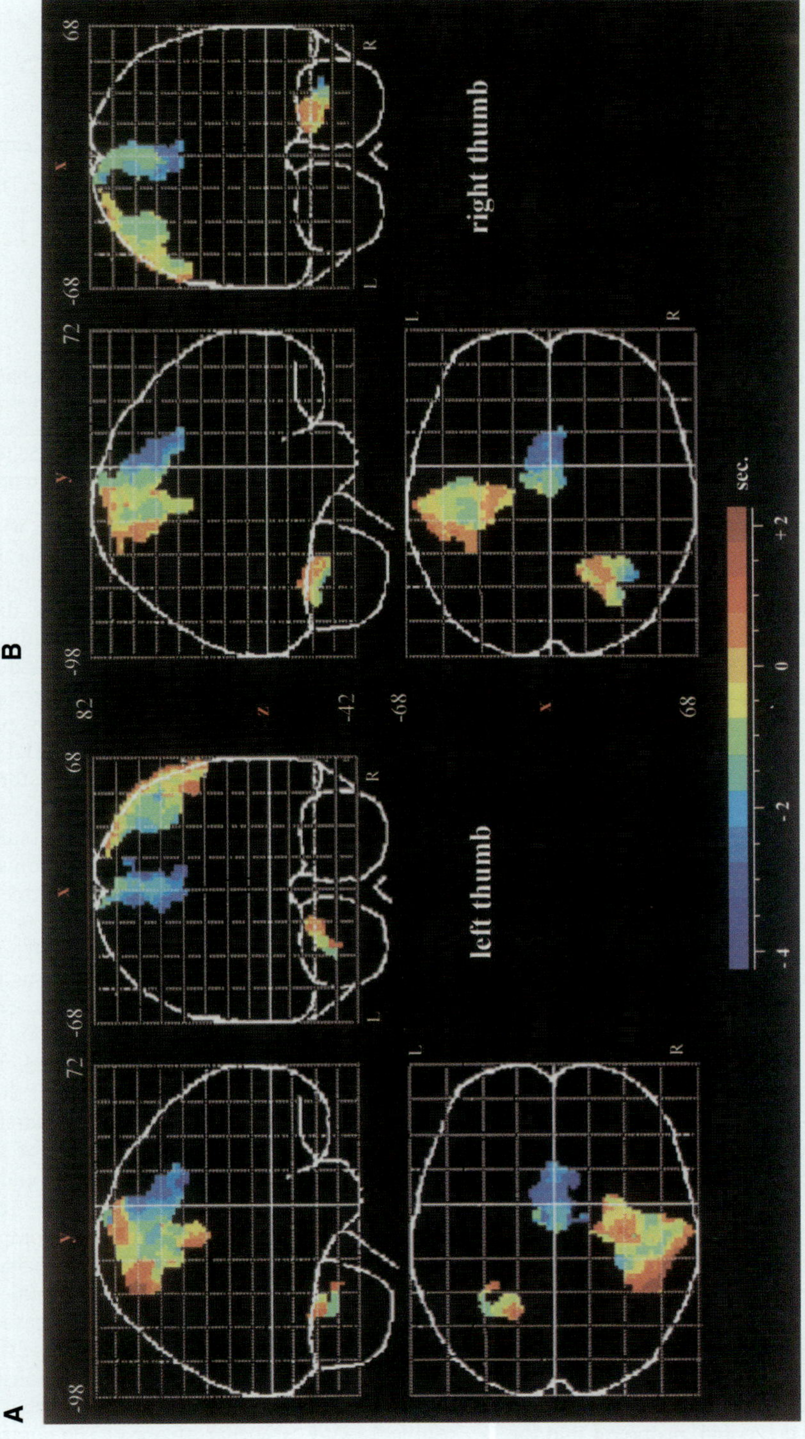

Fig. 12. Delay maps of activation during voluntary movement. Maps of single-voxel hemodynamic response function projected on axial, coronal, and sagital planes (coordinates in millimeters; L, left; R, right) for left (*A*) and right (*B*) thumb movement as a maximum intensity projection of the time point when the projected voxels reached their maximal *t* value (for scaling, see colored bar). Note the sequential delay within the medial prefrontal cortex, the sensorimotor cortex, and the cerebellum. The progress of the cortical activation accounts for approximately 5 mm/s. (*From* Hülsmann E, Erb M, Grodd W. From will to action: sequential cerebellar contribution to voluntary movements. Neuroimage 2003;20:1485–92; with permission.)

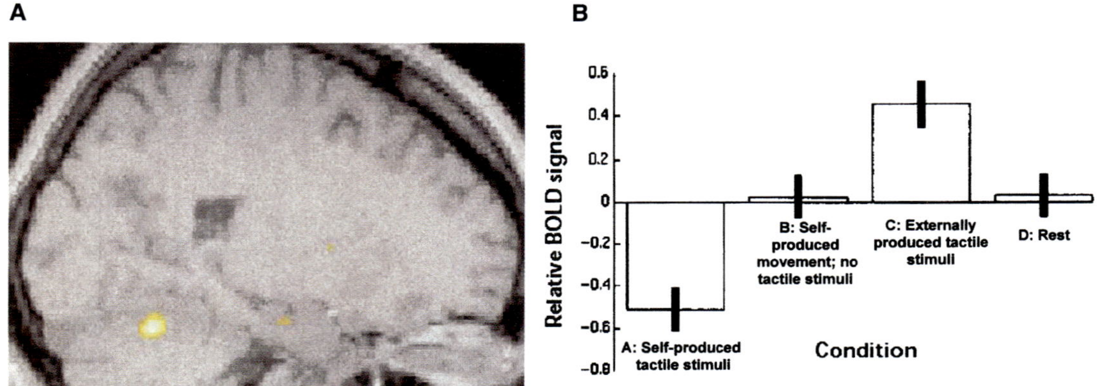

Fig. 13. Cerebellum and tickling cancellation. Significantly decreased activity in the right anterior cerebellar cortex associated with the interaction between the effects of self-generated movement and tactile stimulation for a single subject (*A*) and condition-specific parameter estimates (*B*), which reflect the adjusted blood oxygen level–dependent signal relative to the fitted mean and are expressed as a percentage of whole-brain mean activity. (*From* Blakemore SJ, Wolpert DM, Frith CD. Central cancellation of self-produced tickle sensation. Nat Neurosci 1998;1:635–40; with permission.)

timing functions, cerebellar dysfunctions should therefore impair word recognition. To specify the topography of the assumed cerebellar speech perception mechanism, an fMRI study was performed using the German lexical items "Boden" ([bodn], "floor" in English) and "Boten" ([botn], "messengers" in English) as test materials [43]. The contrast in the sound structure of these two lexical items can be signaled by the length of the wordmedial pause (closure time [CLT], an exclusively temporal measure) or by the aspiration noise of wordmedial "d" or "t" (voice onset time [VOT], an intrasegmental cue). The subjects had to identify both words by analysis of the durational parameter CLT or the VOT aspiration segment. In a subtraction design, CLT categorization as compared with VOT identification yielded a significant hemodynamic response in the right cerebellar hemisphere (neocerebellum Crus I) and in the left frontal lobe inferior to Broca's area (Fig. 16). These findings provide the first evidence for a distinct contribution of the right cerebellar hemisphere to speech perception in terms of encoding of durational parameters of verbal utterances. Verbal working memory tasks, lexical response selection, and auditory imagery of word strings have been reported to elicit activation clusters of a similar location. Conceivably, representation of the temporal structure of speech sound sequences represents the common denominator of cerebellar participation in cognitive tasks acting on a phonetic code.

Recently, Keele and Ivry [44] proposed that the cerebellum may subserve time estimation within the perceptual domain. In accordance with this suggestion, speech perception requiring minute differentiation of time intervals was found to be compromised by cerebellar pathologic findings, because patients performed significantly worse than controls when asked to compare the duration of two successive time intervals (approximately 400 milliseconds), with each bound by pairs of auditory clicks. In a rather recent fMRI study, Mathiak et al [45] suggested that the storage of precise temporal structures relies on a cerebellar-prefrontal loop. They have tested this assumption using a nonspeech task involving duration storage and comparison. The subjects performed two tasks: identifying pauses between tones as "short" or "long" (range: 30–130 milliseconds) and deciding which of two successive pauses was longer. At the level of the cerebellum, the main contrast (discrimination – identification blocks) yielded a single cluster of activation rostral to the horizontal fissure (lateral Crus I) within the right hemisphere (see Fig. 16). The pattern matches the responses found during the encoding of specific temporal aspects of speech sounds [43] and documents cerebellar involvement during an auditory duration short-term memory and comparison task. A distinct right hemisphere cerebellar activation cluster superior to the horizontal fissure emerges when identification was compared with discrimination of pause durations. These findings are in accord with clinical data demonstrating deficient perception of temporal speech cues in subjects with cerebellar atrophy. The comparison to previous findings on speech perception and

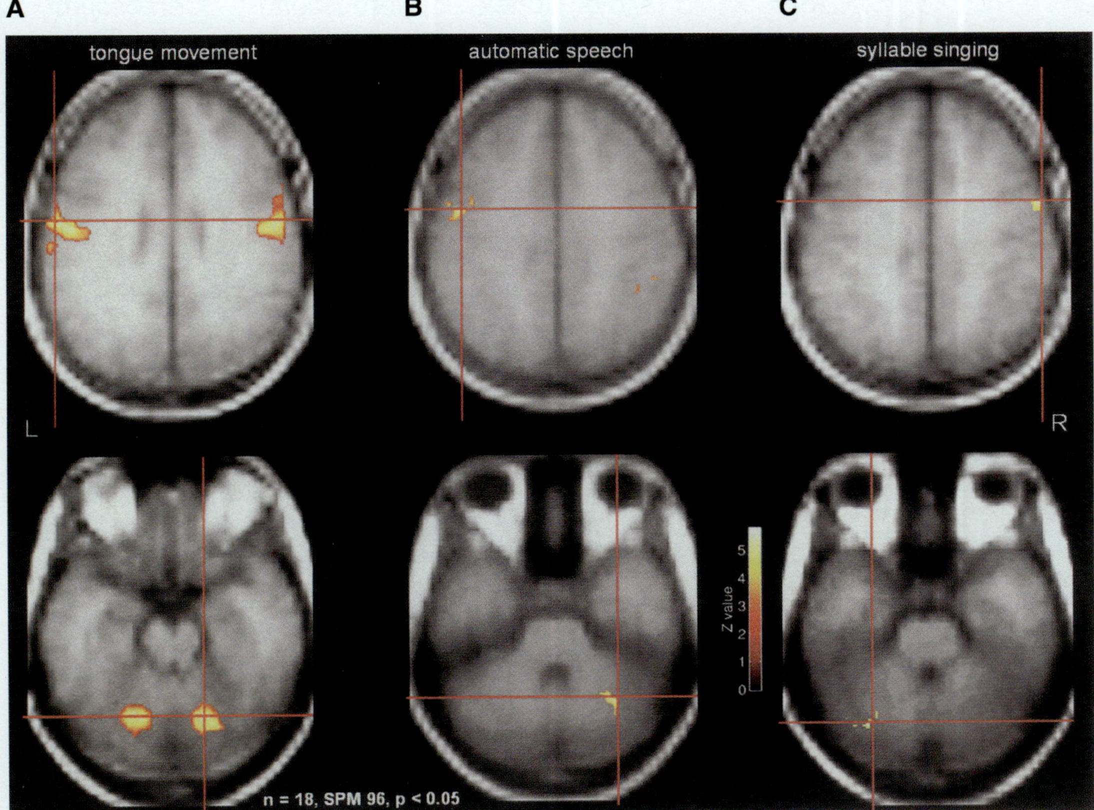

Fig. 14. Cerebellar activation during speech and singing. Functional MRI activation maps (n = 18, Statistical Parameter Mapping = 96; $P < 0.05$) at the level of the primary motor areas (*top row*) and the superior cerebellum (*bottom row*) during tongue movement (*A*), automatic speech (recitation of the name of the month) (*B*), and syllable singing (*C*). Note the shift of cerebellar activation from the right side during speech to the left side during singing. (*From* Ackermann H, Wildgruber D, Daum I, Grodd W. Does the cerebellum contribute to cognitive aspects of speech production? A functional magnetic resonance imaging (fMRI) study in humans. Neurosci Lett 1998;247:187–90; with permission.)

verbal working memory suggests that this operation on intervals is an essential component of language processing.

Clinical perspective and summary

All fMRI findings reported here result exclusively from studies in healthy human subjects and can only be transferred to clinical findings in patients with cerebellar disorders with caution. Nevertheless, mapping of cerebellar function by fMRI now enables us not only to re-establish older anatomic findings of somatotopic representations but to gain new insights in the function of the cerebellum and its intimate relations to cerebral regions serving sensorimotor function, sensory discrimination, and cognitive processing. Consequently, it will change our understanding of neurologic and psychologic failures in patients with inborn errors or neurodegenerative diseases or after neurosurgical procedures.

One consideration concerning the cerebellum that may deserve greater recall than the well-acknowledged differences in size, cellular anatomy, and neuronal organization is the simple fact that the cerebrum is a structure of midline origin. Although connected to bilaterally organized inputs and outputs, the cerebellum possesses complete transverse tissue continuity, which permits unrestricted information flow across the

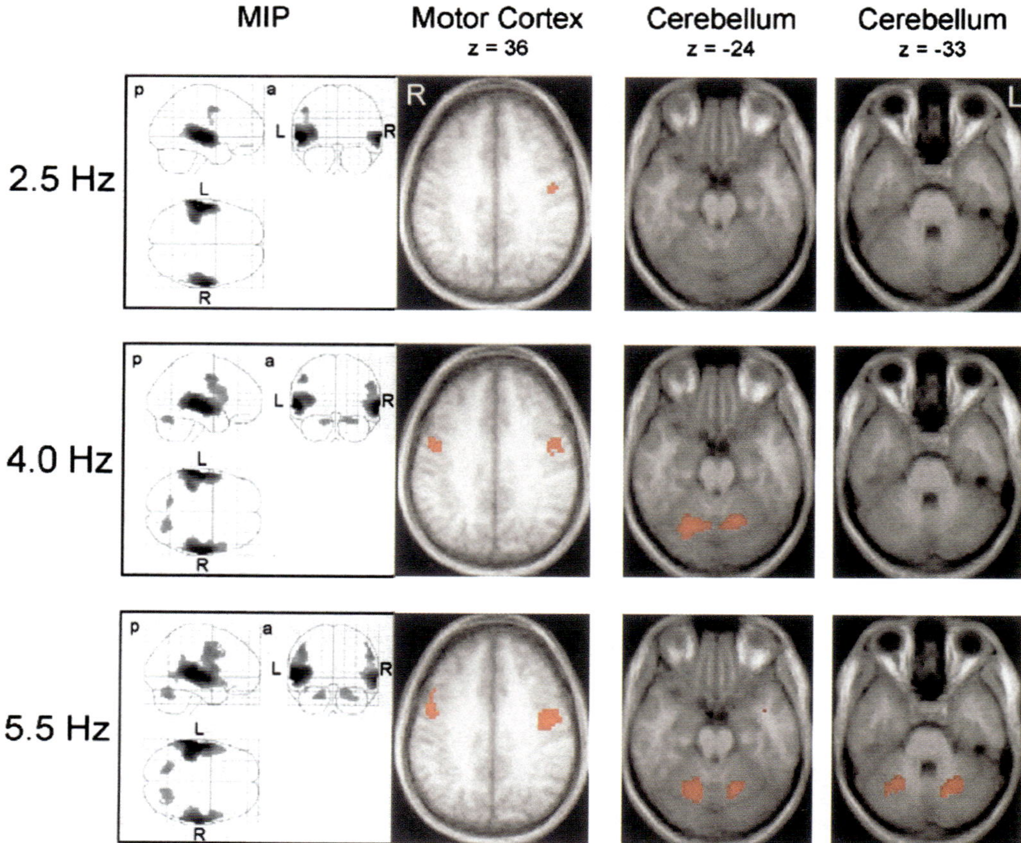

Fig. 15. Cerebellar activation and syllable repetition. Functional MRI activation during covert syllable repetitions at three different frequencies displayed as a maximum intensity projection into a glass brain (*left column*) and superimposed on three transversal planes. The distance to the intercommissural plane is given above the respective columns. Averaged anatomic images across all subjects are used as an anatomic reference ($n = 10$; $P < 0.05$, corrected). Note the appearance of cerebellar activation at 4 Hz and higher. (*From* Wildgruber D, Ackermann H, Grodd W. Differential contributions of motor cortex, basal ganglia, and cerebellum to speech motor control: effects of syllable repetition rate evaluated by fMRI. Neuroimage 2001;13:101–9; with permission.)

hemispheres on all levels. This is important for the functional interpretation of the cerebellum as well as for the judgment of causes for clinical symptoms in cerebellar patients and one reason for the plasticity of symptoms and their fast recovery. In this context, we finally discuss two clinical syndromes of midline cerebellar pathologic change: the posterior vermal split syndrome and the Joubert syndrome.

Bastian et al [46] first described the posterior vermal split syndrome after surgery for removal of fourth ventricle tumors in children. The immediate postoperative clinical symptoms comprise deficits of balance and stepping in tandem gait but only mild abnormalities in self-paced gait, whereas voluntary movement of the fingers, arms, and legs remains normal. All signs resolve within 3 to 4 weeks. These findings are the result of a neurosurgical procedure in which tumor access is achieved by a midline approach through lobules VI through X. Because lobules VI through X receive mainly vestibular and only sparse somatosensory and corticopontine inputs and project to the fastigial nucleus, a splitting of the median region causes a transverse disconnection syndrome across the midline, which results in a disturbance of balance and bilateral coordination of the legs.

Similar underlying pathophysiology could account for the symptomatology of the Joubert

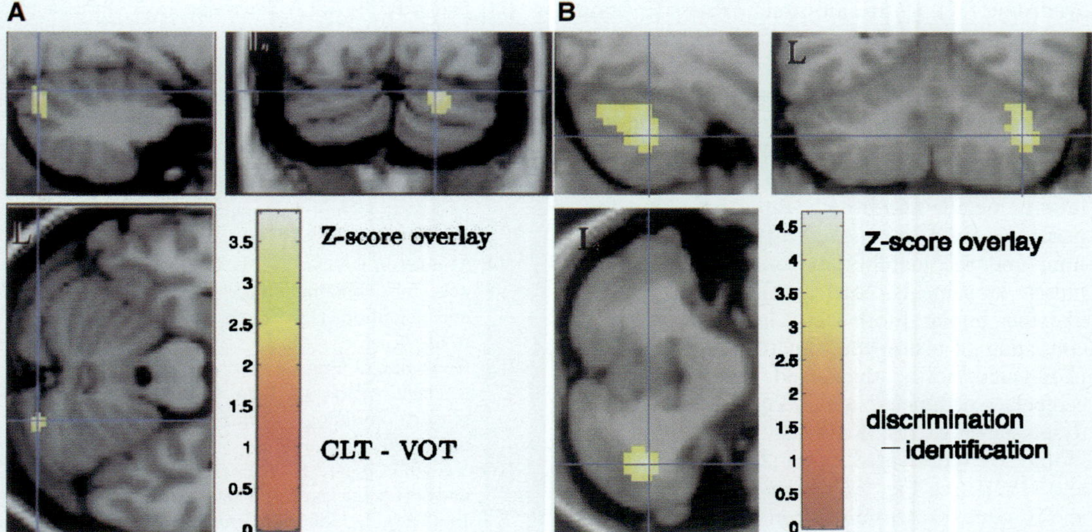

Fig. 16. Cerebellar activation in syllable and temporal discrimination. Syllable discrimination (*A*) and temporal discrimination (*B*) depicted in parasagittal, coronal, and axial views (Z-score overlay on normalized anatomic images with a threshold at $Z > 3.1$ corresponds to $P < 0.001$, uncorrected) both yield right cerebellar activation (lateral aspect of Crus I). (*A*) Decoding of the intersegmental closure time (CLT) versus the voice onset time (VOT). (*B*) Discrimination of pause durations (short versus long) versus stimulus categorization. (*A*: *From*: Mathiak K, Hertrich I, Grodd W, Ackermann H. Cerebellum and speech perception: a functional magnetic resonance imaging study. J Cogn Neurosci 2002;14:902–12; with permission. *B*: *From* Mathiak K, Hertrich I, Grodd W, Ackermann H. Discrimination of temporal information at the cerebellum: functional magnetic resonance imaging of nonverbal auditory memory. Neuroimage 2004;21:154–62; with permission.)

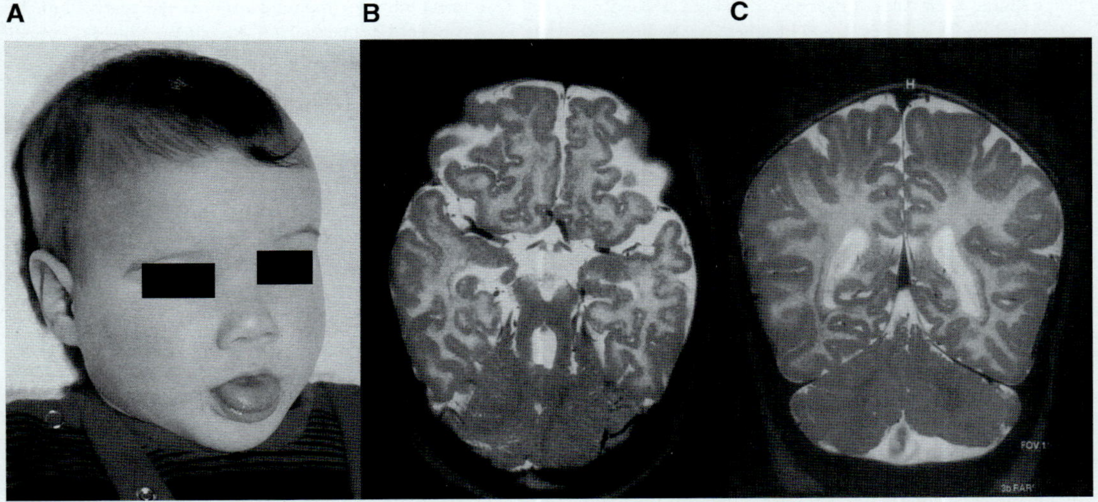

Fig. 17. Joubert syndrome. (*A*) Photograph of a 3-year-old boy with Joubert syndrome. Note the medial rotation of the eyes and the tongue protrusion. T2-weighted MRI scans in axial (*B*) and coronal (*C*) projections depicting the typical "molar tooth sign" in *B* and the missing fusion of the hemispheres because of aplasia of the vermis in *C*. (Courtesy of Prof. E. Boltshauser, Zürich, Switzerland.)

syndrome [47], a rare autosomal recessive brain malformation that is anatomically characterized by the absence or underdevelopment of the cerebellar vermis. Recent observations suggest an absence of the decussatio of the superior cerebellar peduncle and central pontine tracts as well [48]. The most common clinical features in infants include abnormally rapid breathing (hyperpnea), jerky eye movements, mental retardation, and the inability to coordinate voluntary muscle movements. MRI reveals typical features like the "molar tooth sign" in the axial plane, consisting of a deepening of the posterior interpeduncular fossa, thick and straight superior cerebellar peduncles, and vermal hypoplasia or dysplasia (Fig. 17). Knowing that the lips and mouth are represented bilaterally in lobules HVI and HVIII (see Fig. 7), the jerky eye movements and tongue protrusion accompanying the syndrome most likely reflect a lack of transverse continuity in the medial zone of lobules VI through X. Again, one can hypothesize that parallel fiber inputs to Purkinje cells across the midline are a necessary condition for bilateral coordination and for sufficient control of orofacial musculature, a consideration that was suggested by Bolk a century ago [6].

References

[1] Larsell O. Morphogenesis and evolution of the cerebellum. Arch Neurol Psychiatry 1934;31:373–95.

[2] MacLeod C, Zilles K, Schleicher A, Rilling JK, Gibson KR. Expansion of the neocerebellum in Hominoidea. J Hum Evol 2003;44:401–29.

[3] Glickstein M, Yeo C. The cerebellum and motor learning. J Cogn Neurosci 1990;2:69–80.

[4] Flourens P. Recherches expérimentales sur le propriétés et les fonctions du systéme nerveux dans les animaux vertebrés. Arch Gén Med 1824;2:321–70.

[5] Luciani L. Il cervelletto: nuovi studi di Fisiologia normale e patologica. Firenze: Le Monnier; 1891.

[6] Bolk L. Das Cerebellum der Säugetiere: Eine vergleichende anatomische Untersuchung. Nederl. Bydragen Anat 1904;3:1–136.

[7] Comolli A. Per una nuova divisione del cervelletto dei mammiferi. Arch Ital Anat 1910;9:247–73.

[8] Edinger L. Über die Entstehung des Cerebellums. Anat Anz 1910;35:319–23.

[9] Larsell O, Jansen J. The comparative anatomy and histology of the cerebellum: the human cerebellum, cerebellar connections, and cerebellar cortex. Minneapolis: University of Minnesota Press; 1971.

[10] Adrian ED. Afferent areas in the cerebellum connected with the limbs. Brain 1943;66:289–315.

[11] Snider R, Stowell A. Receiving areas of the tactile, auditory and visual systems in the cerebellum. J Neurophysiol 1944;7:331–57.

[12] Hampson JL, Harrison CR, Woolsey CN. Cerebrocerebellar projections and the somatotopic localization of motor function in the cerebellum. Res Publ Assn Nerv Ment Dis Proc 1952;30:299–316.

[13] Dow RS, Moruzzi O. The physiology and pathology of the cerebellum. Minneapolis: University of Minnesota Press; 1958.

[14] Middleton FA, Strick PL. Cerebellar output channels. In: Schmahmann JE, editor. The cerebellum and cognition. New York: Academic Press; 1997. p. 61–82.

[15] Oscarsson O. Functional organization of the spinocerebellar paths. In: Iggo A, editor. Handbook of sensory physiology. Berlin: Springer-Verlag; 1973. p. 340–80.

[16] Voogd J, Bigaré F. Topographical distribution of and corticonuclear fibers in the cerebellum: a review. In: Courville J, de Montigny C, Lamarre Y, editors. The inferior olivary nucleus: anatomy and physiology. New York: Raven Press; 1980. p. 207–34.

[17] Asanuma C, Thach WT, Jones EG. Brain stem and spinal projections of the deep cerebellar nuclei in the monkey, with observations on the brain stem projections of the dorsal column nuclei. Brain Res Rev 1983;5:299–322.

[18] Shambes GM, Gibson JM, Welker W. Fractured somatotopy in granule cell tactile areas of rat cerebellar hemispheres revealed by micromapping. Brain Behav Evol 1978;15:94–140.

[19] Schmahmann JD. The cerebellum and cognition. New York: Academic Press; 1997.

[20] Dichgans J, Diener HC. Clinical evidence for functional compartmentalization of the cerebellum. In: Bloedel JR, Dichgans P, Precht W, editors. Cerebellar functions. Berlin: Springer; 1985. p. 126–47.

[21] Talairach J, Tournoux P. Co-planar stereotatic atlas of the human brain. New York: Thieme; 1988.

[22] Statistical Parametric Mapping Web site. Available at: http://www.fil.ion.ucl.ac.uk/spm. Accessed September 27, 2004.

[23] Brain Innovation B.V. Web site. http://www.Brain-Voyager.com. Accessed September 27, 2004.

[24] Schmahmann JD, Doyon J, Toga AW, Petrides M, Evans AC. MRI atlas of the cerebellum. San Diego: Academic Press; 2000.

[25] Dimitrova A, Weber J, Redies C, Kindsvater K, Maschke M, Kolb FP, et al. MRI atlas of the human cerebellar nuclei. Neuroimage 2002;17: 240–55.

[26] Grodd W, Hülsmann E, Lotze M, Wildgruber D, Erb M. Sensorimotor mapping of the human cerebellum: fMRI evidence of somatotopic organization. Hum Brain Mapp 2001;13:55–73.

[27] Snider RS, Eldred E. Cerebro-cerebellar relationships in the monkey. J Neurophysiol 1951;15: 27–40.

[28] Thickbroom GW, Byrnes ML, Mastaglia FL. Dual representation of the hand in the cerebellum: activation with voluntary and passive finger movement. Neuroimage 2003;18:670–4.

[29] Decety J, Perani D, Jeannerod M, Bettinardi V, Tadary B, Woods R, et al. Mapping motor representations with PET. Nature 1994;371:600–2.

[30] Lotze M, Montoya P, Erb M, Hülsmann E, Flor H, Klose U, et al. Activation of cortical and cerebellar motor areas during executed and imagined hand movements: an fMRI study. J Cogn Neurosci 1999;11:491–501.

[31] Riecker A, Wildgruber D, Mathiak K, Grodd W, Ackermann H. Parametric analysis of rate dependent hemodynamic response functions of cortical and subcortical brain structures during auditorily cued finger tapping: an fMRI study. Neuroimage 2003;18:731–9.

[32] Mink JW, Thach WT. Basal ganglia motor control II. Late pallidal timing relative to movement onset and inconsistent pallidal coding of movement parameters. J Neurophysiol 1991;65:301–3.

[33] Rao SM, Harrington DL, Haaland KY, Bobholz JA, Cox RW, Binder JR. Distributed neural systems underlying the timing of movements. J Neurosci 1997;17:5528–35.

[34] Hülsmann E, Erb M, Grodd W. From will to action: sequential cerebellar contribution to voluntary movements. Neuroimage 2003;20:1485–92.

[35] Blakemore SJ, Wolpert DM, Frith CD. Central cancellation of self-produced tickle sensation. Nat Neurosci 1998;1:635–40.

[36] Wolpert DM, Ghahramani Z, Jordan MI. An internal model for sensorimotor integration. Science 1995;269:1880–2.

[37] Fiez JA, Raichl ME. Linguistic processing. Int Rev Neurobiol 1997;41:233–54.

[38] Courchesne E, Allen G. Prediction and preparation, fundamental functions of the cerebellum. Learn Mem 1997;4:1–35.

[39] Ackermann H, Graber S, Hertrich I, Daum I. Categorical speech perception in cerebellar disorders. Brain Lang 1997;60:323–31.

[40] Ackermann H, Wildgruber D, Daum I, Grodd W. Does the cerebellum contribute to cognitive aspects of speech production? A functional magnetic resonance imaging (fMRI) study in humans. Neurosci Lett 1998;247:187–90.

[41] Wildgruber D, Ackermann H, Grodd W. Differential contributions of motor cortex, basal ganglia, and cerebellum to speech motor control: effects of syllable repetition rate evaluated by fMRI. Neuroimage 2001;13:101–9.

[42] Ackermann H, Hertrich I. The contribution of the cerebellum to speech processing. J Neurolingustics 2000;13:95–116.

[43] Mathiak K, Hertrich I, Grodd W, Ackermann H. Cerebellum and speech perception: a functional magnetic resonance imaging study. J Cogn Neurosci 2002;14:902–12.

[44] Keele SW, Ivry R. Does the cerebellum provide a common computation for diverse tasks? A timing hypothesis. Ann NY Acad Sci 1990;608: 179–207.

[45] Mathiak K, Hertrich I, Grodd W, Ackermann H. Discrimination of temporal information at the cerebellum: functional magnetic resonance imaging of nonverbal auditory memory. Neuroimage 2004;21: 154–62.

[46] Bastian AJ, Minck JW, Kaufmann BA, Thach WT. Posterior vermal split syndrome. Ann Neurol 1998; 44:601–10.

[47] Joubert M, Eisenring JJ, Robb JP, Andermann F. Familial agenesis of the cerebellar vermis. A syndrome of episodic hyperapnoea, abnormal eye movements, ataxia, and retardation. Neurology 1969;19:813–25.

[48] Barkovich AJ. Pediatric neuroimaging. 3rd edition. Philadelphia: Lippincott Williams & Wilkins; 2000.

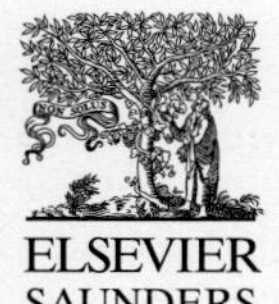

ELSEVIER
SAUNDERS

Neurosurg Clin N Am 16 (2005) 101–114

NEUROSURGERY
CLINICS
OF NORTH AMERICA

Proton magnetic resonance spectroscopic imaging in brain tumor diagnosis

Stephen Gruber, PhD[a,b], Andreas Stadlbauer, PhD[a,b], Vladimir Mlynarik, PhD[a], Brigitte Gatterbauer, MD[c], Karl Roessler, MD[c], Ewald Moser, PhD[a,b,d,*]

[a] *Magnetic Resonance Centre of Excellence, Medical University of Vienna, Lazarettgasse 14, A-1090 Vienna, Austria*

[b] *Department of Medical Physics, Medical University of Vienna, Kompetenzzentrum Hochfeld-MR (MR-Holzhaus), A-1090 Vienna, Lazarettgasse 14, Austria*

[c] *Department of Neurosurgery, Medical University of Vienna, Kompetenzzentrum Hochfeld-MR (MR-Holzhaus), A-1090 Vienna, Lazarettgasse 14, Austria*

[d] *Department of Radiodiagnostics, Medical University of Vienna, Waehringer Guertel 18–20, A-1090 Vienna, Austria*

Over the last 15 years, single-voxel and multi-voxel proton magnetic resonance spectroscopy (^{1}H-MRS) and ^{1}H-magnetic resonance spectroscopic imaging (MRSI) have become useful tools in supporting the understanding and diagnosis of a number of clinical pathologic findings, particularly brain tumors. Several excellent reviews document this progress [1–6]. Primary brain tumors are recognized and characterized not only via the lesion size but also via the pathologic metabolism, although this is quite heterogeneous [7,8]. This limits the use of established (invasive) diagnostic approaches, namely, conventional contrast-enhanced MRI (CE-MRI) at 1.5 T, with a diagnostic accuracy of 30% to 90% depending on tumor type [9,10], and the "gold standard" of brain biopsy. Brain biopsy is a heavily invasive technique with minor morbidity in up to 3.3% of cases, major morbidity in up to 3.6% of cases, a hemorrhage rate up to 8% of cases, and mortality in up to 1.7% of cases, as assessed over a large number of studies [11–15]. Diagnostic accuracy is 91% (low-grade astrocytoma), 83% (anaplastic astrocytoma), and 88% (glioblastoma multiforme). The histologic grade of malignancy, however, is predictable, with an accuracy of only 57% to 61% [16]. Differentiation between brain abscess and cystic or necrotic brain tumor using CT or MRI has not been particularly successful to date [17,18], although Arnold et al [19] have shown similar performance to brain biopsy. Early identification and differentiation of brain abscesses and malignant brain tumors should be followed by the selection of appropriate treatment strategies to improve outcome or the survival rate, particularly in heterogeneous tumors, whether of low or high grade.

This study was financially supported by the Austrian Science Fund (FWF P14715-PSY to E. Moser) and the German Science Foundation (DFG Ga 638/2-1 to O. Ganslandt).

S. Gruber and A. Stadlbauer contributed equally to this work.

* Corresponding author.

E-mail address: ewald.moser@meduniwien.ac.at (E. Moser).

What is Magnetic Resonance Spectroscopy?

MRS is based on the magnetic interaction between tiny magnetic moments (spins) of atomic nuclei of the body and an external (static) magnetic field of the strength B_0 (in tesla), produced by the magnetic resonance scanner. This interaction is modulated by electrons surrounding atomic nuclei, resulting in molecule-specific absorption lines in so-called "nuclear magnetic resonance (NMR) spectra." The original term "nuclear magnetic

1042-3680/05/$ - see front matter
doi:10.1016/j.nec.2004.07.004

resonance" already contains all essential aspects: (1) the atomic nucleus with a detectable spin, (2) the magnetic interaction between spins and external (static and radiofrequency) magnetic fields, and (3) the resonance condition that has to be fulfilled between the frequency of the external magnetic field and the frequency of the spin precession. This magnetic interaction results in a time-dependent (high-frequency) magnetic response of the spin system, which is called free induction decay (FID). The FID contains various frequency components that can be identified via the Fourier transform (FT), resulting in a characteristic pattern or spectrum. Using additional magnetic fields for localization, characteristic spectra may be observed from defined regions in the body. The appearance of these spectra depends on general conditions, that is, which NMR-sensitive nuclei (eg, hydrogen [protons (^{1}H)], carbon [^{13}C], phosphorus [^{31}P]) are to be studied, instrumental (eg, field strength [B_0]) and methodologic parameters (eg, spatial localization or water suppression techniques) and, of course, the biochemical composition and architecture of the tissue studied. Examples may be found in several excellent textbooks on clinical MRS [20,21].

Currently, ^{1}H-MRS is the most frequently used methodology in tumor diagnosis [22]. Because MRS is basically a low-sensitivity method, only metabolites above approximately 0.5 mmol in brain tissue may be detected. Thus, only spectral lines of *N*-acetylaspartate (NAA, at approximately 2.0 ppm), choline (Cho)-containing compounds at approximately 3.2 ppm, total creatine (Cr) and phosphocreatine at approximately 3.0 and 3.9 ppm, myoinositol (mINS, two lines at approximately 3.6 ppm), a mixture of glutamine and glutamate (Glx, overlapping multiplets at approximately 2.0–2.5 ppm and 3.75 ppm, respectively), lactate (Lac, doublet at approximately 1.3 ppm), and lipids (Lip, broad lines at 0.9 and 1.3 ppm) [23,24] may be observed if not always quantified. An example of a single-voxel short–echo time (TE) proton spectrum of human brain tissue is given in Fig. 1, including assignments of spectral lines. For tumor diagnosis, spectral lines of NAA and Cho are of primary importance. NAA is seen as a neuronal marker, which may be reduced if neurons are being replaced by tumor cells, whereas Cho is thought to reflect cell membrane, myelin, and Lip turnover, leading to increased MRS-visible Cho resonances. The lines of Cr are reduced

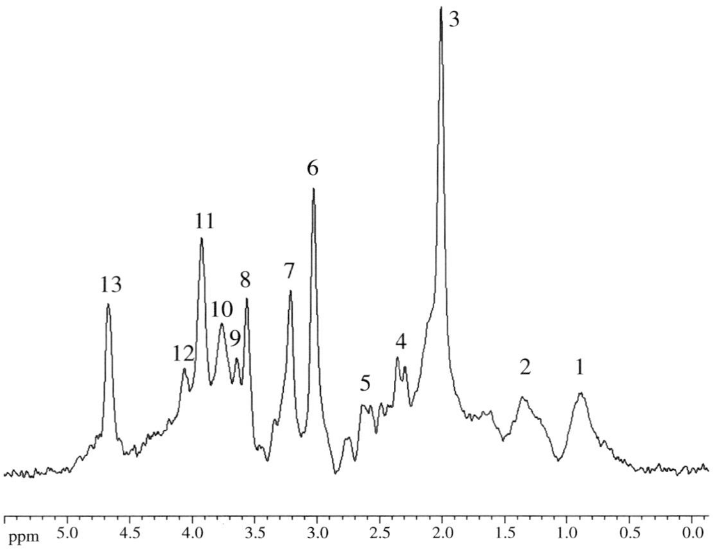

Fig. 1. Single-voxel spectrum from occipital gray matter of a healthy volunteer, obtained at 3 T using a 10-cm surface coil (echo time [TE]/repetition time [TR] = 9/2500 milliseconds, voxel size = 16 cm^3, 384 averages). The spectral lines are assigned as follows: 1, 2 = macromolecules/lipids; 3 = *N*-acetylaspartate (NAA; + N-acetylaspertylglutamate [NAAG] + glucose [Glu] + glutamine [Gln]); 4 = Glu; 5 = NAA; 6 = total creatine (Cr; Cr + phosphocreatine [PCr]); 7 = choline [Cho] (+ myoinositol [mINS]); 8, 9 = mINS; 10 = Glu + Gln; 11 = total Cr; 12 = mINS; 13 = residual water. Note that the excellent signal-to-noise ratio (SNR) is a result of the large voxel size and number of averages, resulting in a measurement time of 16 minutes for a single spectrum as well as the use of a surface coil and very short TE.

in necrotic areas, Lip increases in some high-grade tumors, and Lac is not visible in normal brain but transiently increases in pathologic (anaerobic) metabolism. Automated spectrum-fitting programs (eg, LCModel [25] or VARPRO [26]) and pattern recognition techniques (if a sufficient number of data sets are available [27–29]) may be used to support a diagnosis, because the interpretation of spectra still requires some experience as well as some technical know-how to identify artifacts and to assess the quality of (pathologic) spectra.

Application of proton magnetic resonance spectroscopy and magnetic resonance spectroscopic imaging in brain tumor diagnosis

Several studies and reviews suggest that in vivo ^{1}H-MRS might significantly contribute to brain tumor characterization and staging. Most importantly, ^{1}H-MRS is a noninvasive approach that allows monitoring of metabolic changes as a result of tumor-induced pathologic conditions, with the potential to diagnose the presence of tumors, to differentiate tumors from other pathologic processes of similar appearance (eg, brain abscesses), and to characterize the stage of tumor development. Although the brain metabolites detectable via ^{1}H-MRS in vivo are not tumor specific, distinct metabolic patterns [24] and changes have been reported in ^{1}H-MRS applications in human brain tumors (for recent reviews, see the articles by Burtscher and Holtas [5], Smith et al [22], and Howe and Opstad [6], and Kwock et al [30]).

Most ^{1}H-MRS brain tumor studies to date have been performed at 1.5 T using localized single-voxel spectroscopy or spectroscopic imaging with relatively low spatial resolution (approximately 1–8 cm^{3}) compared with conventional MRI, with resolutions of approximately 1 mm^{3}. This was a common obstacle in early tumor studies [31]. Ricci et al [32] pointed out that the positioning of single-voxel spectra influences the accuracy of findings in tumor ^{1}H-MRS. They reported that from voxels positioned centrally within the lesion, the ^{1}H-MRS findings reflected histologic outcome in only two of nine lesions, whereas including the enhancing edge of the lesions allowed correct classification of seven of eight lesions. High spatial resolution may increase specificity, although at the cost of reduced sensitivity, and thus plays an important role in the clinical application of ^{1}H-MRS in human brain tumor diagnosis and therapy monitoring.

Localized spectroscopy measurements and quantification are straightforward and were approved by the US Food and Drug Administration (FDA) in 1995. One or more cubic voxels are measured within one session, using relatively large (3–8 cm^{3}) volumes. Data can be absolutely quantified using a number of commercially available software tools (eg, LCModel) [25,33]. The relatively large voxel size in single-voxel spectroscopy prevents accurate matching of different anatomic or pathologic structures, however, reducing diagnostic specificity.

In contrast, two-dimensional (2D) or three-dimensional (3D) MRSI enables the collection of spectra from several hundreds or thousand of voxels within one session, although only some may be of diagnostic relevance. Because one large area is measured at one time/session, exact positioning is not critical. Depending on the technique used for spatial encoding, the actual position of the measured voxels can be shifted after data collection using techniques like zero filling or (the mathematically equivalent) voxel shifting [34,35]. Of special interest is the computation of metabolic maps (eg, by integrating the area under a given peak in the spectrum for each voxel) to monitor the spatial distribution of metabolic changes. A number of methods have been proposed for absolute quantification of MRSI data. McLean et al [36] developed an automatic routine overlay for large 2D MRSI data sets to obtain quantitative metabolic maps using the LCModel. At 1.5 T, 0.5 cm^{3} represents the approximate resolution limit within tolerable measurement times of 10 to 15 minutes for 2D chemical shift imaging (CSI) or 50 minutes for 3D MRSI with four slices using head volume coils [37].

Based on matured hardware and software as well as increasing clinical experience, the following clinical applications or studies using in vivo ^{1}H-MRS, as summarized by Howe and Opstad [6], are currently underway: (1) noninvasive diagnosis of a mass or lesion in the brain, (2) tumor grading, (3) noninvasive follow-up of therapeutic response and progression, (4) therapeutic planning, and (5) prognostic information on patient survival.

We proceed to an example of contemporary clinical ^{1}H-MRS, describing a typical measurement session and showing clinical data. These were obtained from a routine clinical 1.5-T scanner installed in a surgical theater using a 2D CSI localization technique with the highest possible spatial resolution and software developed in-house to quantify and visualize metabolic changes in and around tumors and to correlate these MRS-based results with the neuronavigation system. The final section describes cutting-edge achievements in spectroscopic imaging at 3 T. We conclude with an outlook of the prospects for faster data collection, which should increase patient comfort, and even higher field strengths in MRS of the brain.

Description of noninvasive 1.5-T MRI/magnetic resonance spectroscopic imaging sessions

Patients, all with untreated supratentorial gliomas (World Health Organization [WHO] grade II–IV), and matched controls are examined on a 1.5-T clinical whole-body scanner (MAGNETOM Sonata; Siemens Medical, Erlangen, Germany) equipped with the standard head coil. Measurements, data processing, and integration into frameless stereotaxy are performed at the Department of Neurosurgery, University of Erlangen-Nuremberg, Erlangen, Germany.

2D ^{1}H-MRSI experiments are performed in separate sessions after routine MRI for initial lesion diagnosis. Tumor MRI includes (1) an axial turbo spin echo (TSE) sequence (T_2-weighted, 5-mm slices, repetition time [TR]/TE = 4000/98 milliseconds), (2) an axial fluid-attenuated inversion recovery (FLAIR) sequence (5-mm slices, TR/TE = 10,000/103 milliseconds), and (3) pre- and postgadolinium, contrast-enhanced, coronal gradient echo sequences (T_1-weighted, 5-mm slices, TR/TE = 430/12 and 525/17 milliseconds, respectively). In a subsequent MRS session, two localization scans and an axial spin echo (SE) sequence (T_1-weighted) are acquired for MRSI excitation volume location. The T_1-weighted SE sequence is used for matching spectroscopic images to an anatomic 3D MRI set [38]. Typical parameters are TR/TE of 500/15 milliseconds, 256 × 256 matrix size, 16-cm × 16-cm field of view (FOV), 20 slices with no gap, and a slice thickness of 2 mm. The ^{1}H-MRSI slab with point-resolved spectroscopy (PRESS) [39] volume preselection is aligned parallel to the axial localizer slices. Water suppression is achieved using three chemical shift selective (CHESS) [40] pulses before the PRESS excitation. The MRSI parameters are TR/TE of 1600/135 milliseconds, 24 × 24 circular phase-encoding scheme across a 16-cm × 16-cm FOV, 10-mm slice thickness, 50% Hamming filter and two averages, 1000-Hz spectral width, and 1024 complex points of acquisition size. The total spectroscopic data acquisition time is less than 13 minutes, whereas the routine MRI session, including contrast agent application, takes approximately 40 minutes. The nominal voxel size in 2D MRSI is 0.67 cm^3 × 0.67 cm^3 × 1.0 cm^3 (approximately 0.45-cm^3 resolution). Taking into account the effect of the applied k-space filter (50% Hamming filter) [41] on the full-width-at-half-maximum and after zero filling to a 32 × 32 matrix size, the volume of the measured voxels is 0.52 cm^3. The PRESS excitation volume is positioned to cover the whole or at least the bulk of the tumor and as much apparently normal brain tissue as possible.

In a single session 1 day before surgery, a 3D anatomic magnetization–prepared rapid acquisition gradient echo (MPRAGE) sequence is performed with the following parameters: TR/TE of 2020/4.38 milliseconds, 25-cm × 25-cm FOV, 1 mm isotropic, and 160 slices. For registration in a frameless stereotactic system (VectorVisionSky; BrainLab, Heimstetten, Germany) six to eight adhesive skin fiducials are positioned in a scattered pattern on the head surface before imaging. Thus, all MRI and MRSI data may be converted into the same frame of reference with a typical accuracy of 1 mm^3 isotropically.

Data processing

Zero filling to a 32 × 32 matrix size and 2D spatial FT is performed with the manufacturer's data processing software (syngo MR 2002A; Siemens Medical). MRSI raw data sets without any header information are processed with the freely available LINUX-based reconstruction program, CSX, obtained from PB Barker (Baltimore, Maryland). Spectroscopic imaging data are exponentially filtered with a line-broadening factor of 3 Hz, zero filled to 2048 data points, and undergo a FT with respect to the spectral dimension. To remove the residual water peak, we use a high-pass convolution filter (50-Hz stop band) [42]. Magnitude spectra are calculated, the position of NAA is set to 2.02 ppm, and a susceptibility correction is applied. The peak areas for Cho, Cr, and NAA are calculated by integration over the frequency range of 3.34 to 3.14 ppm, 3.14 to 2.94 ppm, and 2.22 to 1.82 ppm, respectively (see Fig. 1). Smooth linear interpolation to a 256 × 256 matrix results in the metabolic maps. Cho and NAA images (Fig. 2) are used to calculate a map of Cho/NAA ratios. Tumor borders are automatically segmented in this Cho/NAA image based on

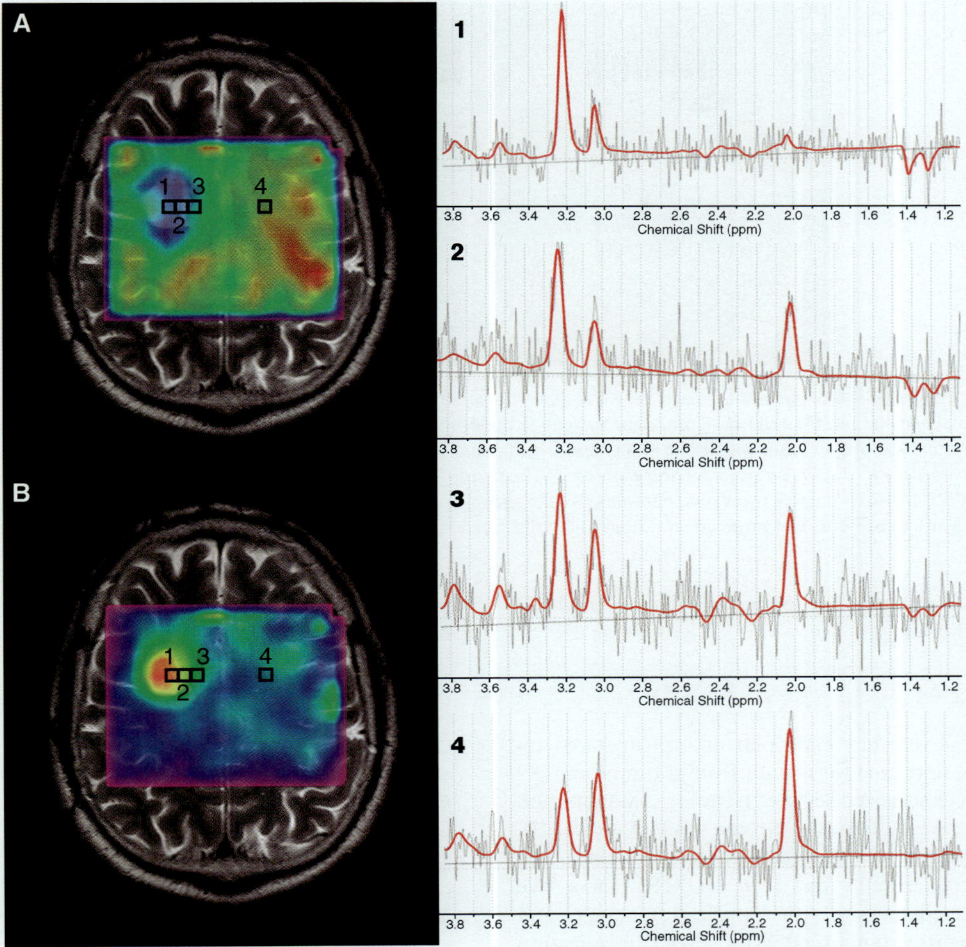

Fig 2. Anatomic images (T2-weighted) overlaid with metabolic maps of a patient with an oligoastrocytoma, World Health Organization grade III. *N*-acetylaspartate map (*A*); choline map (*B*); and spectra of (1) the tumor center, (2) the intermediate zone, (3) the tumor border and (4) contralateral normal brain according to the marked positions in A and B.

the assumption of Gaussian distribution of the Cho/NAA values for normal brain [43].

Coregistration of metabolic and anatomic MRI

Because of the choice of the same FOV and precise alignment of the T_1-weighted SE protocol and the MRSI experiment, direct coregistration of the data of the MRSI slab (10-mm thick) with five slices (each 2-mm thick, no gap) of the anatomic MRI can be achieved [38]. A combined data set consisting of MRI and MRSI data, a so-called "MRI/MRSI hybrid data set," is created and matched exactly to a 3D data set for use with frameless stereotaxy (Fig. 3).

Clinical results at 1.5 T

High-resolution MRSI data of good quality have been obtained from all patients examined. MRSI data analysis, including the calculation of metabolic maps and segmentation as well as the integration of these MRSI results in functional neuronavigation, was successfully performed in most cases. The precision and accuracy of the method have been validated by inspection of the congruency of structural details between the anatomic slices in the hybrid data set and the 3D MPRAGE data set. The total time for performing this procedure was about 1 hour 20 minutes for conventional MRI (SE sequence) and MRSI data acquisition, 30 minutes for MRSI data analysis,

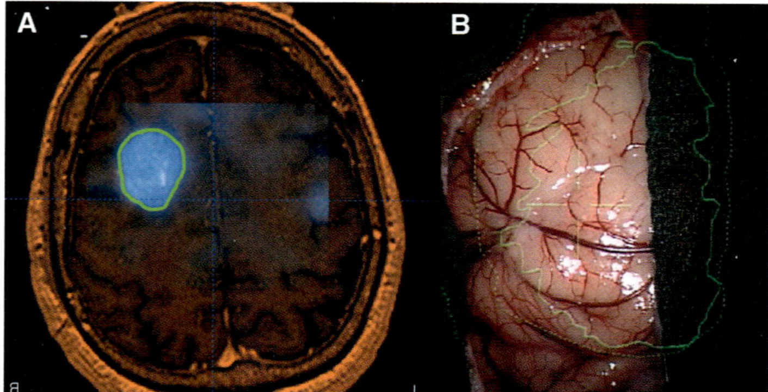

Fig. 3. Image fusion of metabolic maps (MRI/magnetic resonance spectroscopic imaging [MRSI] hybrid data set) and a three-dimensional (3D) MRI data set (same patient as presented in Fig. 2). (*A*) The result is a 3D MRI scan consisting of anatomic (in amber) and metabolic (biochemical, in blue) information for surgical planning. Regions of interest (tumor border) as drawn by the neurosurgeon on the basis of the spectroscopic information are outlined in green. (*B*) Proton (^{1}H)-MRSI–guided frameless stereotaxy: view through the navigation microscope. The maximum and actual tumor borders are outlined in green as dotted and solid lines, respectively.

and 10 minutes for obtaining the MRI/MRSI hybrid data set.

Illustrative case at 1.5 T

A 38-year-old male patient was operated on for the first time for a right frontal tumor in 1999 after a generalized seizure. Histologic examination revealed an oligoastrocytoma (WHO grade II). Two years later, he had new focal seizures and tumor recurrence was seen on MRI scans. We performed surgery with frameless stereotaxy and preoperative functional MRI (fMRI) localization of the motor cortex. During surgery, phase reversal was in complete agreement with the fMRI results and showed the tumor to be one gyrus anterior to the motor cortex. Simultaneously, metabolic maps from ^{1}H-MRSI were integrated into the neuronavigation system (see Fig. 3B) and multiple biopsies were obtained from the tumor borders according to the biochemical information obtained from ^{1}H-MRSI. Intraoperative MRI showed complete tumor removal. The new histopathologic diagnosis documented transformation into an anaplastic oligoastrocytoma (WHO grade III) supported by the ^{1}H-MRSI results [44].

Discussion of clinical results at 1.5 T

^{1}H-MRSI has been used extensively for the evaluation of brain tumors. The major indications for brain tumor spectroscopy have been differential diagnosis, delineation for treatment planning in radiation therapy, stereotactic brain biopsy, and response to treatment. The problem of representation of metabolic changes in brain tumors has been solved using a number of approaches [45–49]. Images of different metabolite ratios (Cho/NAA, Cho/Cr, and Cr/NAA) were used by Li et al [50] for evaluating and characterizing gliomas. De Edelenyi et al [51] showed six major spectral peaks (Cho, Cr, NAA, alanine, Lac or Lip, and Lip) and information contained in T2-weighted MRI in a profile, so-called "nosologic images," and used them for characterization of brain tumors. Fulham et al [46] and McKnight et al [52] showed that images of Cho and NAA are most suitable for tumor spectroscopy. The signal differences between normal brain and tumor are sufficient to show the position of the tumor but not for delineation of the border zone. Also, partial volume effects of cerebrospinal fluid in sulci and ventricles modulate the level of these metabolites in normal brain tissue. This may cause metabolic variations in normal brain regions not related to pathologic changes. In a recent publication, McKnight et al [52] showed that the use of the relative levels of Cho to NAA is also suitable for delineation of the tumor border. They assumed that the relation between Cho and NAA in normal brain could be modeled as a linear function and used this to select voxels as internal controls for quantifying the probability of abnormality at each voxel location in patients with gliomas. In further studies of this group [53,54], they achieved segmentation of brain tumors using this method and the definition of abnormality index contours. These contours were overlaid on anatomic images or on maps of Cho/NAA and used for target delineation in radiation therapy treatment planning [55].

In addition, a number of recent papers described the integration of functional information (eg, magnetoencephalography [MEG] [56–58] and fMRI [59–61]) into frameless stereotaxy (for a review, see the article by Nimsky et al in this supplement). This implementation of functional imaging and navigation, so-called "functional neuronavigation," covers anatomic and functional data and allows the fast identification of eloquent brain areas. Only a few studies have used MRSI to support biopsy target delineation [62–66] or radiation therapy treatment planning [53,55,60]. None of the cited studies integrated MRSI data in a neuronavigation system and performed intraoperative visualization of MRSI data. Preul et al [67] achieved integration of MRSI data (metabolic maps of Cho) of two patients into an image-guided frameless stereotactic system by computing a transformation between the MRSI space and the global MRI space using the targeting volume acquired immediately before MRSI acquisition. Through this approach, they overcame the fact that MRSI lacks detailed structural information. Our strategy for merging MRSI data to a global 3D MRI data set was the full and accurate integration of metabolic images with coregistered anatomic images (MRI/MRSI hybrid data set), resulting in a data set consisting of anatomic and biochemical information [38,43].

Neuronavigation and anatomic image fusion during neurosurgical procedures for appropriate diagnosis and grading of gliomas have also been established at the Vienna Neurosurgical Clinic for a number of years [68–70]. To promote image fusion with functional and metabolic data sets for presurgical, intraoperative, and postoperative treatment planning, we founded an interdisciplinary scientific study group in 2003 ("NEURONET," Vienna Medical University, Neurosurgical Clinic, together with the Departments of Radiodiagnostics, Medical Physics, Nuclear Medicine, and Neurology; the Clinical Institute of Neurology; and the Institute for Biomedical Engineering and Physics). Direct integration of metabolic positron emission tomography (PET) data and 3-T fMRI data for biopsy planning and preservation of functional brain areas was successfully used in a number of patients. The integration of 3-T MRSI data into the intraoperative neuronavigation setting is currently in progress.

Recent developments in three-dimensional spectroscopic imaging at 3 T

Currently, single-voxel MRS and 2D CSI techniques at 1.5 T are routinely used in clinical metabolic brain mapping. Constant technical and methodologic developments made 3 T research systems available during the early 1990s, growing into almost matured clinical systems by 2002. In combination with stronger and faster gradients, 3 T scanners enable the use of more advanced 3D MRSI techniques with clear advantages over standard 1.5-T systems [33,71,72]. Based on these developments, heterogeneous brain tumors may be diagnosed more reliably by reducing partial volume effects (ie, increasing specificity) without excessive loss of sensitivity (ie, signal-to-noise ratio [SNR] critical for quantification).

With the more common availability of high-field scanners ($\geq$3 T), a significant gain in SNR could be obtained in 3D MRSI [71,72]. Additionally, it has been shown that because of an increased homogeneity in smaller voxels, a sufficient SNR can be achieved using a nominal resolution less than 0.5 cm^3, allowing anatomically or pathologically matched "supravoxels" anatomy-matched voxels (AMVs) to be generated after the measurement [73]. High spatial resolution has the potential to increase the specificity of the measured data using AMVs, because partial volume effects are minimized and retrospective voxel averaging (AMV) preserves sensitivity.

To stimulate future applications, we describe recent developments in 3D MRSI at 3 T using very short (11 milliseconds) or long (135 milliseconds) TE protocols to improve tumor diagnosis and grading by ^{1}H-MRSI. Potential benefits of high-resolution 2D or 3D MRSI for clinical applications on human brain tumors and future methodologic improvements are discussed.

Three-dimensional magnetic resonance spectroscopic imaging at 3 T

Healthy volunteers and tumor patients are scanned in single sessions on a 3-T Medspec S300 (Bruker Biospin, Ettlingen, Germany) using the standard birdcage head coil supplied by the manufacturer. Measurements and data processing are performed at the Magnetic Resonance Centre of Excellence, Medical University of Vienna, Vienna, Austria.

A 3D (single-dimension Hadamard spectroscopic imaging [HSI])/2D CSI ^{1}H-MRSI sequence is used [73]. Eight-centimeter left-to-right (LR) by

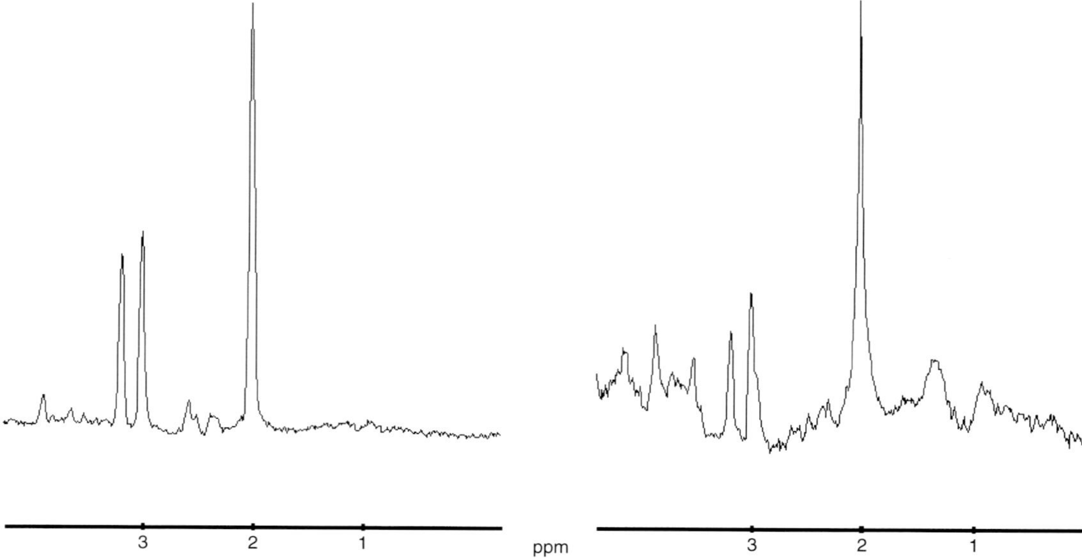

Fig. 4. Anatomy matched voxels spectra of white brain matter (caudal to the ventricles) from two 26-year-old healthy female subjects. (*Left*) One hundred ninety-two zero-filled voxels summed up to 36 cm^3 acquired with point-resolved magnetic resonance spectroscopic imaging (MRSI) (echo time [TE] = 135 milliseconds). (*Right*) One hundred sixty-five zero-filled voxels measured with stimulated echo MRSI (TE = 11 milliseconds). The nominal resolution of both experiments was 0.33 cm^3. Note the different choline/creatine ratios of the short and long TE experiments. Spectra are shown in magnitude mode.

10-cm anterior-posterior (AP) by 3-cm inferior-superior (IS) volumes of interest (VOIs) are excited using the PRESS or stimulated echo (STEAM) localization method with a TE of 135 or 11 milliseconds, respectively, and a TR of 1600 milliseconds. The 16 cm × 16 cm FOV in the LR-AP direction is encoded into a 16 × 16 or 24 × 24 matrix using phase encoding. A total of 1024 complex points are sampled, and a spectral bandwidth of 2500 Hz is used, resulting in an acquisition time of 412 milliseconds. The total measurement time for each session is approximately 27 minutes (patients: nominal resolution of 0.75 cm^3) or 1 hour (healthy volunteers: nominal resolution of 0.33 cm^3). For localization purposes, high-resolution, multislice, rapid acquisition, relaxation-enhanced imaging (RARE, TE/TR = 80/3180 milliseconds) in the axial orientation (512 × 512 matrix size) is performed. Before each experiment, the B_0 field is shimmed in the selected VOI using a fast, automatic stammering technique by mapping along projections pro-

Fig. 5. Anatomic MRI of a brain tumor (*center*) overlaid with the chemical shift imaging grid (red; zero filled to 32 × 32) and the stimulated echo box (*large black rectangle*). (*A*) Four spectra were extracted (position marked by *small black squares* 0.19 cm^3 in size) from the full magnetic resonance spectroscopic imaging data set. (*Top left*) Extracted spectra from the tumor center with poor signal-to-noise ratio (SNR) and residual signal from *N*-acetylaspartate (NAA) only. The extracted spectrum from the right brain hemisphere shows normal-appearing metabolic ratios (*bottom left*). The extracted spectrum from the tumor border (*top right*) and the spectrum from the normal appearing white matter (NAWM) (*bottom right*) at a distance of 2 to 3 cm from the tumor show increased choline (Cho)/NAA ratios. Note the limited SNR in single small voxels not suitable for quantification. (*B*) Four anatomy matched voxels (AMVs) were manually selected: AMV of the tumor center (*top left*) with poor SNR and residual signals from NAA and creatine. The AMV spectrum selected from the right brain hemisphere shows normal-appearing metabolic ratios (*bottom left*, Cho/NAA = 0.28). The selected AMVs from the tumor border (*top right*, marked with red squares) and the AMV spectrum from the NAWM (*bottom right*) show increased Cho/NAA ratios (Cho/NAA = 0.48 and 0.58, respectively).

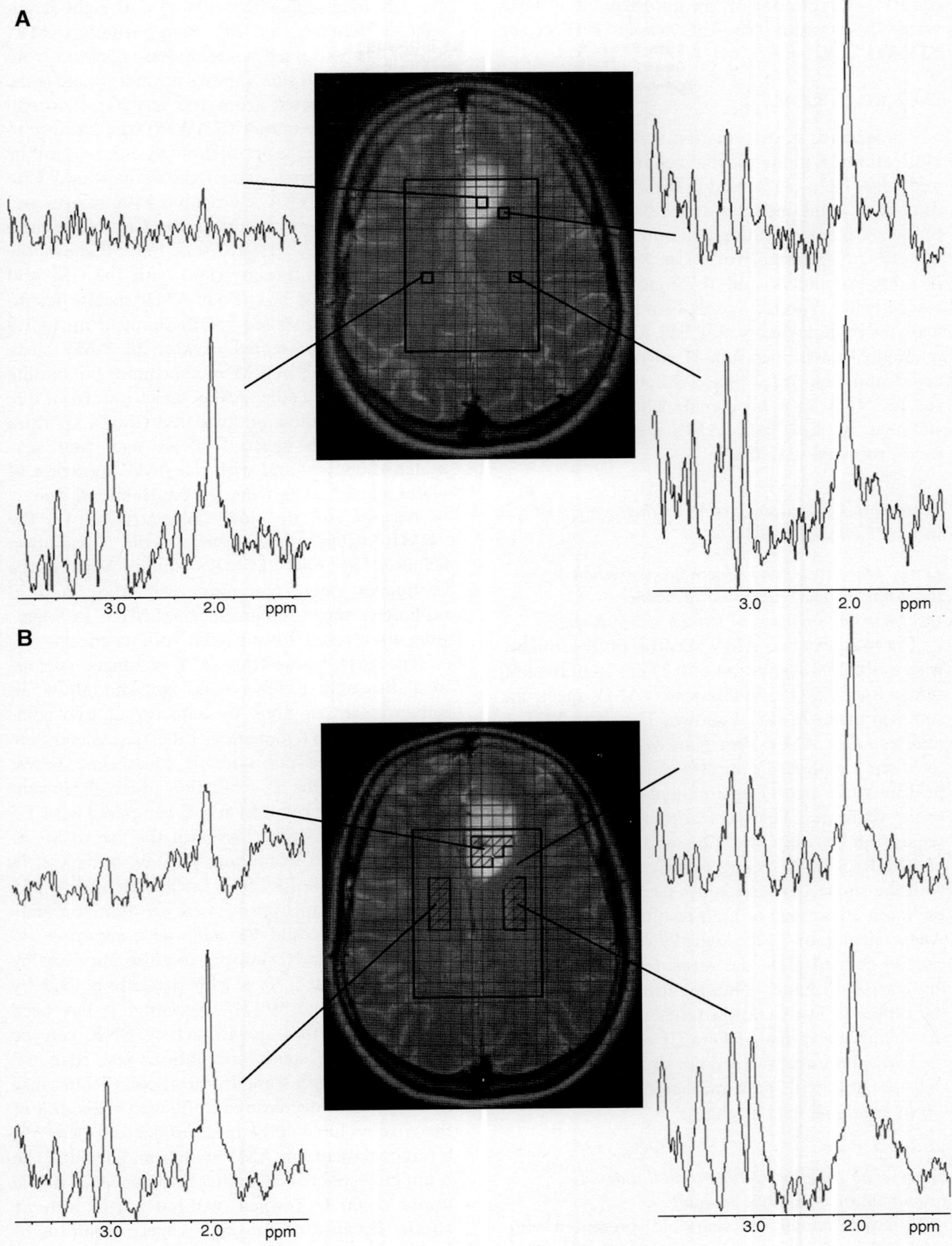
A
3.0
2.0
ppm
3.0
2.0
ppm
B
3.0
2.0
ppm
3.0
2.0
ppm

cedure [74], resulting in an approximately 9 Hz water line width for the whole PRESS or STEAM box.

Data processing at 3 T

Hadarmard transformation is performed in the z-direction (ie, along the magnet and patient axis), and a fast FT is performed in the other two spatial directions. This includes zero filling to 32 × 32 in the x-y plane, resulting in a minimum voxel size of 0.19 cm^3 (nominal voxel size was 0.33 cm^3 for healthy volunteers and 0.75 cm^3 for patients, respectively). Specific voxels forming an anatomically or pathologically matched AMV are chosen manually. Each spectrum is corrected for zero-order and first-order phase shifts and is aligned to the NAA or Cho signal. These spectra are summed, resulting in the AMV spectrum, which is then processed with CSX.

Results at 3 T and discussion of their potential value for clinical diagnosis

Long– and short–echo time high-resolution three-dimensional magnetic resonance spectroscopic imaging of human white matter

Fig. 4 shows two AMV spectra, both acquired with a nominal resolution of 0.33 cm^3. On the left side, a long TE (135 milliseconds) AMV spectrum summed up to 36 cm^3 is shown. The short TE (11 milliseconds) AMV spectrum was summed up to 31 cm^3. Both AMV spectra were obtained from healthy white matter approximately 1 cm caudal to the ventricles. The spectral resolution (note the separation between the Cho and Cr resonance) and SNR of both spectra are excellent compared with the single-voxel reference (see Fig. 1). This is the main advantage of high-resolution ^{1}H-MRSI. Anatomically or pathologically matched voxels can be defined after the measurement, minimizing partial volume contaminations. Because of the different T_2-relaxation times of Cr and Cho, the metabolic ratios of Cho/Cr are different for the two experiments. A quantitative comparison is only possible with data measured with the same TE at the same field strength.

Short–echo time three-dimensional magnetic resonance spectroscopic imaging

A female patient (31 years old) presented with a frontal hyperintense lesion after a horse-riding accident with the primary diagnosis of a possible glioma. Fig. 5A shows four voxels extracted from the left (containing the tumor) and right hemispheres marked on the high-resolution MRI scans. The extracted white matter spectrum from the contralateral side appears normal, whereas the spectrum extracted from the ipsilateral normal appearing white matter (NAWM) (the distance to the tumor border is approximately 2.5 cm) and the tumor border (red voxels) shows increased Cho and decreased NAA. Compared with an age- and sex-matched control subject, the Cho/NAA ratio was increased by 50% to 70%. Fig. 5B shows the same anatomic slice overlaid with the CSI grid and the STEAM box. Four AMV spectra resulting from 10 zero-filled voxels summed up to 1.9 cm^3 each are presented. Again, the AMV spectrum from the NAWM in the tumor-containing hemisphere and the AMV spectrum from the tumor border show an increased Cho/NAA ratio compared with spectra of an age- and sex-matched control and with the AMV spectrum of white matter taken from the contralateral side.

Because of the low concentration of the "NMR-visible" metabolites, the resolution achieved in most ^{1}H-MRS studies was in the centimeter range compared with the standard millimeter range in conventional MRI. Problems thus often result from partial volume effects.

The first whole-body 3 T scanners became available only a few years ago and allow an improvement in SNR by a factor of two compared with 1.5-T systems if other parameters are assumed to be constant. It has been shown, however, that the T_2-relaxation times of relevant metabolites are reduced at 3 T compared with 1.5 T, resulting in signal loss with the use of SE or stimulated echo techniques [75]. Nevertheless, in 3D MRSI with PRESS preselection (TE = 135 milliseconds), an improvement of approximately 23% to 46% could be achieved comparing 1.5 and 3 T [71]. Spectral dispersion also improves by a factor of 2 at 3 T, a gain partially eroded by broader line widths [71]. Recently, it has been demonstrated that a satisfactory SNR can be achieved using spatial resolutions less than 0.5 cm^3 at 3 T with a standard head coil [73] because of a nonlinear decrease in SNR with reduction of the voxel volume in the range of 0.5 to 0.1 cm^3. In a tumor patient, an AMV within an edema in the brain hemisphere contralateral to the MRI-visible tumor could be formed, without partial volume effects, because of the high voxel resolution of 0.33 cm^3 used [73]. Unexpectedly, the edema showed tumor-like metabolic patterns indicating tumor progression. The use of AMVs has the potential to increase the diagnostic value of ^{1}H-MRSI as a result of higher specificity.

In addition, a 3D MRSI sequence with a TE of 11 milliseconds was developed in Vienna to compensate for signal losses caused by the shorter T_2-relaxation times at 3 T [76]. All spectra of the patient (0.75-cm^3 nominal resolution, acquisition time of 27 minutes) showed a satisfactory SNR, except for the spectra extracted from inside the tumor (see Fig. 5, top left). High spatial resolution, as shown in Fig. 4, also reduces susceptibility variations within a voxel, otherwise resulting in broadened and distorted spectral lines; thus, it may be useful to study "difficult" regions in the brain, such as the frontal lobe, temporal lobe, or brain stem [77]. The long acquisition time of approximately 1 hour currently limits the application of this technique to healthy subjects, however.

Outlook

High-field (ie, 3–5 T) in vivo MRI used within current legal limits for patient studies, combined with fast acquisition strategies [78] for time-consuming methods like 3D MRSI [79,80], should significantly improve diagnostic value (via SNR per unit time and spectral dispersion) and patient comfort (total measurement time) and, in addition, render the full combination of anatomic (CE-MRI), functional (blood oxygenation level dependent fMRI) [81], CE-susceptibility weighted imaging [82], perfusion [83], and metabolic imaging with sufficient spatial resolution possible for tumor patients. This combined information, if fully exploited for brain tumor diagnosis, staging, and therapy control, should have a significant impact on patient survival.

For brain research, ultrahigh-field MRI (7 T and higher) should have an impact on a better understanding of brain metabolism and physiology in healthy subjects. Because of increasing technical and methodologic problems (eg, homogeneity, specific absorption rate, shielding) as well as increasing costs, at least for a period of several years, these systems will be used for brain research only.

Acknowledgments

We are grateful to E. Knosp (Vienna, Austria) and R. Fahlbusch (Erlangen, Germany) for their expertise and generous support.

References

[1] Negendank W. Studies of human tumors by MRS: a review. NMR Biomed 1992;5(5):303–24.

[2] Ross B, Michaelis T. Clinical applications of magnetic resonance spectroscopy. Magn Reson Q 1994; 10(4):191–247.

[3] Falini A, Calabrese G, Origgi D, Lipari S, Triulzi F, Losa M, et al. Proton magnetic resonance spectroscopy and intracranial tumours: clinical perspectives. J Neurol 1996;243(10):706–14.

[4] Castillo M, Kwock L, Scatliff J, Mukherji SK. Proton MR spectroscopy in neoplastic and non-neoplastic brain disorders. Magn Reson Imaging Clin N Am 1998;6(1):1–20.

[5] Burtscher IM, Holtas S. Proton magnetic resonance spectroscopy in brain tumours: clinical applications. Neuroradiology 2001;43(5):345–52.

[6] Howe FA, Opstad KS. 1H MR spectroscopy of brain tumours and masses. NMR Biomed 2003; 16(3):123–31.

[7] Segebarth CM, Baleriaux DF, Luyten PR, den Hollander JA. Detection of metabolic heterogeneity of human intracranial tumors in vivo by 1H NMR spectroscopic imaging. Magn Reson Med 1990; 13(1):62–76.

[8] Paulus W, Peiffer J. Intratumoral histologic heterogeneity of gliomas. A quantitative study. Cancer 1989;64(2):442–7.

[9] Alesch F, Pappaterra J, Trattnig S, Koos WT. The role of stereotactic biopsy in radiosurgery. Acta Neurochir Suppl (Wien) 1995;63:20–4.

[10] Mihara F, Numaguchi Y, Rothman M, Sato S, Fiandaca MS. MR imaging of adult supratentorial astrocytomas: an attempt of semi-automatic grading. Radiat Med 1995;13(1):5–9.

[11] Bernstein M, Parrent AG. Complications of CT-guided stereotactic biopsy of intra-axial brain lesions. J Neurosurg 1994;81(2):165–8.

[12] Yu X, Liu Z, Tian Z, Li S, Huang H, Xiu B, et al. Stereotactic biopsy for intracranial space-occupying lesions: clinical analysis of 550 cases. Stereotact Funct Neurosurg 2000;75(2–3):103–8.

[13] Sawin PD, Hitchon PW, Follett KA, Torner JC. Computed imaging-assisted stereotactic brain biopsy: a risk analysis of 225 consecutive cases. Surg Neurol 1998;49(6):640–9.

[14] Field M, Witham TF, Flickinger JC, Kondziolka D, Lunsford LD. Comprehensive assessment of hemorrhage risks and outcomes after stereotactic brain biopsy. J Neurosurg 2001;94(4):545–51.

[15] Kreth FW, Muacevic A, Medele R, Bise K, Meyer T, Reulen HJ. The risk of haemorrhage after image guided stereotactic biopsy of intra-axial brain tumours—a prospective study. Acta Neurochir (Wien) 2001;143(6):539–545; discussion 545–6.

[16] Christy PS, Tervonen O, Scheithauer BW, Forbes GS. Use of a neural network and a multiple regression model to predict histologic grade of

astrocytoma from MRI appearances. Neuroradiology 1995;37(2):89–93.

[17] Klug N, Ellams ID. Advances in neurosurgery, vol. 9. Difficulties in the differential diagnosis of brain abscesses. Berlin: Springer-Verlag; 1981.

[18] Scully RE, Mark EJ, McNeely WF, Ebeling SH, Phillips LD. Case records of the Massachusetts General Hospital. Weekly clinicopathological exercises. Case 20–1997. A 74-year-old man with progressive cough, dyspnea, and pleural thickening. N Engl J Med 1997;336(26):1895–903.

[19] Arnold DL, Shoubridge EA, Villemure JG, Feindel W. Proton and phosphorus magnetic resonance spectroscopy of human astrocytomas in vivo. Preliminary observations on tumor grading. NMR Biomed 1990;3(4):184–9.

[20] de Graaf RA. In vivo NMR spectroscopy. New York: Wiley; 1998.

[21] de Certaines JD, Bovee W, Podo F. Magnetic resonance spectroscopy in biology and medicine. Tarrytown, NY: Pergamon Press; 1992.

[22] Smith JK, Castillo M, Kwock L. MR spectroscopy of brain tumors. Magn Reson Imaging Clin N Am 2003;11(3):415–29 [v–vi].

[23] Bruhn H, Michaelis T, Merboldt KD, Hanicke W, Gyngell ML, Hamburger C, et al. On the interpretation of proton NMR spectra from brain tumours in vivo and in vitro. NMR Biomed 1992;5(5):253–8.

[24] Howe F, Barton SJ, Cudlip SA, Stubbs M, Saunders DE, Murphy M, et al. Metabolic profiles of human brain tumors using quantitative in vivo 1H magnetic resonance spectroscopy. Magn Reson Med 2003;49:223–32.

[25] Provencher SW. Estimation of metabolite concentrations from localized in vivo proton NMR spectra. Magn Reson Med 1993;30(6):672–9.

[26] van der Veen JW, de Beer R, Luyten PR, van Ormondt D. Accurate quantification of in vivo 31P NMR signals using the variable projection method and prior knowledge. Magn Reson Med 1988;6(1): 92–8.

[27] Usenius JP, Tuohimetsa S, Vainio P, Ala-Korpela M, Hiltunen Y, Kauppinen RA. Automated classification of human brain tumours by neural network analysis using in vivo 1H magnetic resonance spectroscopic metabolite phenotypes. Neuroreport 1996;7(10):1597–600.

[28] Preul MC, Caramanos Z, Leblanc R, Villemure JG, Arnold DL. Using pattern analysis of in vivo proton MRSI data to improve the diagnosis and surgical management of patients with brain tumors. NMR Biomed 1998;11(4–5):192–200.

[29] Tate AR, Majos C, Moreno A, Howe FA, Griffiths JR, Arus C. Automated classification of short echo time in in vivo 1H brain tumor spectra: a multicenter study. Magn Reson Med 2003;49(1): 29–36.

[30] Kwock L, Smith JK, Castillo M, Ewend MG, Cush S, Hensing T, et al. Clinical applications of proton MR spectroscopy in oncology. Technol Cancer Res Treat 2002;1(1):17–28.

[31] Negendank WG, Sauter R, Brown TR, Evelhoch JL, Falini A, Gotsis ED, et al. Proton magnetic resonance spectroscopy in patients with glial tumors: a multicenter study. J Neurosurg 1996;84(3):449–58.

[32] Ricci PE, Pitt A, Keller PJ, Coons SW, Heiserman JE. Effect of voxel position on single-voxel MR spectroscopy findings. AJNR Am J Neuroradiol 2000;21(2):367–74.

[33] Gruber S, Frey R, Mlynarik V, Stadlbauer A, Heiden A, Kasper S, et al. Quantification of metabolic differences in the frontal brain of depressive patients and controls obtained by 1H-MRS at 3 tesla. Invest Radiol 2003;38(7):403–8.

[34] Haacke EM, Brown RW, Thompson MR, Venkatesan R. Magnetic resonance imaging: physical principles and sequence design. New York: Wiley; 1999.

[35] von Kienlin M. Empfindlichkeit und Ortsauflösung in der lokalisierten NMR-Spektroskopie. Universität Würzburg: Habilitationsschrift; 1996.

[36] McLean MA, Woermann FG, Barker GJ, Duncan JS. Quantitative analysis of short echo time (1)H-MRSI of cerebral gray and white matter. Magn Reson Med 2000;44(3):401–11.

[37] Nelson SJ, Vigneron DB, Star-Lack J, Kurhanewicz J. High spatial resolution and speed in MRSI. NMR Biomed 1997;10(8):411–22.

[38] Stadlbauer A, Moser E, Gruber S, Nimsky C, Fahlbusch R, Granslandt O. Integration of biochemical tumor images into frameless stereotaxy using a MRI/MRSI hybrid data set. J Neurosurg 2004; 101:287–94.

[39] Bottomley PA, Drayer BP, Smith LS. Chronic adult cerebral infarction studied by phosphorus NMR spectroscopy. Radiology 1986;160(3):763–6.

[40] Haase A. Localization of unaffected spins in NMR imaging and spectroscopy (LOCUS spectroscopy). Magn Reson Med 1986;3(6):963–9.

[41] Vikhoff-Baaz B, Starck G, Ljungberg M, Lagerstrand K, Forssell-Aronsson E, Ekholm S. Effects of k-space filtering and image interpolation on image fidelity in (1)H MRSI. Magn Reson Imaging 2001;19(9):1227–34.

[42] Jacobs MA, Horska A, van Zijl PC, Barker PB. Quantitative proton MR spectroscopic imaging of normal human cerebellum and brain stem. Magn Reson Med 2001;46(4):699–705.

[43] Stadlbauer A, Moser E, Gruber S, Buslei R, Nimsky C, Fahlbusch R, et al. Improved delineation of brain tumors: an automated method for segmentation based on pathologic changes of 1H-MRSI metabolites in gliomas. Neuroimage, in press.

[44] Stadlbauer A, Ganslandt O, Gruber S, Buslei R, Nimsky C, Fahlbusch R, et al. Improved preoperative diagnostics of brain tumors by quantification of 1H-MRSI metabolites. In: International Society of Magnetic Resonance in Medicine. Kyoto; 2004.

[45] Go KG, Kamman RL, Mooyaart EL, Heesters MA, Pruim J, Vaalburg W, et al. Localised proton spectroscopy and spectroscopic imaging in cerebral gliomas, with comparison to positron emission tomography. Neuroradiology 1995;37(3):198–206.

[46] Fulham MJ, Bizzi A, Dietz MJ, Shih HH, Raman R, Sobering GS, et al. Mapping of brain tumor metabolites with proton MR spectroscopic imaging: clinical relevance. Radiology 1992;185(3):675–86.

[47] Mader I, Roser W, Hagberg G, Schneider M, Sauter R, Seelig J, et al. Proton chemical shift imaging, metabolic maps, and single voxel spectroscopy of glial brain tumors. MAGMA 1996;4(2):139–50.

[48] Preul MC, Caramanos Z, Collins DL, Villemure JG, Leblanc R, Olivier A, et al. Accurate, noninvasive diagnosis of human brain tumors by using proton magnetic resonance spectroscopy. Nat Med 1996; 2(3):323–5.

[49] Kamada K, Saguer M, Moller M, Wicklow K, Katenhauser M, Kober H, et al. Functional and metabolic analysis of cerebral ischemia using magnetoencephalography and proton magnetic resonance spectroscopy. Ann Neurol 1997;42(4):554–63.

[50] Li X, Lu Y, Pirzkall A, McKnight T, Nelson SJ. Analysis of the spatial characteristics of metabolic abnormalities in newly diagnosed glioma patients. J Magn Reson Imaging 2002;16(3):229–37.

[51] De Edelenyi FS, Rubin C, Esteve F, Grand S, Decorps M, Lefournier V, et al. A new approach for analyzing proton magnetic resonance spectroscopic images of brain tumors: nosologic images. Nat Med 2000;6(11):1287–9.

[52] McKnight TR, Noworolski SM, Vigneron DB, Nelson SJ. An automated technique for the quantitative assessment of 3D-MRSI data from patients with glioma. J Magn Reson Imaging 2001;13(2): 167–77.

[53] Pirzkall A, McKnight TR, Graves EE, Carol MP, Sneed PK, Wara WW, et al. MR-spectroscopy guided target delineation for high-grade gliomas. Int J Radiat Oncol Biol Phys 2001;50(4):915–28.

[54] Pirzkall A, Nelson SJ, McKnight TR, Takahashi MM, Li X, Graves EE, et al. Metabolic imaging of low-grade gliomas with three-dimensional magnetic resonance spectroscopy. Int J Radiat Oncol Biol Phys 2002;53(5):1254–64.

[55] Nelson SJ, Graves E, Pirzkall A, Li X, Antiniw Chan A, Vigneron DB, et al. In vivo molecular imaging for planning radiation therapy of gliomas: an application of 1H MRSI. J Magn Reson Imaging 2002; 16(4):464–76.

[56] Ganslandt O, Steinmeier R, Kober H, Vieth J, Kassubek J, Romstock J, et al. Magnetic source imaging combined with image-guided frameless stereotaxy: a new method in surgery around the motor strip. Neurosurgery 1997;41(3):621–7; discussion 627–8.

[57] Ganslandt O, Fahlbusch R, Nimsky C, Kober H, Moller M, Steinmeier R, et al. Functional neuronavigation with magnetoencephalography: outcome in 50 patients with lesions around the motor cortex. J Neurosurg 1999;91(1):73–9.

[58] Jannin P, Fleig OJ, Seigneuret E, Grova C, Morandi X, Scarabin JM. A data fusion environment for multimodal and multi-informational neuronavigation. Comput Aided Surg 2000;5(1):1–10.

[59] Jannin P, Morandi X, Fleig OJ, Le Rumeur E, Toulouse P, Gibaud B, et al. Integration of sulcal and functional information for multimodal neuronavigation. J Neurosurg 2002;96(4):713–23.

[60] Nimsky C, Ganslandt O, Kober H, Moller M, Ulmer S, Tomandl B, et al. Integration of functional magnetic resonance imaging supported by magnetoencephalography in functional neuronavigation. Neurosurgery 1999;44(6):1249–55; discussion 1255–6.

[61] Sabbah P, Foehrenbach H, Dutertre G, Nioche C, DeDreuille O, Bellegou N, et al. Multimodal anatomic, functional, and metabolic brain imaging for tumor resection. Clin Imaging 2002;26(1):6–12.

[62] Croteau D, Scarpace L, Hearshen D, Gutierrez J, Fisher JL, Rock JP, et al. Correlation between magnetic resonance spectroscopy imaging and image-guided biopsies: semiquantitative and qualitative histopathological analyses of patients with untreated glioma. Neurosurgery 2001;49(4):823–9.

[63] Dowling C, Bollen AW, Noworolski SM, McDermott MW, Barbaro NM, Day MR, et al. Preoperative proton MR spectroscopic imaging of brain tumors: correlation with histopathologic analysis of resection specimens. AJNR Am J Neuroradiol 2001;22(4):604–12.

[64] Hall WA, Martin A, Liu H, Truwit CL. Improving diagnostic yield in brain biopsy: coupling spectroscopic targeting with real-time needle placement. J Magn Reson Imaging 2001;13(1):12–5.

[65] McKnight TR, von dem Bussche MH, Vigneron DB, Lu Y, Berger MS, McDermott MW, et al. Histopathological validation of a three-dimensional magnetic resonance spectroscopy index as a predictor of tumor presence. J Neurosurg 2002; 97(4):794–802.

[66] Rock JP, Hearshen D, Scarpace L, Croteau D, Gutierrez J, Fisher JL, et al. Correlations between magnetic resonance spectroscopy and image-guided histopathology, with special attention to radiation necrosis. Neurosurgery 2002;51(4):912–9; discussion 919–20.

[67] Preul MC, Leblanc R, Caramanos Z, Kasrai R, Narayanan S, Arnold DL. Magnetic resonance spectroscopy guided brain tumor resection: differentiation between recurrent glioma and radiation change in two diagnostically difficult cases. Can J Neurol Sci 1998;25(1):13–22.

[68] Roessler K, Nasel C, Czech T, Matula C, Lassmann H, Koos WT. Histological heterogeneity of neuroradiologically suspected adult low grade gliomas detected by Xenon enhanced computerized

tomography (CT). Acta Neurochir (Wien) 2003; 138(11):1341–7.

[69] Roessler K, Ungersboeck K, Czech T, Aichholzer M, Dietrich W, Goerzer H, et al. Contour-guided brain tumor surgery using a stereotactic navigating microscope. Stereotact Funct Neurosurg 1997;68(1–4 Part 1):33–8.

[70] Roessler K, Czech T, Dietrich W, Ungersboeck K, Nasel C, Hainfellner JA, et al. Frameless stereotactic-directed tissue sampling during surgery of suspected low-grade gliomas to avoid histological undergrading. Minim Invasive Neurosurg 1998; 41(4):183–6.

[71] Gonen O, Gruber S, Li BS, Mlynarik V, Moser E. Multivoxel 3D proton spectroscopy in the brain at 1.5 versus 3.0 T: signal-to-noise ratio and resolution comparison. AJNR Am J Neuroradiol 2001;22(9): 1727–31.

[72] Gruber S, Li BS, Soher BJ, Mlynarik V, Moser E, Gonen O. Head-to-head performance comparison of 3D multivoxel proton MR spectroscopy: 1.5 vs 3 tesla in the human brain. In: Radiologic Society of North America. Chicago; 2000.

[73] Gruber S, Mlynarik V, Moser E. High-resolution 3D proton spectroscopic imaging of the human brain at 3 T: SNR issues and application for anatomy-matched voxel sizes. Magn Reson Med 2003;49(2): 299–306.

[74] Gruetter R. Automatic, localized in vivo adjustment of all first- and second-order shim coils. Magn Reson Med 1993;29(6):804–11.

[75] Mlynarik V, Gruber S, Moser E. Proton T (1) and T (2) relaxation times of human brain metabolites at 3 tesla. NMR Biomed 2001;14(5):325–31.

[76] Mlynarik V, Gruber S, Stadlbauer A, Starcuk Z, Moser E. Anatomically matched short-echo time spectroscopy of human brain at 3T. In: European Society for Magnetic Resonance in Medicine and Biology, Rotterdam (NL), 2003, Nr. 390.

[77] Ebel A, Maudsley AA. Improved spectral quality for 3D MR spectroscopic imaging using a high spatial resolution acquisition strategy. Magn Reson Imaging 2003;21(2):113–20.

[78] Pruessmann KP, Weiger M, Scheidegger MB, Boesiger P. SENSE: sensitivity encoding for fast MRI. Magn Reson Med 1999;42(5): 952–62.

[79] Posse S, Tedeschi G, Risinger R, Ogg R, Le Bihan D. High speed 1H spectroscopic imaging in human brain by echo planar spatial-spectral encoding. Magn Reson Med 1995;33(1):34–40.

[80] Dydak U, Pruessmann KP, Weiger M, Tsao J, Meier D, Boesiger P. Parallel spectroscopic imaging with spin-echo trains. Magn Reson Med 2003;50(1): 196–200.

[81] Barth M, Nobauer-Huhmann IM, Reichenbach JR, Mlynarik V, Schoggl A, Matula C, et al. High-resolution three-dimensional contrast-enhanced blood oxygenation level-dependent magnetic resonance venography of brain tumors at 3 tesla: first clinical experience and comparison with 1.5 tesla. Invest Radiol 2003;38(7):409–14.

[82] Law M, Yang S, Wang H, Babb JS, Johnson G, Cha S, et al. Glioma grading: sensitivity, specificity, and predictive values of perfusion MR imaging and proton MR spectroscopic imaging compared with conventional MR imaging. AJNR Am J Neuroradiol 2003;24(10):1989–98.

[83] Ugurbil K, Adriany G, Andersen P, Chen W, Garwood M, Gruetter R, et al. Ultrahigh field magnetic resonance imaging and spectroscopy. Magn Reson Imaging 2003;21(10):1263–81.

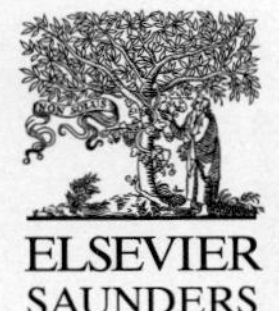
ELSEVIER
SAUNDERS

Neurosurg Clin N Am 16 (2005) 115–134

NEUROSURGERY
CLINICS
OF NORTH AMERICA

Diffusion tensor magnetic resonance imaging of brain tumors

L. Celso Hygino Cruz, Jr, MD[a], A. Gregory Sorensen, MD[b,*]

[a]*Clínica de Diagnóstico por Imagem, Multi-Imagem Ressonância Magnética, Av. das Amerëricas 4666, Centro Médico Barrashopping, Rio de Janeiro, Brazil*

[b]*Department of Radiology, Massachusetts General Hospital, Athinoula A. Martinos Center for Biomedical Imaging, Division of Health Sciences and Technology, Haravrd-MIT, Building 149m 13th Street, Boston, MA 02421, USA*

Primary neoplasms of the central nervous system (CNS) have a prevalence between 15,000 and 17,000 new cases annually in the United States, and when metastatic lesions are included, brain tumors are estimated to cause the deaths of 90,000 patients every year [1,2]. Gliomas remain the most common primary CNS tumor, accounting for 40% to 50% of cases [3] and 2% to 3% of all cancers [4]. Despite new techniques of treatment, patient survival still remains low, varying between 16 and 53 weeks [5].

For more than 40 years [6], nuclear magnetic resonance has been used to analyze and assess brain tumors. It is generally accepted that conventional MRI, typically T1- and T2-weighted imaging, tends to underestimate the extent of the tumor, which can, in turn, lead to suboptimal treatment [7]. New functional MRI (fMRI) sequences, such as diffusion imaging, perfusion imaging, and spectroscopic imaging, have been widely used to evaluate such tumors. In this review, diffusion tensor imaging (DTI), one of the newer methods, is described, particularly the ability of DTI to aid in differentiating a tumor from surrounding edema and infiltrating tumor [8] and, to some extent, to grade brain tumors [9].

Diffusion MRI

Physical basis

The random or Brownian movement of water molecules is the basis of diffusion. In the brain, the presence of tissue structures restricts free water motion [10–12], for example, rendering the diffusion of water molecules higher in the ventricles than in the parenchyma. MRI makes it possible to estimate the diffusivity of water molecules.

Because some pathologic processes seem to change the characteristic of the brain diffusion [13], diffusion-weighted imaging (DWI) has become increasingly popular over the past few years. In typical clinical practice, diffusion imaging is used to assess acute cerebral ischemia [14–17], where the water mobility acutely decreases after the onset of ischemia. The mechanisms to explain the decrease in diffusion coefficients are still controversial. Failure of the Na^+/K^+ adenosine triphosphatase pump is believed to play an important role in this process, however, leading many to term this state as *cytotoxic edema* [17,18]. Diffusion imaging has also been successfully applied to the evaluation of other neurologic conditions, such as multiple sclerosis [19–22], encephalitis [23], and Creutzfeldt-Jakob disease [24].

Most diffusion measurements today are made using a variant of the diffusion-weighted sequence first described by Stejskal and Tanner [25]. Their initial approach described a spin echo (SE) sequence together with two equal and opposite extra gradient pulses [25]; the amount of signal loss can be related to the magnitude of diffusion. For practical purposes, an echo planar imaging (EPI), SE, T2-weighted sequence is used, causing reduction of motion artifacts and speeding the time of acquisition [26]. Stejskjal and Tanner's [25] approach uses two magnetic pulses or gradients to label the spins: the application of the first diffusion gradient causes a dephasing of water protons;

* Corresponding author.
E-mail address: sorensen@nmr.mgh.harvard.edu (A.G. Sorensen).

doi:10.1016/j.nec.2004.07.007

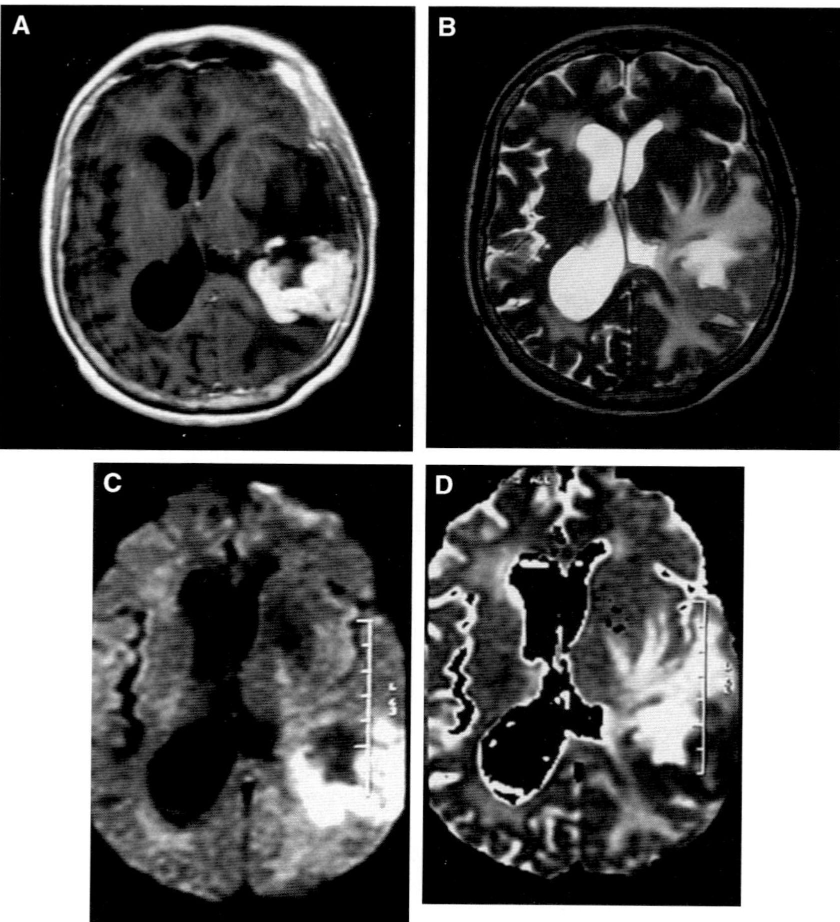

Fig. 1. A 75-year-old woman with a glioblastoma multiforme. (*A*) Contrast-enhanced, axial, T1-weighted image shows an enhancing necrotic mass surrounded by an abnormal hyperintense area on the axial T2-weighted image (T2WI). (*B*) These abnormal hyperintense T2WI areas can represent peritumoral edema or infiltrating tumor. The tumor is isohypointense on the T2WI, indicating high cellularity; this is also demonstrated as restricted diffusion on the diffusion-weighted image (*C*) and apparent diffusion coefficient map (*D*).

because they move randomly, not all water protons are in place for rephrasing from the application of the second diffusion gradient. Thus, there is a signal decrease that depends on how far the water molecules move [13]. The net signal on the final diffusion-weighted image is therefore influenced by the T2 tissue effect and by the tissue diffusion characteristics. By acquiring an image with little diffusion weighting and another image with substantial diffusion weighting, the apparent diffusion coefficient (ADC) can be calculated on a voxel-by-voxel basis, allowing the generation of a map that reflects solely the diffusion influence, excluding the T2 effects, which prevents misinterpretation from the so-called "T2 shine-through" effect [13,26].

Diffusion-weighted MRI in brain tumors

Although most of this review focuses on DTI, a few words about the more common, nontensor (or "trace-weighted") DWI approaches are appropriate. DWI has been used to assess brain tumors, and although it has had limited success as a definitive prognostic tool, its proponents suggest that in certain settings, it can increase the sensitivity and specificity of MRI in the evaluation of brain tumors by providing information about

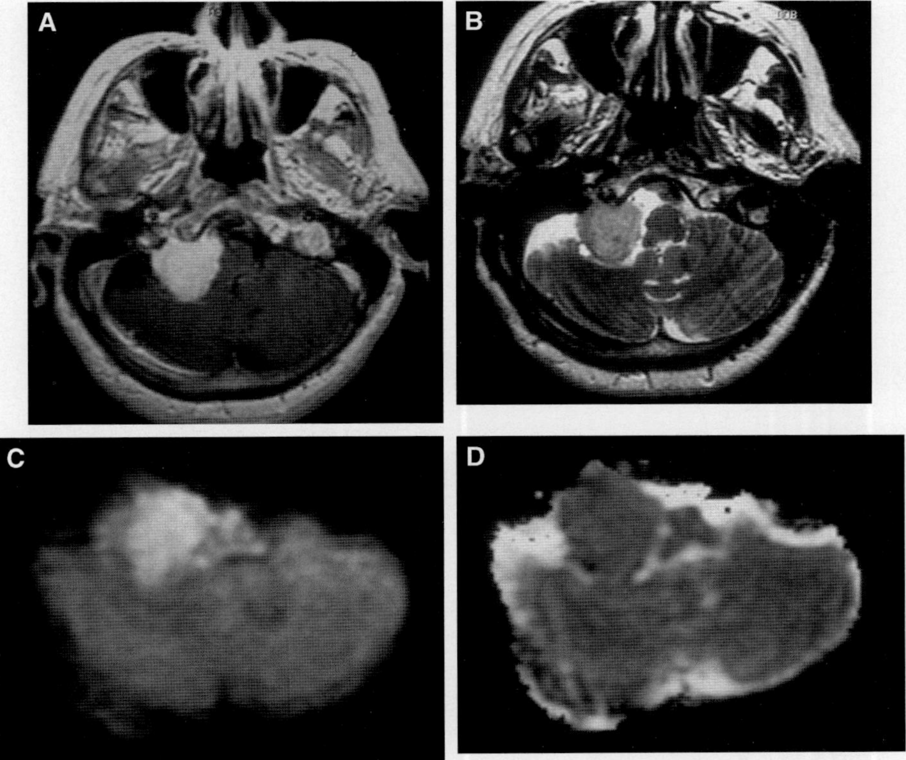

Fig. 2. An 84-year-old woman with a meningioma. An axial, postcontrast-enhanced, T1-weighted image (*A*) and an axial T2-weighted image (*B*) show an extra-axial enhancing lesion in the right cerebellopontomedullary angle cistern. Axial diffusion-weighted imaging (*C*) shows "T2-shine through," whereas the apparent diffusion coefficient map (*D*) demonstrates isointense signal intensity suggesting cellularity similar to that of brain tissue.

tumor cellularity, which may, in turn, improve prediction of tumor grade. Some also suggest that DWI can provide information about peritumoral neoplastic cell infiltration [8,9,27–31].

One example of a specific helpful arena in which DWI may be helpful is the distinction between brain abscesses and necrotic and cystic neoplasms on MRI. DWI can provide a sensitive and specific method for differentiating tumor from abscess in certain settings [32–35]. The abscesses have a high signal on DWI and a reduced ADC within the cavity. This restricted diffusion is thought to be related to the characteristic of the pus in the cavity. Because pus is a viscous fluid that consists of inflammatory cells, debris, and macromolecules like fibrinogen [36], this may, in turn, lead to reduced water mobility, lower ADC, and bright signal on DWI. Conversely, necrotic and cystic tumors display a low signal on DWI (similar to the cerebrospinal fluid [CSF] in the ventricles), with an increased ADC as well as isointense or hypointense DWI signal intensity in the lesion margins [34]. Although these findings can be helpful, they are, of course, not absolute; under certain conditions, restricted diffusion has been documented in hemorrhagic metastases, radiation necrosis, and cystic astrocytoma [37].

DWI is also an effective way of differentiating an arachnoid cyst from epidermoid tumors [38]. Both lesions present the same T1 and T2 signal intensity characteristic of CSF. On DWI, epidermoid tumors are hyperintense, because they are solidly composed, whereas arachnoid cysts are hypointense, demonstrating high diffusivity [38]. The ADC values of epidermoid tumors are similar to those of the brain parenchyma, whereas the ADC values of arachnoid cysts are similar to those of CSF [39]. As a result, DWI can be used to assess follow-up of surgically resected epidermoid tumors, proving efficacious in the detection of residual lesions [40].

Another use for DWI has been to attempt to assist in determination of the margins of tumors in

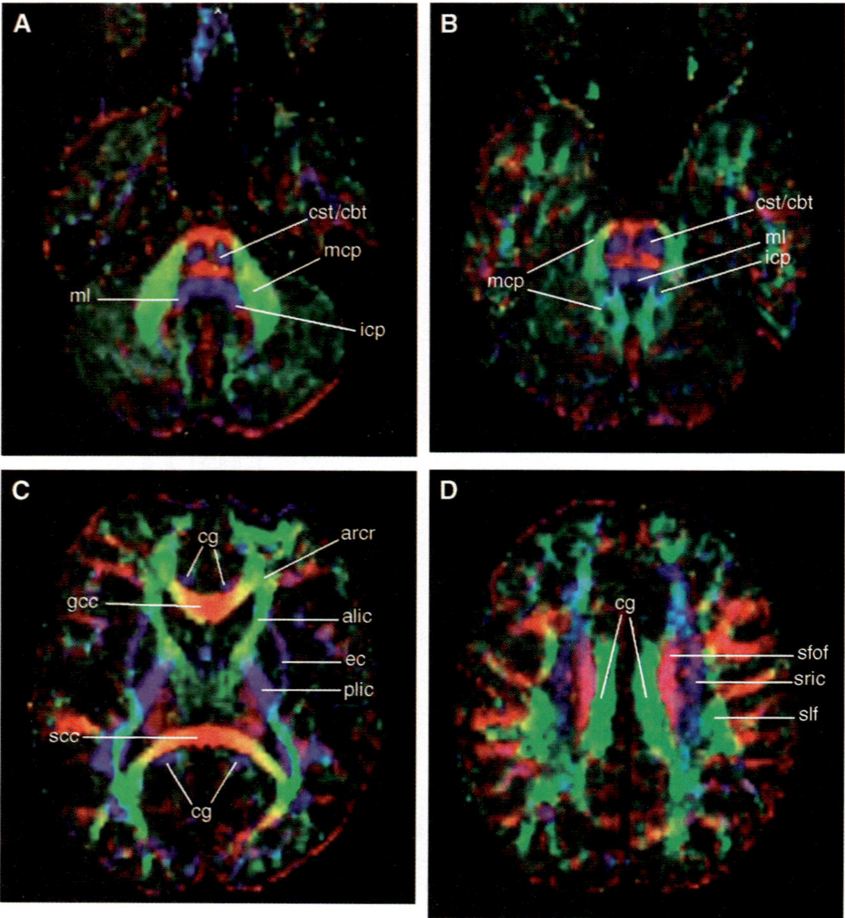

Fig. 3. Diffusion tensor imaging color-coded map of a healthy volunteer. Locations of white matter tracts are assigned on color maps. The direction of the main fiber tracts is represented by red (right-left), green-yellow (anterior-posterior), and blue (superior-inferior). Several main fiber tracts visible on color maps are annotated on the basis of anatomic knowledge. (*A–D*) Axial fractional anisotropic (FA) color maps. (*E–H*) Coronal FA color maps. (*I, J*) Sagittal FA color maps. Mcp, middle cerebral peduncle; cst, corticospinal tract; cbt, corticobulbar tract; ml, medial lemniscus; icp, inferior cerebellar peduncle; cg, cingulum; cc, corpus callosum; gcc, genu of corpus callosum; scc, splenium of corpus callosum; arcr, anterior region of corona radiata; alic, anterior limb of internal capsule; plic, posterior limb of internal capsule; ec, external capsule; sric, superior region of internal capsule; sfof, superior fronto-occipital fasciculus; ifof, inferior fronto-occipital fasciculus; slf, superior longitudinal fasciculus; ilf, inferior longitudinal fasciculus.

the brain. High-grade tumors tend to spread diffusely across the brain, moving along the fiber tracts [41,42]. Some studies have demonstrated the capability of DWI to discriminate the tumor, the infiltrating tumor, the peritumoral edema, and the normal brain parenchyma [8,9,14,43]. Other studies did not find any advantages of this method with regard to the evaluation of tumor extensions [44–46], however, likely because of the difficulty of finding any border even on histopathologic examination of some tumors.

Perhaps most helpfully, DWI has been shown to assist in assessing the cellularity of tumors [44]. In some studies, high-grade tumors have been found to have low ADC values (Fig. 1). This suggests a correlation between the ADC values and tumor cellularity [46,47], with lower ADC values suggesting high-grade lesions [46,48]. In some studies, however, ADC values found in high- and low-grade gliomas have overlapped somewhat [46]. Lymphoma, a highly cellular tumor, has hyperintensity on DWI and reduced ADC values [49],

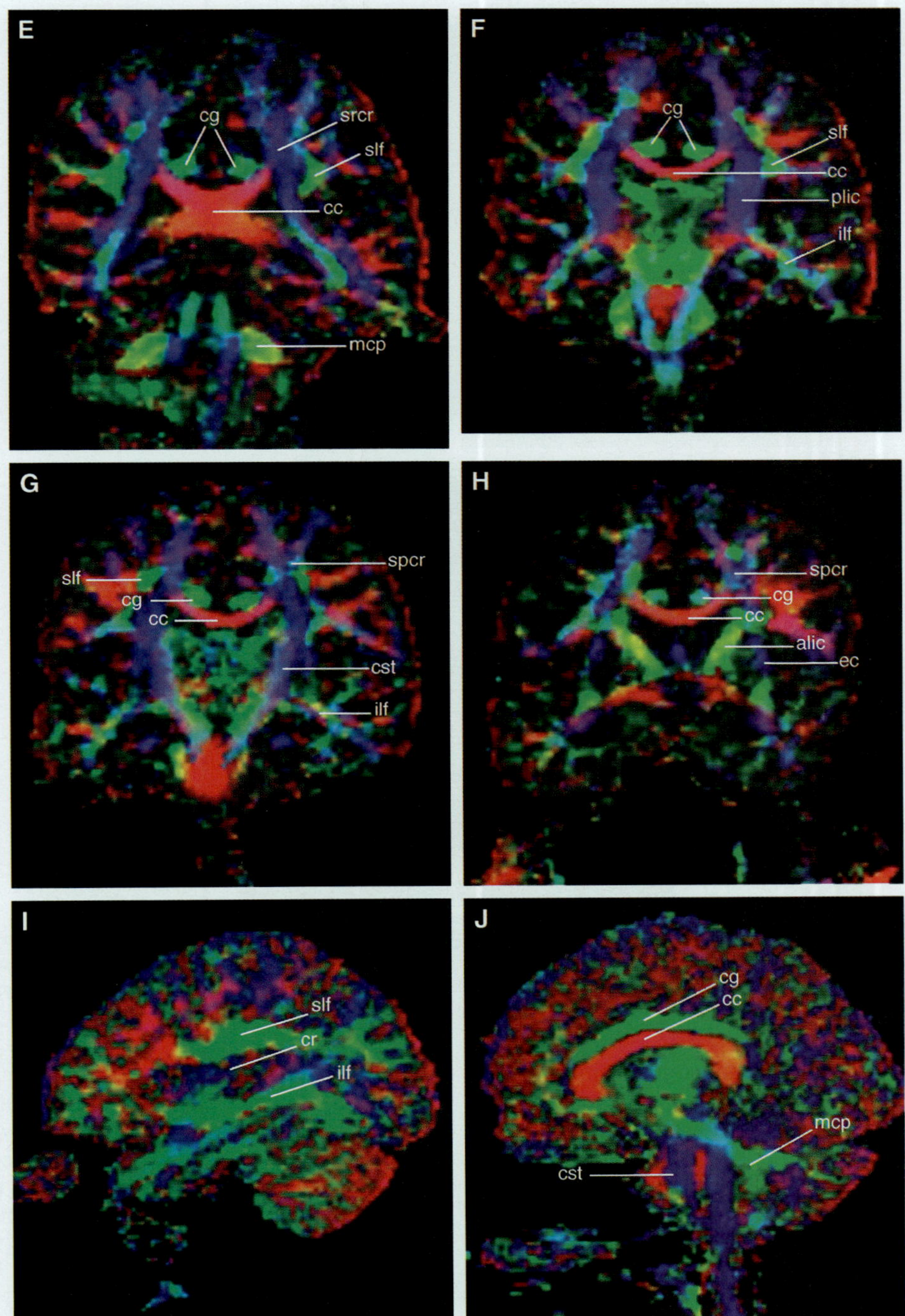

Fig. 3 (*continued*)

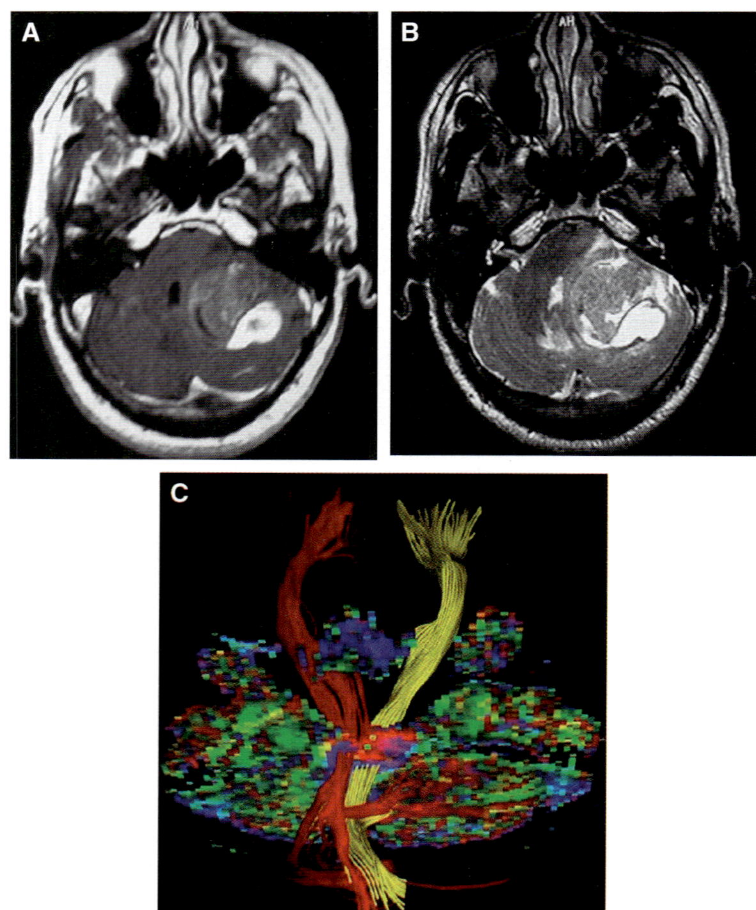

Fig. 4. A 47-year-old man with medulloblastoma. A heterogeneous mass with intratumoral hemorrhage (*A*) surrounded by peritumoral vasogenic edema (*B*) is located in the right cerebellum hemisphere. This mass causes compression and distortion of the fourth ventricle. (*C*) Tractography demonstrates contralateral displacement of the corticospinal tract without clear evidence of invasion or disruption of these fibers.

and it may be in differentiating lymphoma from other CNS lesions that DWI has its greatest value. Although meningiomas also have a restricted diffusion, displaying low ADC values (Fig. 2) [46], they rarely present difficulty in diagnosis. Metastases with perilesional edema have higher ADC values than a primary brain tumor with peritumoral edema, and some have suggested that this may allow better differentiation [28].

Finally, DWI may be useful for posttreatment assessment, demonstrating acute postoperative procedure–induced changes [50] but, more importantly, possibly providing an early surrogate marker for the efficacy of the chemotherapeutic treatment [51,52], because such treatments may cause cytotoxic or vasogenic edema that DWI can differentiate and monitor. DWI also has been suggested as a tool for monitoring the effectiveness of radiation therapy [2] In summary, DWI has a limited prognostic role but may become an important tool in assessing the response to radiation therapy and chemotherapy [2] as well as the complications related to each type of therapy [53,54].

Diffusion tensor MRI

Physical basis

The movement of water occurs in all three directions and is assumed to behave in a manner that physicists can describe using a Gaussian approximation. When water molecules diffuse equally in all directions, this is termed *isotropic diffusion*. This phenomenon is typical in the ventricles, and at the resolution of standard MRI, also seems to be the case in the gray matter. In the white matter, however, free water molecules diffuse anisotropically, that is, the water diffusion is not equal in all three orthogonal directions [55,56,61]. This is likely because tissue structures cause impediment of the water motion; these structures likely include the cell membranes but, more importantly, the myelin sheath surrounding myelinated white matter [57]. Put another way, isotropic diffusion can be graphically represented as a sphere [58], whereas anisotropic diffusion can be graphically expressed as an ellipsoid [58], with water molecules moving farther along the long axis of a fiber bundle and less movement perpendicularly [59].

To estimate the nine tensor matrix elements required for a Gaussian description of water mobility, the diffusion gradient must be applied to at least six noncollinear directions (only six of the nine elements are unique under this assumption) [60]. The eigenvalues represent the three principal diffusion coefficients measured along the three coordinate directions of the ellipsoid [59]. The eigenvectors represent the directions of the tensor [60]. Because interpreting a tensor representation can be difficult, scalar metrics have been proposed to simplify DTI data [57]. For example, fractional anisotropy (FA) measures the fraction of the total magnitude of diffusion anisotropy. FA values vary from complete isotropic diffusion (graded as 0) up to complete anisotropic diffusion (graded as 1) [57,58].

In addition to assessment of the diffusion in a single voxel, DTI has been used to attempt to map the white matter fiber tracts. This is typically done by connecting a given voxel to the appropriately adjacent voxel in accordance with the direction that the voxel's principal eigenvector is oriented [62,63]. A color-coded map of fiber orientation can also be determined by DTI [64]. A different color has been attributed to represent a different fiber orientation along the three orthogonal spatial axes: in the standard convention, red stands for the left-to-right direction of x-oriented fibers, blue stands for the superior-to-inferior direction of y-oriented fibers, and green stands for the anterior-to-posterior direction of z-oriented fibers (Fig. 3) [64,65].

Diffusion tensor MRI in brain tumors

Often, a primary aim of surgical brain tumor treatment is complete lesion resection without harming vital brain functions [66,67]. Because it is generally accepted that conventional MRI underestimates the real extent of the brain tumor, given its ability to verify neoplastic cells that infiltrate peritumoral areas of abnormal T2-weighted signal intensity [68], many practitioners are uncomfortable using only conventional MRI

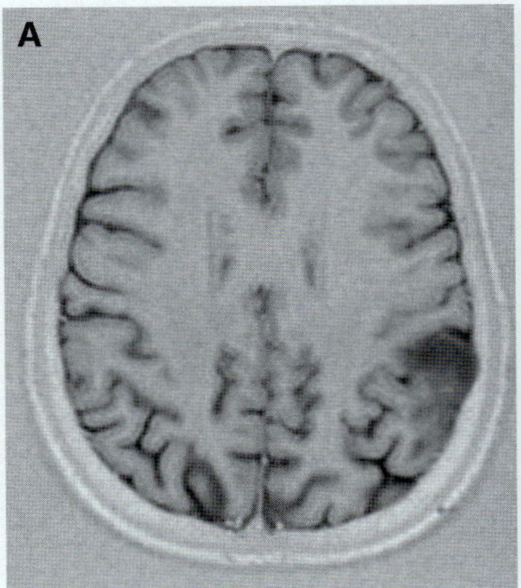

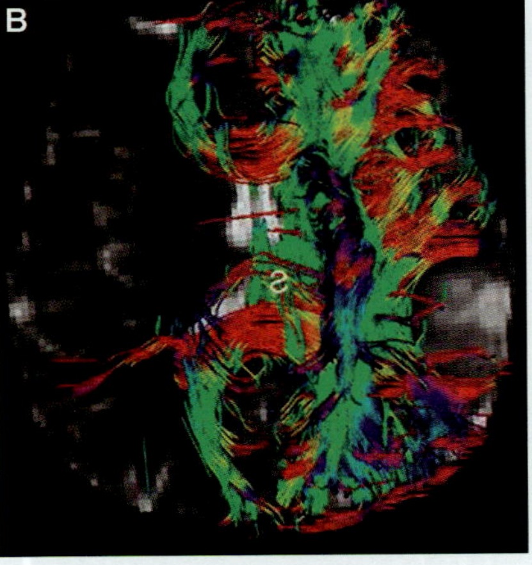

Fig. 5. A 42-year-old man with a diagnosis of a low-grade astrocytoma presented with early onset of focal seizures. (*A*) The MRI examination demonstrates an expansive lesion in the perirolandic area, which does not have hyperperfusion. (*B*) The mass lesion causes displacement of the main fiber tracts adjacent to the tumor, which is well demonstrated on tractography. There seems to be no invasion or disruption of these tracts.

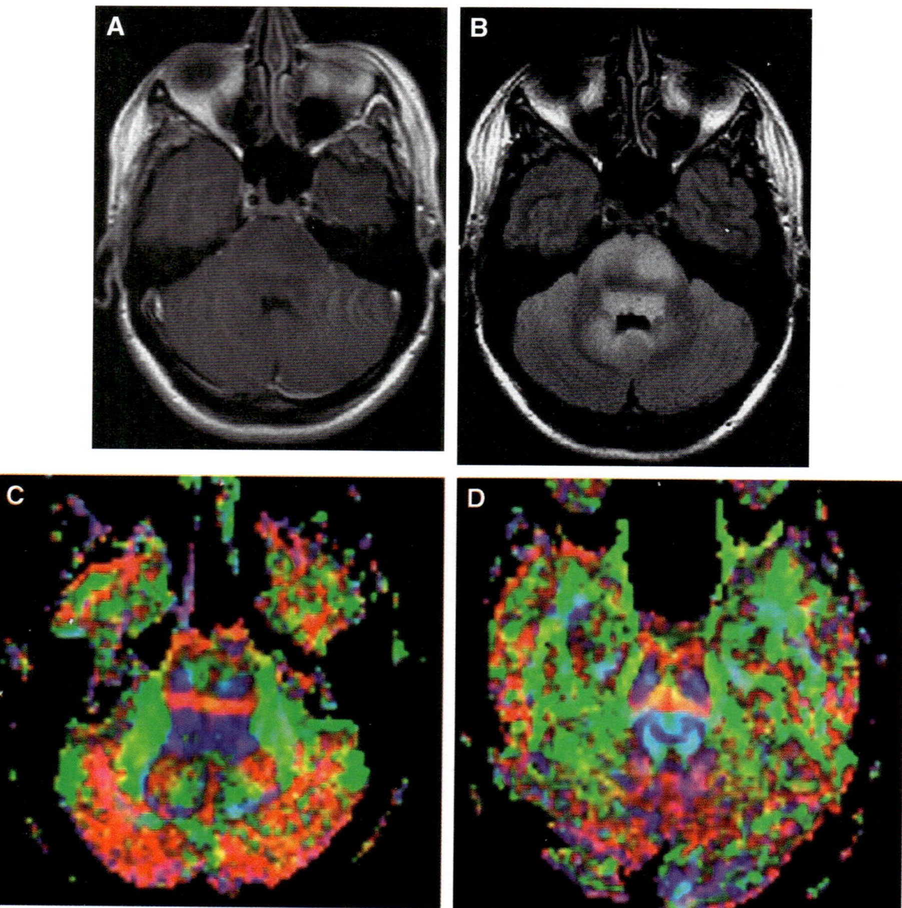

Fig. 6. An invading brain stem lesion that extends to the right cerebellum hemisphere though the middle cerebellar peduncle in a 40-year-old man who presented with left sixth cranial nerve palsy. The diagnosis of gliomatosis cerebri was made after a biopsy. The lesion does not enhance on the postcontrast T1-weighted image (*A*), has hyperintense signal on the T2-weighted image (*B*), and causes minimum expansion of the brain stem. Magnetic resonance spectroscopy shows a high myoinositol peak, a moderately high choline peak, and a subtle reduction on the *N*-acetylaspartate peak (not shown). The diffusion tensor imaging–fractional anisotropy maps (*C–F*) and tractography (*G, H*) demonstrate that the main brain stem fiber tracts are preserved. This is probably explained by the fact that gliomatosis cerebri is a diffusely invading lesion that preserves the normal underlying cytoarchitectural pattern because it does not destroy the nerve fibers.

approaches. By examining the microscopic tissue environment, DTI may be able to delineate the tumor versus the infiltrating tumor between the peritumoral edema and normal brain parenchyma more accurately, which, in turn, may help to optimize the treatment of patients [69]. Although this remains to be proven, it does appear from straightforward inspection that DTI seems to be able to illustrate the relation of a tumor to the nearby main fiber tracts (Fig. 4). Because of this, many have begun to suggest that DTI might be used to aid in surgical planning [70] as well as radiotherapy planning [71] and to monitor tumor recurrence and the response to the treatment [72]. Examples of these applications are given below.

Tumor grading

As mentioned previously, DWI (nontensor diffusion) seems to provide some utility in tumor grading by assessment of tumor cellularity. To

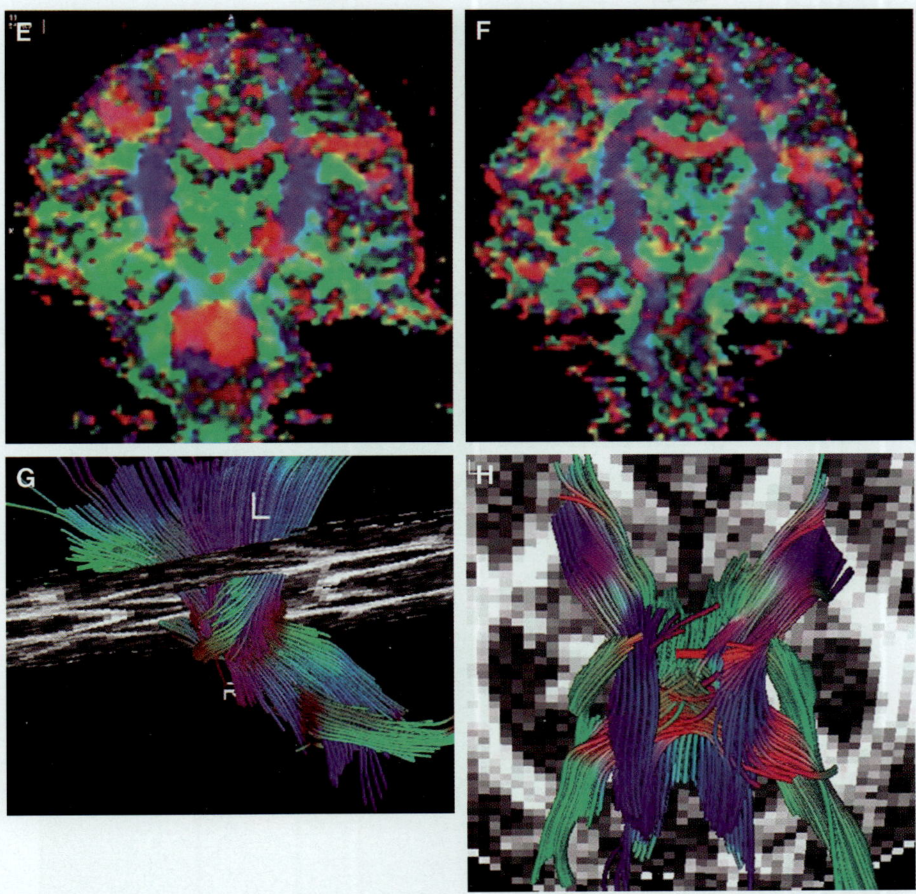

Fig. 6 (*continued*)

date, the additional information provided by DTI has not been shown to correlate with tumor cellularity [73], although in one series that evaluated epidermoid tumors with DTI, FA values were high, probably because of the high packing density of the cells and their solid-state cholesterol [74].

Presurgical planning

Much more enthusiasm has been shown for using DTI to illustrate the relation of a tumor to neighboring white matter tracts, with initial reports suggesting that this may be feasible [74]. DTI seems to be the only noninvasive method of obtaining information about the fiber tracts and is able to suggest them three dimensionally, although the validity of these suggestions remains to be studied carefully. Many practitioners accept an underlying assumption that the chief cause of anisotropy is related to the white matter bundles; with this assumption, the involvement of the white matter tracts can often be clearly identified in brain tumor patients by using anisotropic maps (the FA maps are the most widely used) and so-called "diffusion tractography," where images of the mathematically described connections between voxels are generated.

White matter involvement by a tumor can be arranged into five different categories as follows:

1. Displaced: maintained normal anisotropy relative to the contralateral tract in the corresponding location but situated in an abnormal T2-weighted signal intensity area or presenting in an abnormal orientation
2. Invaded: slightly reduced anisotropy without displacement of white matter architecture, remaining identifiable on orientation maps
3. Infiltrated: reduced anisotropy but remaining identifiable on orientation maps

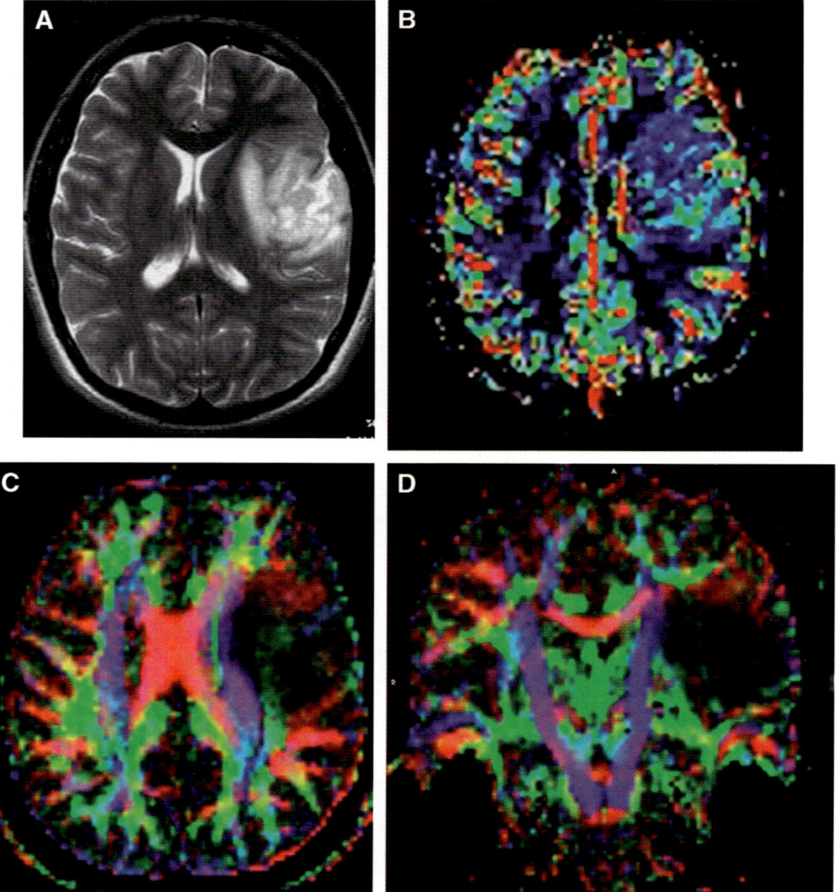

Fig. 7. A nonenhancing insular anaplastic astrocytoma lesion in a 56-year-old man (*A*), in which the relative cerebral blood volume map (*B*) demonstrates some areas of hyperperfusion within the lesion. There is infiltration of the corticospinal tract and corona radiata as well as of the superior longitudinal fasciculus on the axial (*C*) and coronal (*D, E*) diffusion tensor imaging (DTI)–fractional anisotropy maps and of the left corticospinal fibers tracts on tractography (*F*). DTI shows reduced anisotropy, but the main tracts remain identifiable on tractography.

4. Disrupted: marked reduced anisotropy and unidentifiable on orientation maps
5. Edematous: maintained normal anisotropy and normally oriented but located in an abnormal T2-weighted signal intensity area [75]

The neoplastic cells and the peritumoral edema cause changes in the brain structure; typically, measurement of diffusion anisotropy from the normal brain parenchyma up to near the tumor demonstrates a decrease in FA values [1].

Displacement rather than destruction of white matter fibers around low-grade gliomas has been described [71,76]. Low-grade neoplasms (Fig. 5) are well-circumscribed lesions that do not cause invasion or destruction of fiber tracts. These lesions tend to produce a deviation of surrounding white matter fibers. A study described a case in which the corticospinal tract (CST) had been infiltrated by an oligodendroglioma, although it spared the motor strip and the posterior limb of the internal capsule [77]. Displacement rather than infiltration of the adjacent white matter tracts has also been described in cerebral metastases [71] and meningiomas [78].

The main fiber tracts are invaded in cases of gliomatosis cerebri (Fig. 6), which has a specific histopathologic behavior. The neoplastic cells form parallel rows among nerve fibers, preserving

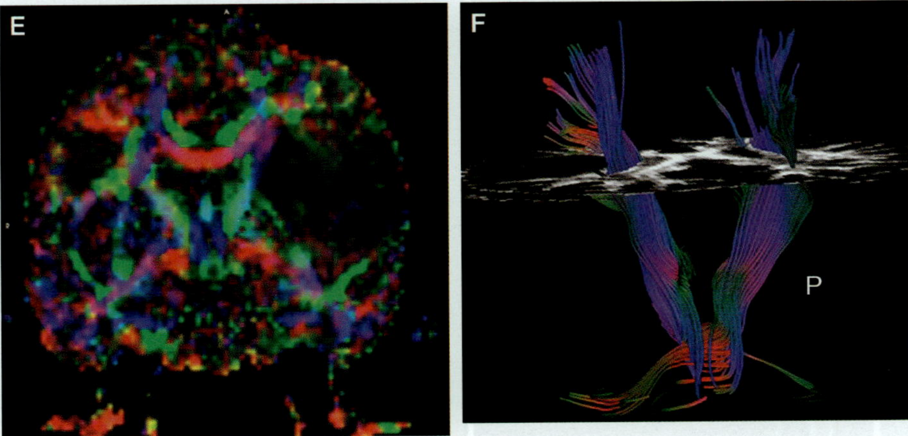

Fig. 7 (*continued*)

them; however, there is destruction of myelin sheaths. Thus, the anisotropy is slightly reduced when compared with normal subjects but greater than it is when compared with high-grade gliomas. The main fiber tracts remain identifiable on orientation maps and on the tractography.

The anisotropy in the T2-weighted hyperintense area that surrounds the tumor is reduced because of infiltration of neoplastic cells. Compared with the contralateral hemisphere in patients with high-grade gliomas (but not with low-grade gliomas or cerebral metastases) (Fig. 7), the anisotropy is also low in the white matter areas adjacent to tumors that look normal on T2-weighted images [71]. The same situation can be observed in lymphoma (Fig. 8). When compared with the abnormal white matter adjacent to metastases, Jellison et al [79] demonstrated decreased anisotropy of the abnormal white matter that surrounds the gliomas (Fig. 9). FA values decrease in the abnormal area that surrounds high-grade tumors on T2-weighted imaging. This presumably happens because of increased water content and tumor infiltration. A major brain structural disorganization then occurs [72]. Further study is necessary in this arena, because conflicting results have been described, with no difference found in FA value analyses of abnormal white matter adjacent to high-grade gliomas and metastases [72] in some studies.

The tract disruption mostly found in high-grade tumors (Fig. 10) may be caused by peritumoral edema, tumor mass effect, and tumor infiltration effect [71,78]. The anisotropic maps and tractography show destruction or discontinuation of the fiber tracts because of local tumor cell invasion (Fig. 11).

Metastatic lesions are surrounded by abnormal T2-weighted imaging that may consist of vasogenic edema. The edematous areas have reduced FA values. This fact can be explained by the increase in water content rather than by destruction or infiltration of nerve fibers. DTI did not help to differentiate apparently normal white matter from edematous brain and enhancing peritumoral margins [69]. The drop in FA values of the area infiltrated by cell tumors is lower than in the peritumoral edema [1,70,75]. DTI can distinguish the edematous areas with intact fibers mostly found in metastases (Fig. 12) from the disrupted fibers mostly found in high-grade gliomas [80].

In short, DTI is gaining support as a preoperative MRI method of evaluating brain tumors closely related to eloquent regions [75]. DTI seems to be particularly advantageous for certain types of surgical planning, optimizing the surgical evaluation of brain tumors near white matter tracts. Formal studies demonstrating that DTI can successfully prevent postoperative complications have yet to be performed, but preliminary data look promising [80].

Combination of diffusion tensor imaging with functional MRI

Intracranial neoplasms may involve the functional cortex and the corresponding white matter tracts. The preoperative identification of eloquent areas through noninvasive methods, such as blood

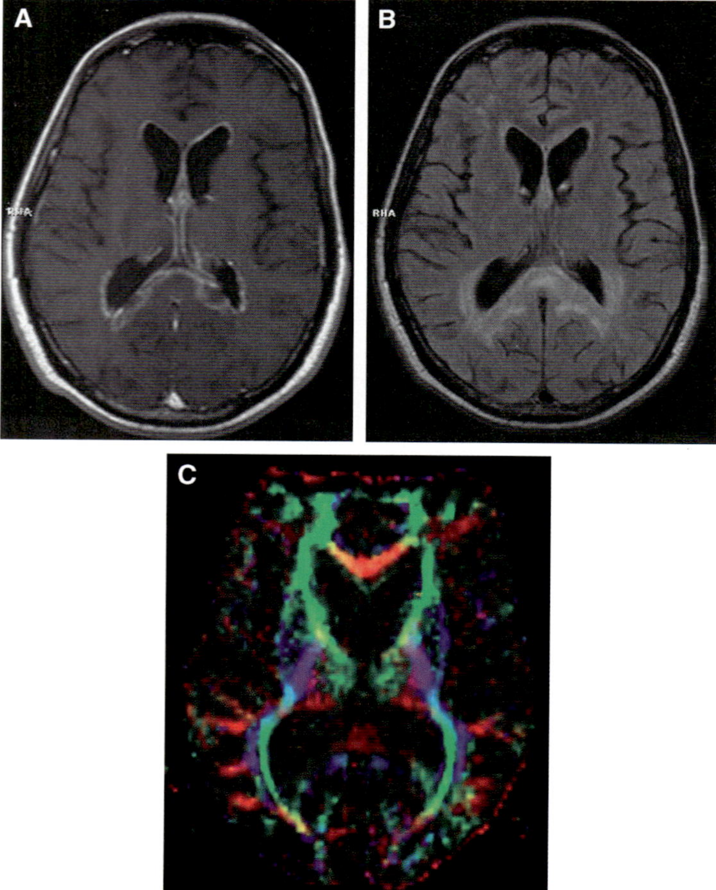

Fig. 8. A 50-year-old man with a histopathologic diagnosis of lymphoma complained of mental disturbance, cognitive impairment, and seizures. A contrast-enhanced, axial, T1-weighted image (*A*) demonstrates an enhancing lesion that involves the corpus callosum, surrounded by peritumoral edema/infiltrating lesion (*B*) associated with subependymal enhancement caused by cerebrospinal fluid dissemination. The axial fractional anisotropy color-coded map (*C*) demonstrates the infiltrating aspect of the lesion. The anisotropy in the splenium of the corpus callosum is markedly reduced.

oxygen level dependent (BOLD) fMRI and DTI tractography, offers some advantages; not only can it reduce the time of surgery in some instances, but it may minimize some intraoperative cortical stimulation methods, such as identification of the language cortex [80].

Until recently, preoperative and perioperative methods to evaluate brain function of patients with brain tumors were restricted to cortex activation. Increasingly, investigators are beginning to combine fMRI with DTI. The attraction is that fMRI can be an accurate and noninvasive method for mapping functional cerebral cortex, identifying eloquent areas in the cortex and displaying their relation to the lesion [81], whereas DTI may be able to identify the main fiber tracts to be avoided during surgery so as to safely guide a tumor resection [1]. Consequently, the combination of DTI tractography and fMRI might allow us to map an entire functional circuit precisely [82]. Even though fMRI locates eloquent cortical areas, determination of the course and integrity of the fiber tracts remains essential to the surgical planning [80,83].

This identification of the fiber tracts can facilitate the decision-making process regarding the likelihood of an operation [1]. As a result, neurosurgeons may have more information to

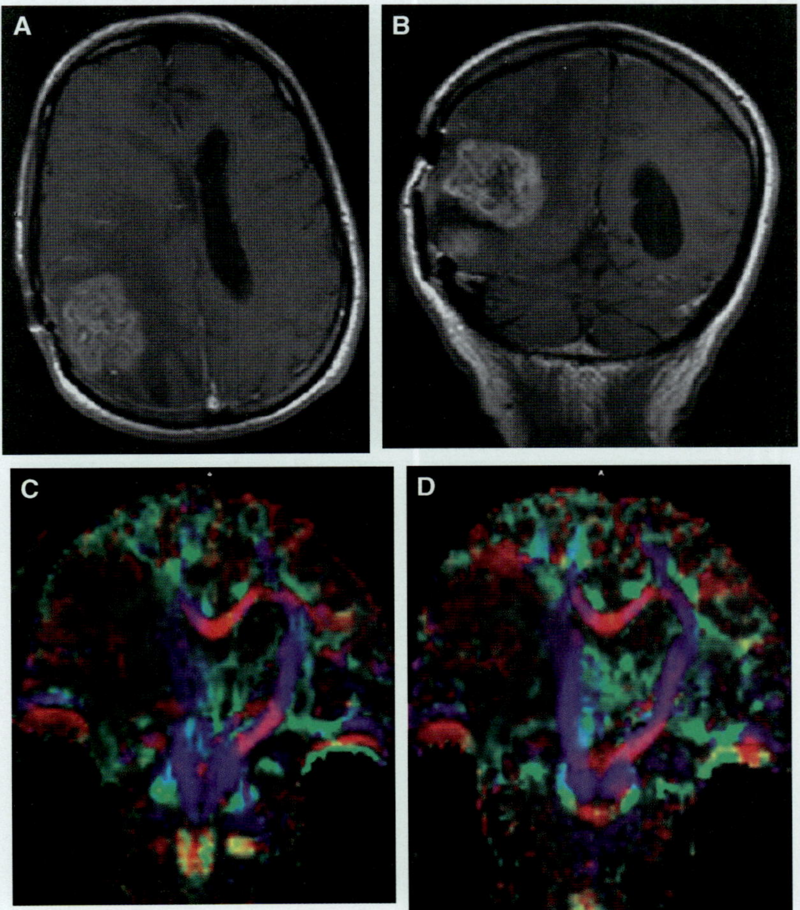

Fig. 9. (*A, B*) An expansive and infiltrating lesion in a 73-year-old man with left hemiparesis and seizures, with the diagnosis of glioblastoma multiforme. The lesion has hyperperfusion, markedly elevated choline and lactate/lipid peaks, and a low of *N*-acetylaspartate peak. (*C, D*) Coronal diffusion tensor imaging–fractional anisotropy maps show that the lesion dislocates and infiltrates the corticospinal tract and the superior longitudinal fasciculus. There is also distortion of the corpus callosum.

inform the choice of surgical approach to be taken. This better evaluation of risks by neurosurgeons is possible if they can know the spatial relation between the tumor and major fiber tracts [63] and thereby avoid postoperative neurologic deficit [2,83]. This remains to be proven in randomized trials, however.

Many investigators hope that the combined use of fMRI and DTI tractography might define the structural basis of functional connectivity in normal and pathologic brains [84]. As a consequence of the mass effect and changes in the structure of the brain caused by tumor, the identification of eloquent areas through conventional MRI results is, so to speak, impossible. Because fMRI is able to depict the exact location of the motor cortex in many instances, it should be possible to delineate the CST by DTI tractography. In one previous report [78], the authors used the motor cortex identified by fMRI as a starting point to trace the CST by DTI tractography. This approach could eventually be extended to other tracts as well.

The neurosurgical navigation system is a real-time device that provides a probe-guided intraoperative MRI (iMRI) display of the brain [85]. This system has already been widely used and is able to combine the information of fMRI [80,85] with that of DTI tractography [82,86], or even of both together [78,81].

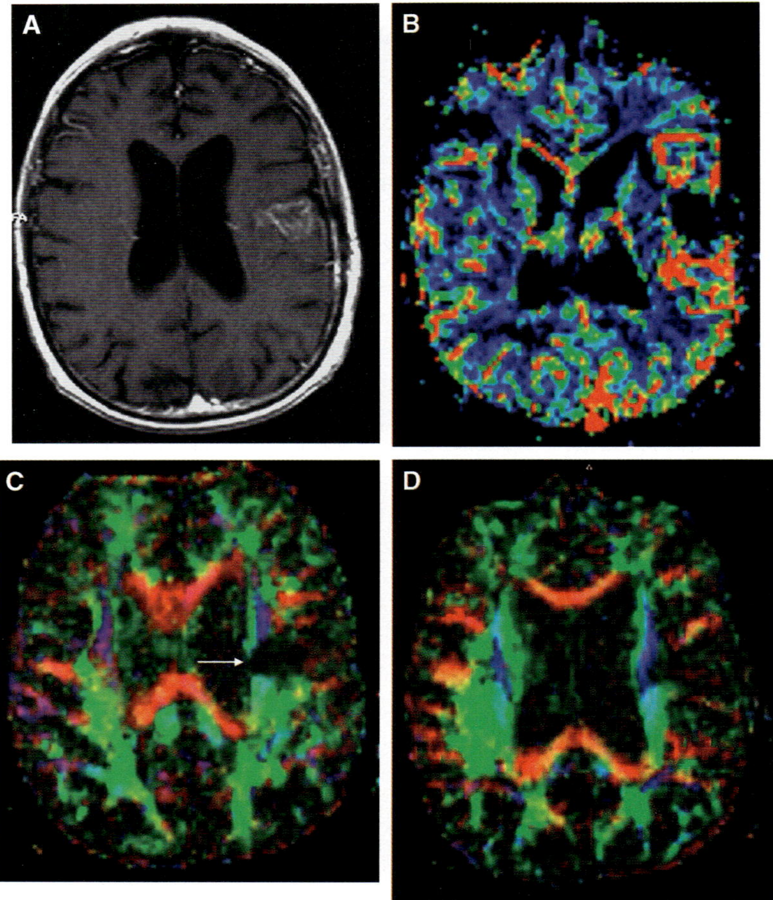

Fig. 10. A 56-year-old man with an anaplastic astrocytoma presented with right hemiparesis. The contrast-enhanced T1-weighted image (*A*) shows a left frontal lesion that has hyperperfusion on the relative cerebral blood volume map (*B*) (note the black signal caused by excessive enhancement with resulting T1 effect). (*C, D*) The axial diffusion-tensor imaging–fractional anisotropy maps demonstrate disruption of the left corona radiata (*arrow*).

Intraoperative utility of diffusion tensor imaging

iMRI has been used to guide a brain tumor resection. Such image-guidance systems can help to determine the optimal placement for the craniotomy.

Because surgical manipulations and maneuvers alter the anatomic position of brain structures and the tumor [87], morphologic changes of the brain may also occur between the time of the preoperative MRI examinations and the time of the surgery [88]. For this reason, the exact location of brain tumors based on preoperative examinations may not be the same. Because of this, iMRI has been proposed as a possible way to enable neurosurgeons to optimize their surgical approaches by avoiding critical structures and the adjacent normal brain parenchyma [87]. Some reports suggest that in 65% to 92% of the cases in which neurosurgeons believed they have performed a complete and thorough tumor resection, iMRI still depicts a lesion to be resected [89,90]. This is particularly relevant in low-grade gliomas, because studies suggest that total resection leads to a higher probability of cure. During surgery, however, such lesions can be difficult to differentiate from the normal brain parenchyma.

iMRI can be performed together with some functional sequences, such as fMRI [85] and diffusion imaging [82]. In one study, intraoperative diffusion imaging was performed during

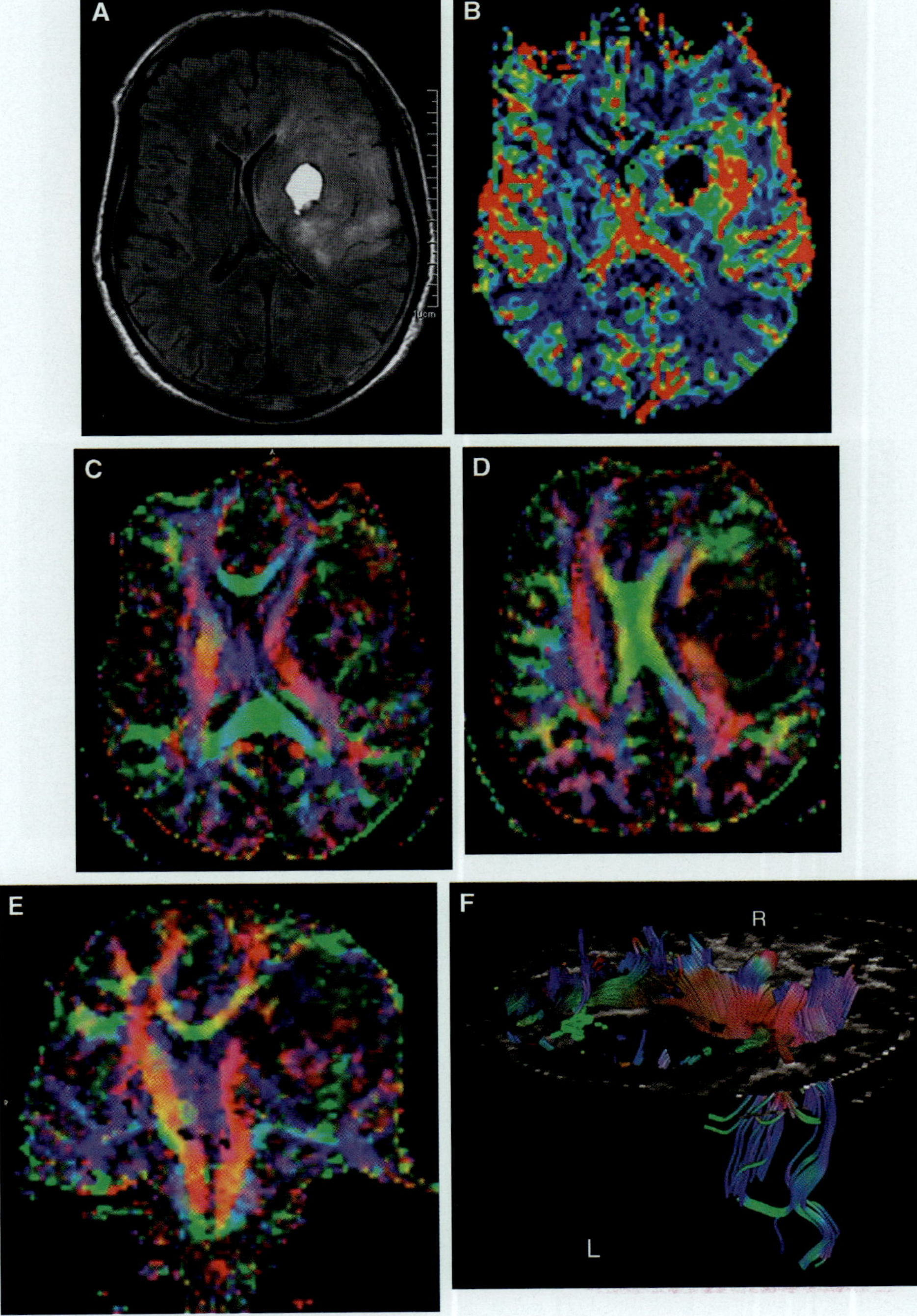

Fig. 11. A 57-year-old man with glioblastoma multiforme presented with right hemiparesis and seizures. An expansive, infiltrating, and enhancing left insular lesion with intratumoral hemorrhage (*A*) and hyperperfusion (*B*) is demonstrated. Axial (*C, D*) and coronal (*E*) diffusion tensor imaging–fractional anisotropy maps and tractography (*F*) show dislocation and disruption of the main fiber tracts, such as the anterior and posterior portions of the internal capsule and the superior longitudinal fasciculus.

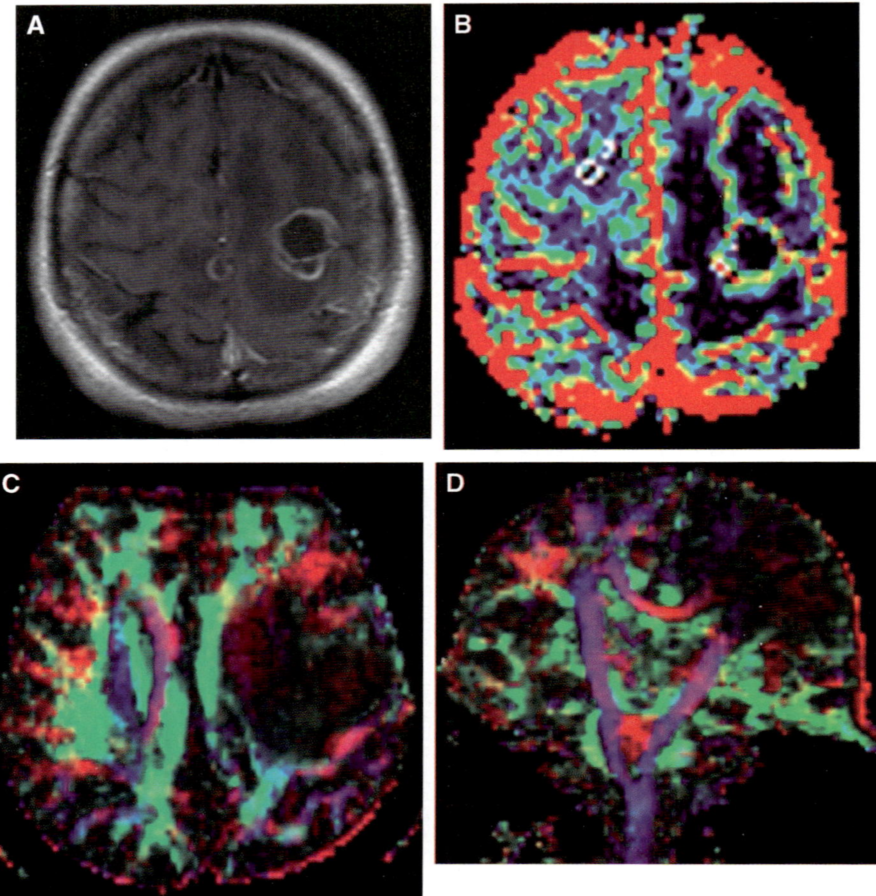

Fig. 12. A 50-year-old woman with new onset of seizures and a history of breast cancer. A round rim-enhancing lesion with a necrotic center (*A*) and hyperperfusion (*B*) is surrounded by peritumoral edema consisting of breast cancer metastasis. Axial (*C*) and coronal (*D*) diffusion tensor imaging–fractional anisotropy (FA) maps show the edematous changes in the FA values. Thus, it is difficult to identify the main fiber tracts within the vasogenic edema. This does not necessarily mean that these fibers are infiltrated with tumor or disrupted, however.

neurosurgery for the resection of a tumor using an interventional MRI system [82].

Intraoperative development of hyperacute cerebral ischemia had been previously detected in two patients, and this was confirmed later by a follow-up MRI examination. DTI, together with a neuronavigation system, was performed in a third patient as an integral part of an image-guided tumor resection. After processing the DTI data, DTI tractography was performed. The relation of the tumor to the anatomy of the white matter fiber tracts adjacent to it was clearly and plainly demonstrated in a case of oligodendroglioma. The fiber tracts were displaced, without being infiltrated or disrupted by the tumor. The complete tumor resection was performed without any postoperative neurologic deficit. Although anecdotal, such reports suggest that intraoperative diffusion imaging may provide important clinical information, adding substantially to the intraoperative information available about the pathologic state of the brain parenchyma and the structure of white matter.

Diffusion tensor imaging in brain tumor therapy

DTI may play a role in the management of patients undergoing radiation therapy and chemotherapy. By adding information about the location of white matter tracts, DTI tractography might be used successfully alongside fMRI for radiosurgery planning. In theory, this should allow a reduction of the dose applied as well as a reduction in the volume of normal brain irradiated with a high dose, hopefully reducing necrosis [71].

DTI may also help in the early detection of white matter injuries caused by chemotherapy and radiation therapy. A report showed a correlation between the reduction of FA values, young age at treatment, an increased interval since the beginning of treatment, and the poor intellectual outcome in patients with medulloblastoma [91]. The possibility of using FA or other DTI changes as a biomarker for neurotoxicity is enticing.

Limitations

Although initial reports suggest advantages of DTI in the evaluation of patients with brain tumors, these reports are largely single-center, uncontrolled, preliminary findings. Therefore, these results must be cautiously interpreted. Furthermore, there remain substantial technical hurdles, with the rapid evolution of MRI systems making ever more powerful approaches possible. Such improvements are particularly welcome, given the limited signal-to-noise ratio of diffusion overall. For example, the limited spatial resolution of EPI approaches may lead to reduced sensitivity. The method herein assessed is only capable of depicting the prominent fiber tracts [70,92], and more advanced approaches (eg, diffusion spectrum imaging) may be much more useful in the future. Susceptibility artifacts can cause image distortion that prevents DTI data from being accurately analyzed [70], and numerous other technical challenges remain. Nevertheless, these initial data are promising.

Summary

DTI seems to offer the possibility of adding important information to presurgical planning. Although experience is limited, DTI seems to provide useful local information about the structures near the tumor, and this seems to be useful in planning. In the future, DTI may provide an improved way to monitor intraoperative surgical procedures as well as their complications. Furthermore, evaluation of the response to treatment with chemotherapy and radiation therapy might also be possible. Although DTI has some limitations, its active investigation and further study are clearly warranted.

References

[1] Landis SH, Murray T, Bolden S. Cancer statistics, 1998. CA Cancer J Clin 1998;48:6–29.

[2] Berens ME, Rutka JT, Rosenblum ML. Brain tumor epidemiology, growth, and invasion. Neurosurg Clin N Am 1990;1:1–18.

[3] Koeller KK, Henry JM. Superficial gliomas: radiologic-pathologic correlation. Radiographics 2001; 21:1533–56.

[4] Hunt D, Treasure P. Year of life lost due to cancer in East Anglia 1990–1994. Cambridge: East Anglian Cancer Intelligence Unit, Institute of Public Health; 1998.

[5] Brain MRC Tumor Working Party. Prognostic factor for high-grade malignant glioma: development of a prognostic index. A report of the Medical Research Council Brain Tumor Working Party. J Neurooncol 1990;9:47–55.

[6] Damadian R. Tumor detection by nuclear magnetic resonance. Science 1971;171:1151–3.

[7] Tovi M. MR imaging in cerebral gliomas analysis of tumor tissue components. Acta Radiol Suppl 1993; 384:1–24.

[8] Brunberg JA, Chenevert TL, McKeever PE, Ross DA, Junck LR, Muraszko KM, et al. In vivo MR determination of water diffusion coefficients and diffusion anisotropy: correlation with structural alteration in gliomas of the cerebral hemispheres. AJNR Am J Neuroradiol 1995;16:361–71.

[9] Tien RD, Felsberg GJ, Friedman H, Brown M, MacFall J. MR imaging of high-grade cerebral gliomas: value of diffusion-weighted echo-planar pulse sequence. AJR Am J Roentgenol 1994;162:671–7.

[10] Holodny AI, Ollenschlager M. Diffusion imaging in brain tumor. Neuroimaging Clin N Am 2002;12: 107–24.

[11] Le Bihan D, Breton E, Lallemand D, Aubin MI, Vignaud J, Laval-Jeantet M. Diffusion and perfusion in intravoxel incoherent motion MR imaging. Radiology 1988;168:497–505.

[12] Turner R, Le Bihan D, Maier J, Vavrek R, Hedges LK, Pekar J. Echo-planar imaging of intravoxel incoherent motion. Radiology 1990;177: 407–14.

[13] Barboriak DP. Imaging of brain tumors with diffusion-weighted and diffusion tensor MR imaging. Magn Reson Imaging Clin N Am 2003;11:379–401.

[14] Maier SE, Gudbjartsson H, Patz SL, Hsu L, Lovblad KO, Edelman RR, et al. Line scan diffusion imaging: characterization in healthy subjects and stroke patients. AJR Am J Roentgenol 1998;171: 85–93.

[15] Warach S, Chien D, Li W, Ronthal M, Edelman RR. Fast magnetic resonance diffusion-

weighted imaging of acute human stroke. Neurology 1992;42:1717–23.

[16] Sunshine JL, Tarr RW, Lanzieri CF, Landis DM, Selman WR, Lewin JS. Hyperacute stroke: ultrafast MR imaging to triage patients prior to therapy. Radiology 1999;212:325–32.

[17] Beauchamp NJ, Uluğ AM, Passe TJ, van Zijl PC. MR diffusion imaging in stoke: review and controversies. Radiographics 1998;18:1269–83.

[18] Schaefer PW. Applications of DWI in clinical neurology. J Neurol Sci 2001;186(Suppl 1):S25–35.

[19] Larsson HB, Thomsen C, Frederiksen J, Stubgaard M, Henriksen O. In vivo magnetic resonance measurement in the brain of patients with multiple sclerosis. Magn Reson Imaging 1993;10:7–12.

[20] Horsfield MA, Lai M, Webb SL, Barker GJ, Tofts PS, Turner R, et al. Apparent diffusion coefficients in benign and secondary progressive multiple sclerosis by nuclear magnetic resonance. Magn Reson Med 1996;36:393–400.

[21] Castriota-Scanderberg A, Tomaiuolo F, Sabatini U, Nocentini U, Grasso MG, Caltagirone C. Demyelinating plaques in relapsing-remitting and secondary progressive multiple sclerosis: assessment with diffusion MR imaging. AJNR Am J Neuroradiol 2000; 21:862–8.

[22] Tsuchiya K, Hachiya J, Maehara T. Diffusion-weighted MR imaging in multiple sclerosis: comparison with contrast-enhanced study. Eur J Radiol 1999;10:7–12.

[23] Tsuchiya K, Katase S, Yoshino A, Hachiya J. Diffusion-weighted MR imaging of encephalitis. AJR Am J Roentgenol 1999;173:1097–9.

[24] Na DL, Suh CK, Choi SH, Moon HS, Seo DW, Kim SE, et al. Diffusion-weighted magnetic resonance imaging in probable Creutzfeldt-Jakob disease. Arch Neurol 1999;56:951–7.

[25] Stejskal E, Tanner J. Spin diffusion measurements: spin echos in the presence of time-dependent field gradient. J Chem Phys 1965;42:288–92.

[26] Romero JM, Schaefer PW, Grant PE, Becerra L, Gonzáles RG. Diffusion MR imaging of acute ischemic stroke. Neuroimaging Clin N Am 2002;12: 35–53.

[27] Eis M, Els T, Hoehn-Berlage M, Hossman KA. Quantitative diffusion MR imaging of cerebral tumor and edema. Acta Neurochir Suppl (Wien) 1994;60:344–6.

[28] Krabbe K, Gideon P, Wang P, Hansen U, Thomsen C, Madsen F. MR diffusion imaging of human intracranial tumours. Neuroradiology 1997; 39:483–9.

[29] Le Bihan D, Douek P, Argyropoulou M, Turner R, Patronas N, Fulham M. Diffusion and perfusion magnetic resonance imaging in brain tumors. Top Magn Reson Imaging 1993;5:25–31.

[30] Tsuruda JS, Chew WM, Moseley ME, Norman D. Diffusion-weighted MR imaging of extraaxial tumors. Magn Reson Med 1991;19:316–20.

[31] Yanaka K, Shirai S, Kimura H, Kamezaki T, Matsumura A, Nose T. Clinical application of diffusion-weighted magnetic resonance imaging to intracranial disorders. Neurol Med Chir 1995;16:361–71.

[32] Guo AC, Provenzale JM, Cruz LCH Jr, Petrella JR. Cerebral abscesses: investigation using apparent diffusion coefficient maps. Neuroradiology 2001;43: 370–4.

[33] Bergui M, Zhong J, Bradac GB, Sales S. Diffusion-weighted images of intracranial cyst-like lesions. Neuroradiology 2001;439(10):824–9.

[34] Chang SC, Lai PH, Chen WL, Weng HH, Ho JT, Wang JS. Diffusion-weighted MRI features of brain abscess and cystic or necrotic brain tumors: comparison with conventional MRI. Clin Imaging 2002; 26(4):227–36.

[35] Chan JH, Tsui EY, Chau LF Chow KY, Chan MS, Yuen MK, et al. Discrimination of an infected brain tumor from a cerebral abscess by combined MR perfusion and diffusion imaging. Comput Med Imaging Graph 2002;26(1):19–23.

[36] Ebisu T, Tanaka C, Umeda M, Kitamura M, Naruse S, Higuichi T, et al. Discrimination of brain abscess from necrotic or cystic tumors by diffusion-weighted echo planar imaging. Magn Reson Imaging 1996;14(9):1113–6.

[37] Hartmann M, Jansen O, Heiland S, Sommer C, Munkel K, Sartor K. Restricted diffusion within ring enhancement is not pathognomonic for brain abscess. AJNR Am J Neuroradiol 2001;22(9):1738–42.

[38] Tsuruda JS, Chew WM, Moseley ME, Norman D. Diffusion-weighted MR imaging of the brain: value of differentiating between extra-axial cysts and epidermoid tumors. AJNR Am J Neuroradiol 1990; 155:1049–65.

[39] Chen S, Ikawa F, Kurisu K, Arita K, Takaba J, Kanou Y. Quantitative MR evaluation of intracranial epidermoid tumors by fast fluid-attenuated inversion recovery imaging and echo-planar diffusion-weighted imaging. AJNR Am J Neuroradiol 2001;22(6):1089–96.

[40] Laing AD, Mitchell PJ, Wallace D. Diffusion-weighted magnetic resonance imaging of intracranial epidermoid tumors. Aust Radiol 1999;43:16–9.

[41] Burger PC, Heinz ER, Shibata T, Kleihues P. Topographic anatomy and CT correlations in the untreated glioblastoma multiforme. J Neurosurg 1988; 68:698–704.

[42] Johnson PC, Hunt SJ, Drayer BP. Human cerebral gliomas: correlation of postmortem MR imaging and neuropathologic findings. Radiology 1989;170: 211–7.

[43] Yoshiura T, Wu O, Zaheer A, Reese TG, Sorensen AG. Highly diffusion-sensitized MRI of brain: dissociation of gray and white matter. Magn Reson Med 2001;45:734–40.

[44] Stadnik TW, Chaskis C, Michotte A, Shabana WM, van Rompaey K, Luypaert R, et al. Diffusion-weighted MR imaging of intracerebral masses:

comparison with conventional MR imaging and histologic findings. AJNR Am J Neuroradiol 2001;22: 969–76.

[45] Castillo M, Smith JK, Kwock L, Wilber K. Apparent diffusion coefficients in the evaluation of high-grade cerebral gliomas. AJNR J Neuroradiol 2001; 22(1):60–4.

[46] Kono K, Inoue Y, Nakayama K, Shakudo M, Morino M, Ohata K, et al. The role of diffusion-weighted imaging in patients with brain tumors. AJNR Am J Neuroradiol 2001;22:1081–8.

[47] Sugahara T, Korogi Y, Kochi M, Ikushima I, Shigematu Y, Hirai T, et al. Usefulness of diffusion-weighted MRI with echo-planar technique in the evaluation of cellularity in gliomas. J Magn Reson Imaging 1999;9:53–60.

[48] Noguchi K, Watanabe N, Nagayoshi T, Kanazawa T, Toyoshima S, Shimizu M, et al. Role of diffusion-weighted echo-planar MRI in distinguishing between brain abscess and tumor: a preliminary report. Neuroradiology 1999;41:171–4.

[49] Guo AC, Cummings TJ, Dash RC, Provenzale JM. Lymphomas and high-grade astrocytomas: comparison of water diffusibility and histologic characteristics. Radiology 2002;224(1):177–83.

[50] Singh S, Leeds N. Postoperative diffusion imaging in the setting of craniotomies for brain masses: incidence of ischemia. Presented at the American Society of Neuroradiology 40th Annual Meeting. Vancouver, May 10–12, 2002.

[51] Kauppienen RA. Monitoring cytotoxic tumour treatment response by diffusion magnetic resonance imaging and proton spectroscopy. NMR Biomed 2002;15(1):6–17.

[52] Chenevert TL, Stegman LD, Taylor JM, Robertson PL, Greenberg HS, Rehemtulla A, et al. Diffusion magnetic resonance imaging: an early surrogate marker of therapeutic efficacy in brain tumors. J Natl Cancer Inst 2000;92(24): 2029–36.

[53] Valk PE, Dillon WP. Radiation injury of the brain. AJNR Am J Neuroradiol 1991;12(1):45–62.

[54] Fujikawa A, Tsuchiya K, Katase S, Kurosaki Y, Hachiya J. Diffusion-weighted MR imaging of carmofur-induced leukoencephalopathy. Eur Radiol 2001;11(12):2602–6.

[55] Chenevert TL, Brunberg JA, Pipe JG. Anisotropic diffusion in human white matter: demonstration with MR techniques in vivo. Radiology 1990;177: 401–5.

[56] Moseley ME, Cohen Y, Kucharczyk J, Mintorovitch J, Asgari HS, Wendland. Diffusion-weighted MF. MR imaging of anisotropic water diffusion in cat central nervous system. Radiology 1990;176:439–45.

[57] Melhem ER, Mori S, Mukundan G, Kraut MA, Pomper MG, Van Zijl PCM. Diffusion tensor MR imaging of the brain and white matter tractography. AJR Am J Roentgenol 2002;178(1):3–16.

[58] Ito R, Mori S, Melhem ER. Diffusion tensor MR imaging and tractography. Neuroimaging Clin N Am 2002;12(1):1–19.

[59] Pierpaoli C, Jezzard P, Basser P, Barnett A, Di Chiro G. Diffusion tensor MR imaging of the human brain. Radiology 1996;201:637–48.

[60] Basser PJ, Mattiello J, LeBihan D. Estimation of the effective self-diffusion tensor from the NMR spin echo. J Magn Reson B 1994;103:247–54.

[61] Shimony JS, McKinstry RC, Akbudak E, Aranovitz JA, Snyder AZ, Lori NF, et al. Quantitative diffusion-tensor anisotropy brain MR imaging: normative human data and anatomic analysis. Radiology 1999;212:770–84.

[62] Basser PJ, Pajevic S, Pierpaoli C, Duda J, Aldroubi A. In vivo fiber tractography using DT-MRI data. Magn Reson Med 2000;44:625–32.

[63] Mamata H, Mamata Y, Westin CF, Shenton ME, Kikinis R, Jolesz FA, et al. High-resolution line scan diffusion tensor MR imaging of white matter fiber tract anatomy. AJNR Am J Neuroradiol 2002;23: 67–75.

[64] Douek P, Turner R, Pekar J, Patronas N, Le Bihan D. MR color mapping of myelin fiber orientation. J Comput Assist Tomogr 1991;15(6):923–9.

[65] Pajevic S, Pierpaoli C. Color schemes to represent the orientation of anisotropic tissues from diffusion tensor data: application to white matter fiber tract mapping in the human brain. Magn Reson Med 1999;42:526–40.

[66] Maldjian JA, Schulder M, Liu WC, Mun IK, Hirschorn D, Murthy R, et al. Intraoperative functional MRI using a real-time neurosurgical navigation system. J Comput Assist Tomogr 1997;21: 910–2.

[67] Schulder M, Maldjian JA, Liu WC, Holodny AI, Kalnin AT, Mun IK, et al. Functional image-guided surgery of intracranial tumors located in or near the sensorimotor cortex. J Neurosurg 1998;89:412–8.

[68] Tovi M. MR imaging in cerebral gliomas analysis of tumor tissue components. Acta Radiol Suppl 1993; 384:1–24.

[69] Sha S, Bastin ME, Whittle IR, Wardlaw JM. Diffusion tensor MR imaging of high-grade cerebral gliomas. AJNR Am J Neuroradiol 2002;23: 520–7.

[70] Mori S, Frederiksen K, Van Zijl PCM, Stieltjes B, Kraut MA, Slaiyappan M, et al. Brain white matter anatomy of tumor patients evaluated with diffusion tensor imaging. Ann Neurol 2002;51:377–80.

[71] Price SJ, Burnet NG, Donovan T, Green HAL, Pena A, Antoun NM, et al. Diffusion tensor imaging of brain tumors at 3T: a potential tool for assessing white matter tract invasion. Clin Radiol 2003;58: 455–62.

[72] Lu S, Ahn D, Johnson G, Cha S. Peritumoral diffusion tensor imaging of high-grade gliomas and metastatic brain tumors. AJNR Am J Neuroradiol 2003;24:937–41.

[73] Gauvain KM, McKinstry RC, Mukherjee P, Perry A, Neil JJ, Kaufman BA, et al. Evaluating pediatric brain tumor cellularity with diffusion-tensor imaging. AJR Am J Roentgenol 2001;177:449–54.

[74] Koot RW, Jagtab AP, Akkerman EM, Heeten GJD, Majoie CBLM. Epidermoid of the lateral ventricle: evaluation with diffusion-weighted and diffusion tensor imaging. Clin Neurol Neurosurg 2003;105: 270–3.

[75] Witwer BP, Moftakhar R, Hasan KM, Deshmukh P, Haughton V, Field A, et al. Diffusion-tensor imaging of white matter tracts in patients with cerebral neoplasm. J Neurosurg 2002;97:568–75.

[76] Weishmann UC, Symms MR, Parker GJM, Clark CA, Lemieux L, Barker GJ, et al. Diffusion tensor imaging demonstrates deviation of fibers in normal appearing white matter adjacent to a brain tumour. J Neurol Neurosurg Psychiatry 2000;68: 501–3.

[77] Holodny AI, Schwartz TH, Ollenschleger M, Liu WC, Schulder M. Tumor involvement of the corticospinal tract: diffusion magnetic resonance tractography with intraoperative correlation. J Neurosurg 2001;95(6):1082.

[78] Holodny AI, Ollenschleger M, Liu WC, Schulder M, Kalnin AJ. Identification of the corticospinal tracts achieved using blood-oxygen-level-dependent and diffusion functional MR imaging in patients with brain tumors. Am J Neuroradiol 2001;22:83–8.

[79] Jellison NJ, Wu Y, Field AS, Hasan KM, Alexander AL, Badie B. Diffusion tensor imaging metrics for tissue characterization: discriminating vasogenic edema from infiltrating tumor. Presented at the American Society of Neuroradiology 41st Annual Meeting. Washington, DC, April 27–May 1, 2003.

[80] Tummala RP, Chu RM, Liu H, Truwit C, Hall WA. Application of diffusion-tensor imaging to magnetic-resonance-guided brain tumor resection. Pediatr Neurosurg 2003;39:39–43.

[81] Schulder M, Maldjian JA, Liu W-C, Holodny AI, Kalnin AT, Mun IK, et al. Functional image-guided survey of intracranial tumors located in or near the sensorimotor cortex. J Neurosurg 1998;89:412–8.

[82] Krings T, Reiges MH, Thiex R, Gilsbach JM, Thron A. Functional and diffusion-weighted magnetic resonance images of space-occupying lesions affecting the motor system: imaging the motor cortex and pyramidal tracts. J Neurosurg 2001;95(5): 816–24.

[83] Mamata Y, Mamata H, Nabavi A, Kacher DF, Pegolizzi RS Jr, Schwartz RB, et al. Intraoperative diffusion imaging on a 0.5 Tesla interventional scanner. J Magn Reson Imaging 2001;13:115–9.

[84] Guye M, Parker GJM, Symms M, Boulby P, Wheeler-Kingshott CAM, Salek-Haddadi A, et al. Combined functional MRI and tractography to demonstrate the connectivity of the human primary motor cortex in vivo. Neuroimage 2003;19: 1349–60.

[85] Maldjian JA, Schulder M, Liu W-C, Mun I-K, Hirschorn D, Murthy R, et al. Intraoperative functional MRI using a real-time neurosurgical navigation system. J Comput Assist Tomogr 1997;21(6): 910–2.

[86] Krings T, Coenen VA, Axer H, Reinges MHT, Holler M, von Keyserlingk DG, et al. In vivo 3D visualization of normal pyramidal tracts in human subjects using diffusion weighted magnetic resonance imaging and a neuronavigator system. Neurosci Lett 2001;307:192–6.

[87] Jolesz FA, Talos I-F, Schwartz RB, Mamat H, Kacher DF, Hynynen K, et al. Intraoperative magnetic resonance imaging and magnetic resonance imaging-guided therapy of brain tumors. Neuroimaging Clin N Am 2002;12:665–83.

[88] Martin AJ, Hall WA, Liu H, Pozza CH, Michel E, Casey SO, et al. Brain tumor resection: intraoperative monitoring with high-field-strength MR imaging—initial results. Radiology 2000;215:221–8.

[89] Bradley WG. Achieving gross total resection of brain tumors: intraoperative MR imaging can make a big difference. AJNR Am J Neuroradiol 2002;23: 348–9.

[90] Albert FK, Forsting M, Sartor K, Adams HP, Kunze S. Early post-operative magnetic resonance imaging after resection of malignant glioma: objective evaluation of residual tumor growth and its influence on regrowth and prognosis. Neurosurgery 1994;34:45–61.

[91] Khong P-L, Kwong DL, Chan GCF, Sham JST, Cham F-L, Ooi G-C. Diffusion-tensor imaging for the detection and qualification of treatment-induced white matter injury in children with medulloblastoma: a pilot study. AJNR Am J Neuroradiol 2003;24:734–40.

[92] Yamada K, Kizu O, Mori S, Ito H, Nakamura H, Yuen S, et al. Brain fibertracking with clinically feasible diffusion-tensor MR imaging: initial experience. Radiology 2003;227:295–301.

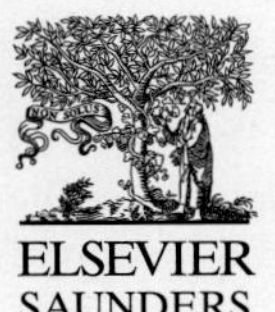
ELSEVIER
SAUNDERS

Neurosurg Clin N Am 16 (2005) 135–141

NEUROSURGERY
CLINICS
OF NORTH AMERICA

A low-field intraoperative MRI system for glioma surgery: is it worthwhile?

Dennis S. Oh, MD*, Peter M. Black, MD, PhD

Department of Neurosurgery, Brigham and Women's Hospital, Harvard Medical School, 75 Francis Street, Boston, MA 02115, USA

A decade ago, intraoperative MRI was regarded as a novelty and somewhat of a luxury. In the past few years, it has steadily moved toward becoming a standard of practice in the surgery of tumors located in critical areas of the brain. More and more neurosurgical centers are acquiring the equipment and setting up the facilities for intraoperative MRI–guided surgery. These facilities differ in several respects, including the design of the machine, the strength of the magnet, the operating room (OR) environment, and the surgical equipment required for performing surgery [1,2]. Each has its own set of advantages and disadvantages, and no single system has gained universal use yet as these systems continue to evolve. It has become clear, however, that intraoperative MRI has revolutionized the practice of neurosurgery, particularly in the management of brain tumors. It has enabled us to localize tumor margins and important neural structures precisely such that neurologic complications are avoided while ensuring maximal, if not total, tumor resection.

Intraoperative MRI has proven to be exceedingly useful in a variety of procedures. In transsphenoidal pituitary surgery, it has been shown to help localize the lesion, identify important surrounding structures, and, most notably, increase the amount of tumor removed [3]. The ability to verify whether there is residual tumor during surgery and to determine where it is in the resection cavity has been crucial in avoiding the common problem of residual tumor in the sella or suprasellar area. Intraoperative MRI has also been used in the evacuation of hypertensive hematomas in the basal ganglia and thalamus [4,5], with the benefit of adequate removal of hematoma in a minimally invasive fashion and observations of better neurologic outcome. Epilepsy surgery is another area in which intraoperative MRI has made a difference [6–8]. Temporal lobe resection is made more accurate in terms of removing the epileptogenic focus while maintaining the integrity of uninvolved brain tissue. Other areas of neurosurgery that have been elevated by intraoperative MRI include cyst aspiration, catheterization, and tumor resection in children [9,10]; laminectomies; thermal ablations; and functional neurosurgery [11].

Although the applications of intraoperative MRI continue to expand, its most important role is in glioma surgery. The difference it makes in achieving surgical goals for glioma patients, particularly those with low-grade types, has driven the development and growing use of intraoperative MRI.

Challenges in cortical surgery and rationale for intraoperative imaging

Inability of the eye to discern tumor

There are several reasons why intraoperative MRI is extremely helpful in glioma surgery. Many of these tumors do not have distinct capsules. As a result, the human eye is unable to discern where tumor ends and viable brain begins. This holds true even with the aid of magnification. Such a problem leads to inadequate resection of the

* Corresponding author.
E-mail address: dennis.oh@tch.harvard.edu (D.S. Oh).

1042-3680/05/$ - see front matter
doi:10.1016/j.nec.2004.07.010

tumor, because surgeons, not wanting to cause neural damage, tend to keep the resection to what is clearly gross glioma tissue. Conversely, it may also be that without clear margins, the process of resection could inadvertently cross over to functioning brain tissue, thereby causing undue neurologic damage. There are some gliomas that are radiographically evident but barely discernible in the surgical field. For all these concerns, intraoperative MRI has proven to be the best answer thus far.

By using instant feedback from intraoperative images, one is able to tell exactly what is brain and what is tumor. Coupled with neuronavigational software, the surgeon is made aware of where his or her instrument is in the surgical space. As a result, any minute piece of residual tumor in the most obscure corner of the resection cavity can be easily pinpointed by the surgeon and removed even when his or her own eyes tell him or her that it is all brain along the walls of the surgical cavity. Some tumors do not appear on T1-weighted images but show up nicely on T2-weighted or fluid-attenuated inversion recovery images. It is thus important to use all available sequences to define the tumor.

Brain shift

One of the most important neuronavigational issues that intraoperative MRI addresses is the occurrence of brain shift. It is common knowledge that after the dura is opened, factors, such as egress of cerebrospinal fluid, gravity, and brain edema, change the position of intracranial structures [12]. The shifting occurs throughout surgery, and the direction and magnitude of deformation are difficult to predict. The displacements have been documented to reach 1 cm [13,14] and can easily lead to directional errors. Such intracranial shifting becomes even more pronounced after initial tumor resection, when the surrounding brain collapses toward the resection cavity. It is for these reasons that other neuronavigational systems that make use of preoperatively acquired images fall short of the objectives of precise lesion localization.

Brain shifting also creates tremendous problems for locating small pockets of residual tumor after initial resection. Without intraoperative updating of images, one cannot even tell whether there is still tumor remaining in the resection area. Correlating points in the resection walls to images in a frameless stereotactic system cannot accurately determine complete resection even if the limits of the resection cavity seem to correspond to the borders of the tumor in the preoperatively acquired images. With intraoperative MRI, residual tumor is readily visualized and can be easily targeted with a coupled neuronavigational system.

Relation to important cortex

The surgical challenge is doubled when the tumor is located near eloquent cortex. Oftentimes, gliomas arise near the speech area or adjacent to the motor strip, making it difficult to be aggressive in taking out tumor. Being intrinsic tumors, gliomas are intimately related to surrounding brain tissue, and their borders are frequently irregular and tend to blend into brain. In such situations, information and feedback on the surgical field are essential for complete resection without injury to important cortex.

The identification of speech, motor, or visual areas can be facilitated by functional MRI, diffusion tensor imaging (Fig. 1) [15,16], and awake cortical mapping. Information from these modalities can be combined and superimposed on the intraoperative images and the surgical field for precise and comprehensive neuronavigation (see Fig. 1). This setup helps to reduce unnecessary hesitancy on the part of the surgeon by eliminating the guesswork that is otherwise involved in determining tumor edges and the continually shifting brain structures. It may not always be possible to achieve complete tumor removal, but

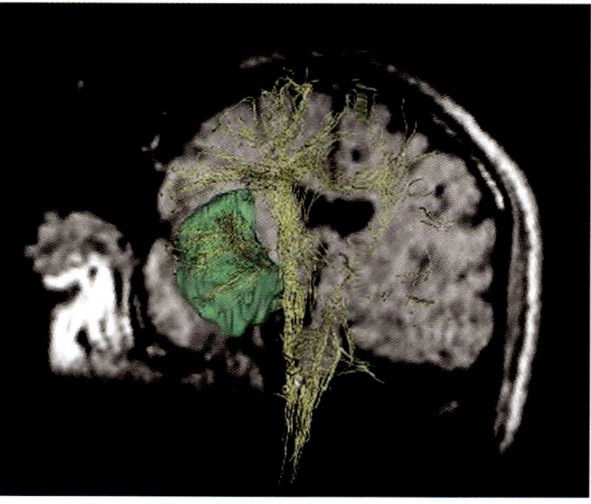

Fig. 1. Intraoperative image showing tumor (green) with added information on white matter tracts (yellow) derived from diffusion tensor imaging. (Courtesy of Ion-Florin Talos, MD, Boston, MA.)

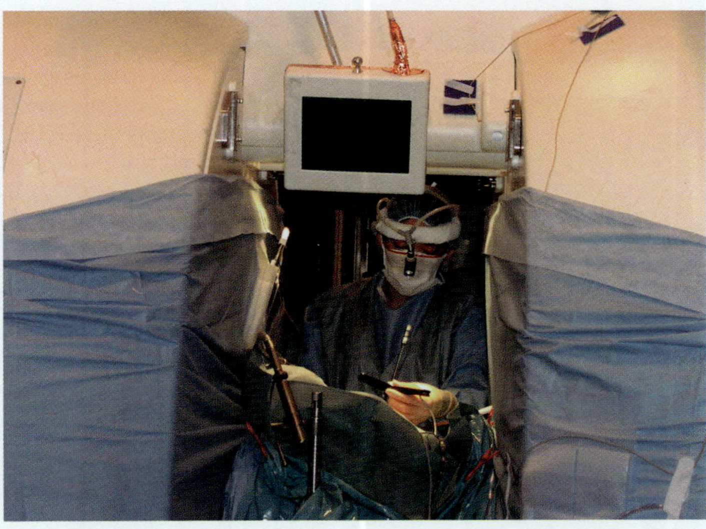

Fig. 2. Surgeon in magnet bore. 3-D slicer probe (held by surgeon) serves as a pointer for localization of tumor and structures. Overhead LCD monitor displays updated images and exact position of probe within the surgical field.

intraoperative MRI together with mapping techniques can take us to the edge of maximal resection just before it causes neurologic complications by removing all guesswork as to the location of tumor and functional cortex. The role of intraoperative MRI in defining the tumor margins and updating the positions of intracranial structures is invaluable in achieving the goals of surgery for tumors in important areas of the brain.

Extent of resection and survival

The issue of optimal resection is made paramount by the likelihood that greater resection leads to longer survival for patients with gliomas. Although there are reports that express doubt over the relation between resection and length of survival of patients [17], most agree on the recent evidence that a more thorough resection translates to longer survival time for patients with low-grade and high-grade gliomas [18–22]. With this in mind, it becomes clear that every effort must be made to maximize our ability to achieve complete tumor resection. In this regard, among all the recent advances in neurosurgery, intraoperative MRI is proving to be the most important innovation because it has enabled us to perform surgical resection to standards that are more exacting than ever.

Brigham and Women's Hospital Magnetic Resonance Therapy Unit experience with gliomas

The Magnetic Resonance Therapy (MRT) Unit at the Brigham and Women's Hospital houses General Electric's (Schenectady, New York) "double-donut" intraoperative MRI system in a dedicated OR setup. It uses a 0.5-T magnet system within which surgery is performed. The patient remains in the same position throughout surgery between the immobile magnets. This system avoids the troubles involved in moving the patient or equipment during surgery, although it does somewhat limit the space for the surgeon. The machine is coupled to a computer-based optical tracking system that allows interactive imaging and navigation through the use of a probe [23]. Overhead liquid crystal display monitors positioned atop the surgical space display the interaction between the probe and the brain image (Fig. 2). The surgical instruments are MRI-compatible.

Most cases that have been treated at this center have been gliomas. Of the 871 procedures done at the MRT Unit from June 1995 to January 2004, 618 (71%) have involved gliomas. This great proportion bespeaks the particular utility of intraoperative MRI in assisting glioma surgery. For reasons cited earlier, gliomas pose certain challenges to the surgeon that are best addressed with the use of intraoperative MRI. Indeed, a good number of these tumors were otherwise regarded

Table 1
Types of tumor in the intraoperative MRI

Tumor type	No. of cases
Astrocytoma grade 1	16 (2.6%)
Astrocytoma grade 2	104 (16.8%)
Astrocytoma grade 3	142 (23.0%)
Glioblastoma multiforme	106 (17.2%)
Oligodendroglioma	127 (20.6%)
Anaplastic oligodendroglioma	20 (3.2%)
Mixed glioma	33 (5.3%)
Anaplastic mixed glioma	22 (3.6%)
Ganglioglioma	20 (3.2%)
Oligoastrocytoma	14 (2.3%)
Anaplastic oligoastrocytoma	5 (0.8%)
Pleomorphic xanthoastrocytoma	4 (0.6%)
Ependymoma	4 (0.6%)
Central neurocytoma	1 (0.2%)
Total	618

as difficult to resect because of their location or previous incomplete resection [14]. The uneasiness, if not unwillingness, that one may otherwise have in a case if it were not done using intraoperative MRI is greatly reduced.

There were 142 cases of anaplastic astrocytoma (23.0%), the most common tumor operated on in the MRT Unit. This was followed by oligodendroglioma, which numbered 127 cases (20.6%). Glioblastoma multiforme and low-grade astrocytoma were also often encountered, with 106 cases (17.2%) and 104 cases (16.8%), respectively. The rest of the diagnoses were pilocytic astrocytoma, mixed glioma, oligoastrocytoma, ganglioglioma, pleomorphic xanthoastrocytoma, ependymoma, and central neurocytoma (Table 1). Of the 618 cases of intraoperative MRI–guided glioma surgery, there were 517 tumor resections and 101 biopsies.

The mean age of the patients who underwent surgery with intraoperative MRI was 41 years. The youngest was a 2-year-old boy with ganglioglioma, and the oldest was an 85-year-old woman with glioblastoma multiforme.

Extent of tumor resection

Several efforts have been made to quantify the added degree of resection afforded by intraoperative MRI through updated images and navigational data. Frequently, when it appeared that all the tumor had been taken out, intraoperative imaging showed residual tumor that needed additional resection (Fig. 3). Several reports indicate that additional resection on the basis of intraoperative MRI findings of residual tumor occur in 48% to 67% of cases [24–26]. Repeated imaging and subsequent resections are performed until the objectives of resection are achieved. The rate of total resection is consequently increased by greater than 20%; as a result, total resection is achieved in close to 90% of cases [6,27,28]. In situations in which complete resection is not possible without causing harm to the patient, the objective is to leave the least amount of residual tumor. Intraoperative MRI helps to bring the resection to this limit and produces a decrease in residual tumor from 32% to 4% for low-grade gliomas and from 29% to 10% for high-grade gliomas [29].

Safety and complications

Our experience has been that the surgery with intraoperative MRI is exceedingly safe and does not carry risks on top of those related to surgery in a conventional OR setting. Wirtz et al [22] reported no complications related to the imaging procedure in 242 cases. The potential complications in intraoperative MRI are similar in incidence to those in the conventional OR setting [11]. In fact, it improves our chances of avoiding postoperative hematoma complications by detecting any hematoma formation early. The reliability of intraoperative MRI in immediately detecting hemorrhagic complications has been reported [30]. In all our cases, an additional Heme sequence is performed before closing the scalp to check for any accumulation of blood in the operative site as well as elsewhere in the intracranial cavity.

As to prevention of neurologic complications, intraoperative MRI combined with cortical mapping techniques gives an unprecedented level of patient safety. In a study done at our center, 90% of patients who underwent the operation for low-grade gliomas were functionally intact after surgery [31]. The rest had temporary hemiparesis or a mild proprioceptive deficit.

Comparison with other modalities

Image-guided frameless or frame-based stereotactic systems enjoy widespread use in neurosurgery. These systems allow accurate localization of tumors and guide the surgical approach through tracking systems that employ neuronavigational software. However, their accuracy can only be as

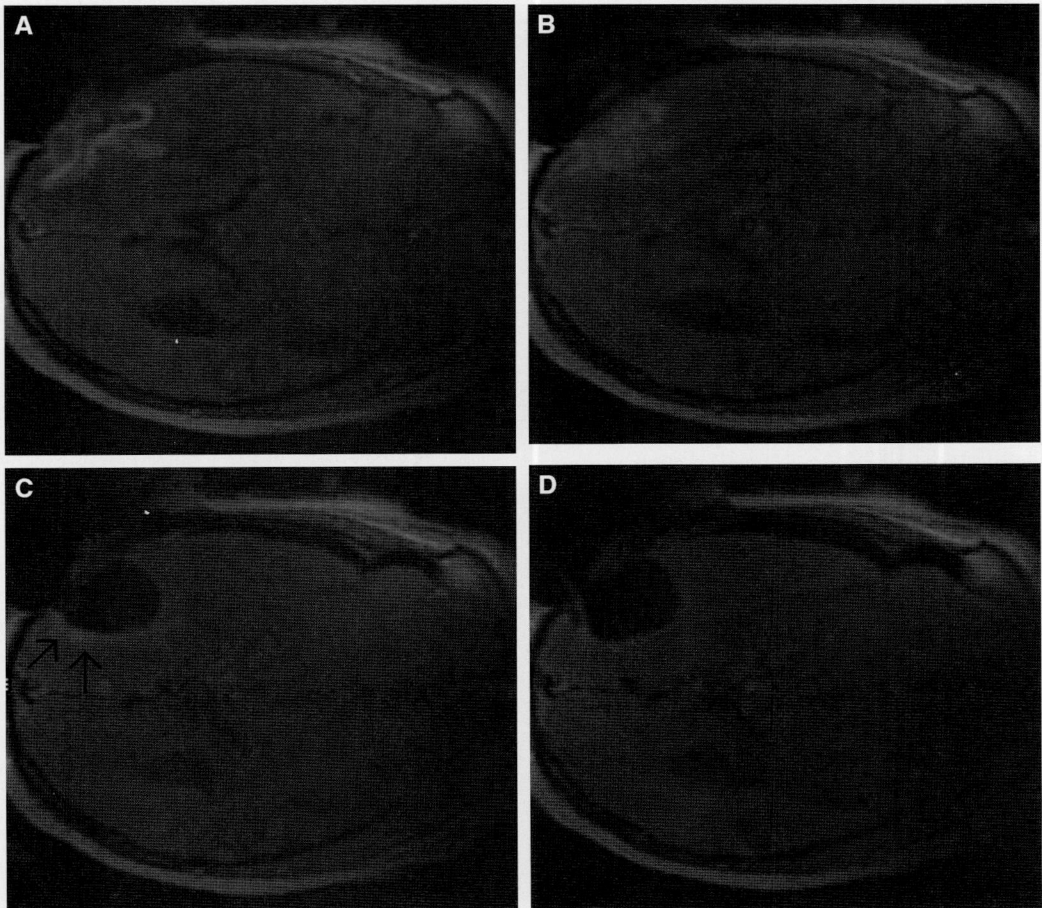

Fig. 3. (*A*) Intraoperative image of glioma before the start of resection. (*B*) Updated image after some resection. (*C*) Near-complete resection. Note residual tumor (*arrows*) that could have been missed without the aid of intraoperative MRI. (*D*) Complete resection.

good as the images on which they are based. Because the images are acquired before surgery and remain static, any change in the position of intracranial structures during surgery can affect navigational precision. Indeed, enough has been said in the literature about brain shift affecting the accuracy of such systems.

The same is not true, however, about other systems that use intraoperative ultrasonography, intraoperative CT, and x-ray fluoroscopy. They have the ability to update images during surgery and enable real-time or near–real-time navigation to obviate the concern over brain shift. They also do not require special instruments and equipment like most intraoperative MRI systems do. Each has its own set of drawbacks, however. Fluoroscopy and CT imaging are unable to provide multiplanar images, only two-dimensional images, and the image quality for soft tissues is poor. In addition, imaging can be limited by concerns over radiation exposure for the patient, surgeon, and surgical assistants. With intraoperative MRI, good-resolution multiplanar images can be easily acquired and the process can be repeated as many times as required until the goals of resection are achieved. As for ultrasonography, images are real time, easy to acquire, and good for cystic lesions. Intraoperative ultrasound is poor in delineating the borders of solid tumors, however, and is limited in its capacity to visualize small tumors. This limitation is particularly troublesome when looking for residual pieces of tumor during the course of resection. Although all these modalities currently have intrinsic limitations in their intraoperative use, there are efforts to combine their strengths to address their individual problems, such as using ultrasonographic data to update preoperatively acquired images in image-guided stereotactic systems.

Summary

As intraoperative MRI expands its presence, its use will undoubtedly increase in glioma surgery. The foregoing discussion makes it clear that its benefits are unsurpassed by any other existing system. Because of their radiographic characteristics and gross appearance, gliomas are particularly suited for intraoperative MRI–guided surgery. It enables us to localize gliomas and define tumor margins precisely when, during surgery, the difference between tumor and brain is not easy to discern. The images generated during surgery serve as a detailed and updated map within which navigation is performed with utmost precision. Its significance is further highlighted when dealing with tumors in eloquent areas of the brain, where uncertainties over the location of tumor in relation to important brain structures can hinder the removal of tumor. By providing accurate positional information and in conjunction with cortical mapping techniques, intraoperative MRI enhances the confidence of the surgeon to go forward with resection or to stop when reaching important cortex. It allows us to perform the resection to the desired limit without causing injury to nearby important structures, thereby preventing postoperative neurologic deficits.

The tracking system guides us in targeting each minute part of the tumor with unprecedented accuracy, and the ability to update images makes possible the constant evaluation of the progress of surgery. This near–real-time imaging can eliminate the errors brought about by the brain shifting that occurs throughout surgery. It also serves the important purpose of verifying the presence and position of any remaining tumor in the operative field. By means of sequential imaging, additional resection can be performed on any remaining tumor until imaging shows completion. The unwanted occurrence of finding residual tumor on a postoperative scan is thus practically eliminated. As a result, the surgical goal of complete or optimal resection can be achieved without any guesswork. Ultimately, what this means for the glioma patient is increased likelihood of longer survival brought about by a more thorough tumor resection.

Intraoperative MRI addresses many of the surgical challenges posed by gliomas. As it becomes more available, there will come a point when the prevailing persuasion will be that some poorly defined tumors near eloquent cortex should not be operated on without intraoperative MRI. In the final analysis, not only is intraoperative MRI worthwhile but it will, in all likelihood, become a standard of care for many glioma cases.

References

[1] Lipson A, Gargollo P, Black P. Intraoperative magnetic resonance imaging: considerations for the operating room of the future. J Clin Neurosci 2001;8(4):305–10.

[2] Jolesz F, Morrison P, Koran S, Kelley R, Hushek S, Newman R, et al. Compatible instrumentation for intraoperative MRI: expanding resources. J Magn Reson Imaging 1998;8(1):8–11.

[3] Martin C, Schwartz R, Jolesz F, Black P. Transsphenoidal resection of pituitary adenomas in an intraoperative MRI unit. Pituitary 1999;2(2):155–62.

[4] Bernays R, Kollias S, Romanowski B, Valavanis A, Yonekawa Y. Near-real-time guidance using intraoperative magnetic resonance imaging for radical evacuation of hypertensive hematomas in the basal ganglia. Neurosurgery 2000;47(5):1081–9.

[5] Tyler D, Mandybur G. Interventional MRI-guided stereotactic aspiration of acute/subacute intracerebral hematomas. Stereotact Funct Neurosurg 1999; 72(2–4):129–35.

[6] Buchfelder M, Fahlbusch R, Ganslandt O, Stefan H, Nimsky C. Use of intraoperative magnetic resonance imaging in tailored temporal lobe surgeries for epilepsy. Epilepsia 2002;43(8):864–73.

[7] King D, Baltuch G. Magnetic resonance imaging and temporal lobe epilepsy. Acta Neurol Scand 1998;98(4):217–23.

[8] Walker D, Talos F, Bromfield E, Black P. Intraoperative magnetic resonance for the surgical treatment of lesions producing seizures. J Clin Neurosci 2002; 9(5):515–20.

[9] Vitaz T, Hushek S, Shields C, Moriarty T. Intraoperative MRI for pediatric tumor management. Acta Neurochir Suppl (Wien) 2003;85:73–8.

[10] Vitaz T, Hushek S, Shields C, Moriarty T. Interventional MRI-guided frameless stereotaxy in pediatric patients. Stereotact Funct Neurosurg 2002;79(3–4): 182–90.

[11] Hall W, Liu H, Martin A, Truwit C. Intraoperative magnetic resonance imaging. Top Magn Reson Imaging 2000;11(3):203–12.

[12] Nabavi A, Black P, Gering D, Westin C, Mehta V, Pergolizzi R Jr, et al. Serial intraoperative MR imaging of brain shift. Neurosurgery 2001;48:787–98.

[13] Roberts S, Hartov A, Kennedy F, Miga M, Paulson K. Intraoperative brain shift and deformation: a quantitative analysis of cortical displacement in 28 cases. Neurosurgery 1998;43:749–60.

[14] Black P, Alexander E III, Martin C, Moriarty T, Nabavi A, Wong T, et al. Craniotomy for tumor treatment in an intraoperative magnetic resonance imaging unit. Neurosurgery 1999;45:423–31.

[15] Westin C, Maier S, Mamata H, Nabavi A, Jolesz F, Kikinis R. Processing and visualization for diffusion tensor imaging. Med Image Anal 2002;6:93–108.

[16] Talos F, O'Donnell L, Westin C, Warfield S, Wells W III, Yoo S, et al. Diffusion tensor and functional MRI fusion with anatomical MRI for image-guided neurosurgery. Ellis RE, Peters TM, editors. In: Proceedings of the Sixth International Conference on Medical Image Computing and Computer-Assisted Intervention. Springer-Verlag: Heidelberg, Germany; 2003. p. 407–15.

[17] Whittle I. Surgery for gliomas. Curr Opin Neurol 2002;15(6):663–9.

[18] Johannesen T, Langmark F, Lote K. Progress in long-term survival in adult patients with supratentorial low-grade gliomas: a population-based study of 993 patients in whom tumors were diagnosed between 1970 and 1993. J Neurosurg 2003;99(5):854–62.

[19] Sakata K, Hareyama M, Komae T, Shirato H, Watanabe O, Watarai J, et al. Supratentorial astrocytomas and oligodendrogliomas treated in the MRI era. Jpn J Clin Oncol 2001;31(6):240–5.

[20] Fernandez-Hidalgo O, Vanaclocha V, Vieitez J, Aristu J, Rebollo J, Gurpide A, et al. High-dose BCNU and autologous progenitor cell transplantation given with intra-arterial cisplatinum and simultaneous radiotherapy in the treatment of high-grade gliomas: benefit for selected patients. Bone Marrow Transplant 1996;18(1):143–9.

[21] Berger M, Rostomily R. Low grade gliomas: functional mapping resection strategies, extent of resection, and outcome. J Neurooncol 1997;34:85–101.

[22] Wirtz C, Knauth M, Staubert A, Bonsanto M, Sartor K, Kunze S, et al. Clinical evaluation and follow-up results for intraoperative magnetic resonance imaging in neurosurgery. Neurosurgery 2000;46(5):1112–20.

[23] Jolesz F, Nabavi A, Kikinis R. Integration of interventional MRI with computer-assisted surgery. J Magn Reson Imaging 2001;13(1):69–77.

[24] Wirtz C, Tronnier V, Bonsanto M, Knauth M, Staubert A, Albert F, et al. Image-guided neurosurgery with intraoperative MRI: update of frameless stereotaxy and radicality control. Stereotact Funct Neurosurg 1997;68(1–4 Part 1):39–43.

[25] Bohinski R, Kokkino A, Warnick R, Gaskill-Shipley M, Kormos D, Lukin R. Glioma resection in a shared-resource magnetic resonance operating room after optimal image-guided frameless stereotactic resection. Neurosurgery 2001;48(4):731–42.

[26] Staubert A, Pastyr O, Echner G, Oppelt A, Vetter T, Schlegel W, et al. An integrated head-holder/coil for intraoperative MRI in open neurosurgery. J Magn Reson Imaging 2000;11(5):564–7.

[27] Buchfelder M, Ganslandt O, Fahlbusch R, Nimsky C. Intraoperative magnetic resonance imaging in epilepsy surgery. J Magn Reson Imaging 2000;12(4):547–55.

[28] Knauth M, Wirtz C, Tronnier V, Staubert A, Kunze S, Sartor K. Intraoperative magnetic resonance tomography for control of extent of neurosurgical operations [German]. Radiologe 1998;38(3):218–24.

[29] Schneider J, Trantakis C, Schulz T, Dietrich J, Kahn T. Intraoperative use of an open mid-field MR scanner in the surgical treatment of cerebral gliomas [German]. Z Med Phys 2003;13(3):214–8.

[30] Rohde V, Rohde I, Thiex R, Kuker W, Ince A, Gilsbach J. The role of intraoperative magnetic resonance imaging for the detection of hemorrhagic complications during surgery for intracerebral lesions: an experimental approach. Surg Neurol 2001;56(4):266–74.

[31] Chabrerie A, Ozlen F, Nakajima S, Leventon M, Atsumi H, Grimson E, et al. Three-dimensional image reconstruction for low-grade glioma surgery. Neurosurg Focus 1998;4(4).

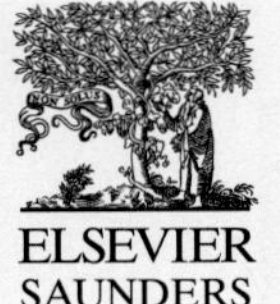
ELSEVIER
SAUNDERS

Neurosurg Clin N Am 16 (2005) 143–154

NEUROSURGERY CLINICS OF NORTH AMERICA

Intraoperative magnetic resonance imaging at 0.12 T: is it enough?

Michael Schulder, MD*, Jeffrey Catrambone, MD, Peter W. Carmel, MD, DMSc

Department of Neurological Surgery, New Jersey Medical School, 90 Bergen Street, Suite 8100, Newark, NJ 07103–2499, USA

Intraoperative MRI (iMRI) was first demonstrated by Black and his group [1] at the Brigham and Women's Hospital. With partners at General Electric Medical Systems (Waukesha, Wisconsin), a 0.5-T magnet was built in a specially designed operating room (OR) suite apart from the OR complex. Other investigators and manufacturers followed in their wake, using magnets of varying strengths and with different requirements for alteration of the OR to accommodate a powerful magnet [2,3] or of a radiology suite to become an occasional OR [4,5].

These brilliant technical innovations did share certain limitations from the perspective of the neurosurgeon. They moved the OR to an unfamiliar location or provided limited access to the surgical field, required complicated patient movements to allow for intraoperative imaging, had limited patient positions available, necessitated the manufacture of MRI-compatible instrumentation, or required special personnel to operate the systems. In addition, costs of these iMRI systems and their installation typically reached at least several million dollars. The PoleStar system was designed as a tool for intracranial neurosurgery, in conjunction with neurosurgeons, to make iMRI an accessible technique for anyone performing brain surgery.

* Corresponding author.
E-mail address: schulder@umdnj.edu (M. Schulder).

PoleStar intraoperative MRI

Specifications

The PoleStar N-10 (Odin Medical Technologies [OMT], Yokne'am, Israel) is built around a 0.12-T permanent magnet [6]. The magnet poles are vertically oriented with a gap of 25 cm. The gradient coils are located on the outside of the magnet, allowing the system to be parked under a standard OR table (Fig. 1). These gradients, equivalent in power to those in diagnostic MRI (dMRI), allow the PoleStar N-10 to provide useful images despite the low magnet strength. A limited field of view (FOV) of 16 cm × 14 cm × 14 cm, enough to encompass essentially any surgical field in practice, is imaged. The gantry (magnet and gradient coils) is moved by electrical motors controlled with a simple handheld device. The MRI computer, cooler, and gradients are in an adjacent room (a small storage room converted for this purpose).

An optical surgical navigation tool is integrated with the PoleStar N-10. Infrared-emitting cameras track passive reflecting spheres on a bayonet-shaped probe, similar to those used in commercially available "frameless stereotaxy" [7]. The magnet is automatically registered with the aid of a magnetic reference frame (MRF) that is attached to one of the magnet poles. A patient reference frame (PRF) is secured to the dedicated MRI-compatible head holder. By thus maintaining a known spatial relation between the surgical field and the acquired image, the navigation probe continues to be spatially accurate throughout the procedure. Movement of the patient's head relative to the head holder renders the navigation

1042-3680/05/$ - see front matter
doi:10.1016/j.nec.2004.07.005

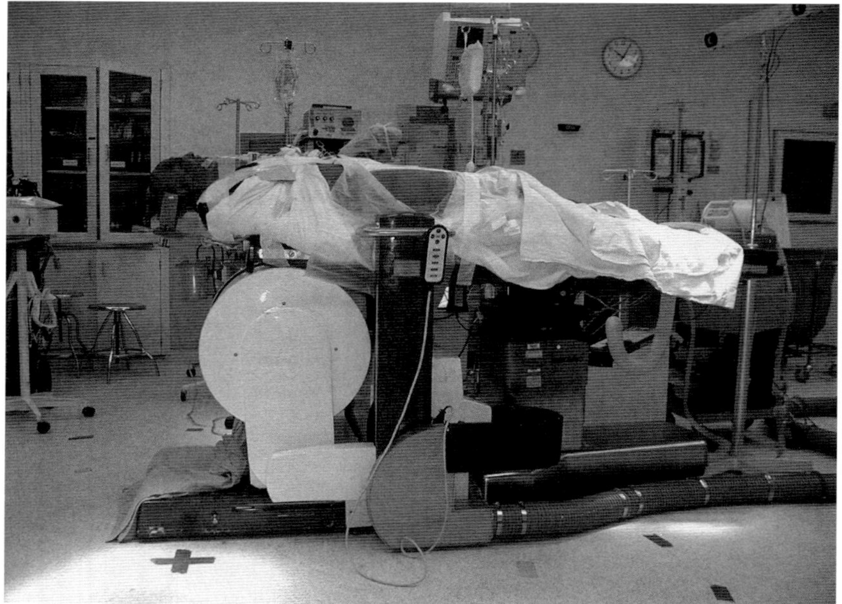

Fig. 1. PoleStar N-10 under operating room table.

accurate, in which case, repeat imaging and securing of the head holder corrects the problem.

The 5-G line of the PoleStar N-10 forms a near-hemisphere with a radius of 1.5 m, slightly elongated in the axis of the magnet poles. In practice, ferromagnetic instruments (eg, periosteal elevators or other hand tools) may be brought within 20 cm or so of the magnet poles without a significant attraction being felt. If, by any chance, an instrument is attracted to the magnet, it is pulled to the poles (ie, away from the patient's head). More complex tools, such as high-speed drills, operating microscopes, and ultrasonic aspirators, may be used in routine fashion. It is recommended that equipment needed for life support be MRI-compatible (eg, anesthesia machine, monitors), however. In most centers, the anesthesiologists have experience with such equipment from use in dMRI scanners.

No magnetic OR shielding is needed for the PoleStar N-10 thanks to the low magnetic field strength. Conversely, radiofrequency shielding

Table 1
Specifications of the PoleStar N-10 and N-20 units

Model Parameter	Odin PoleStar N-10	Odin PoleStar N-20
Magnet type	Permanent	Permanent
Field strength	0.12 T	0.12 T
5-G fringe field (radial/axial, m)	1.5	2.2
Shimming	Passive, active	Passive, active
Gradient subsystem		
Strength (mT/m)	25	22
Rise time to 20 mT/m/ms	<1	<1
Gradient cooling	Coolant circulation	Coolant circulation
FOV, ellipsoid (diameters, cm)	10 × 15	20 × 15
Magnets gap (cm)	25	27
Front end (gantry and magnet) weight (kg)	450	670
Gantry-driving mechanism	Electrical	Combined, electrical and hydraulic
Front end low position height (cm)	95	103
Gap between gradient coils (shoulders, cm)	48	58

is necessary to allow for imaging without radiofrequency interference (RFI) from unfiltered electrical sources. An innovative solution devised by OMT uses a pneumatically operated local shield, which is closed over the patient and magnet for imaging and left opened most of the time for surgery. This method obviates the need for potentially costly room shielding and permits more routine work flow throughout iMRI-guided surgery [8].

Early experience with the PoleStar N-10, however favorable overall, exposed some limitations of the system. The limited FOV was disorienting to some surgeons; the 25-cm magnet gap made lateral head turning problematic; and the posterior fossa was difficult to image, with only the cerebellopontine angle visible with the patient in a lateral decubitus position. In general, positioning was often a chore; the anterior skull base could be hard to image, especially in patients with large shoulders, and the image quality could be variable, especially when imaging during surgery [9]. To address these concerns, OMT has recently released a newer version of their iMRI, the PoleStar N-20. This new system has a 0.15-T magnet. It is slightly larger and heavier than its predecessor, but its wider magnet gap, expanded FOV, and other structural changes were designed to make its positioning and use generally easier and more reliable than with the PoleStar N-10. The PoleStar iMRI system, marketed by Medtronic Surgical Navigation Technologies (Louisville, CO), costs approximately $1,000,000 to purchase and install. The specifications of the PoleStar N-10 and N-20 are summarized in Table 1.

Stereotactic accuracy

We assessed the accuracy of the integrated infrared navigational tool, as previously reported [10]. A water-covered phantom was imaged in axial and coronal planes, and the onscreen distance from the virtual probe tip from the target center was measured. Measurements were taken in the center and periphery of the images as well as on images acquired in the center and upper limit of the magnetic field. Accuracy was about 2 mm or less overall, mirroring in essence the results obtained with frameless stereotactic instruments [11,12]. Accuracy was consistent in different imaging planes and throughout the magnetic field. There was a trend for greater accuracy in the center of the images compared with the periphery, but this was not statistically significant. These results are summarized in Table 2.

Table 2
Stereotactic accuracy of the PoleStar N-10 navigational tool

Plane	Range (mm)	Mean (mm)
Axial	0.5–4.3	1.8
Coronal	0.3–4.3	2.1

Surgical experience

Technique

The PoleStar N-10 is easily powered on, and the imaging program is begun. This can be done by the surgeon or an assistant. A dedicated physician extender, such as a physician's assistant or nurse, goes a long way toward ensuring the smooth operation of this or any other iMRI system. The OR table is reversed to allow room for the magnet. To begin, the PoleStar is powered on and removed from the protective cage while the patient is placed under anesthesia and lined. After patient positioning, the system is wheeled into place and parked under the head of the OR table. The patient should be placed in such a way that the magnet poles do not collide with the head or the PRF and that

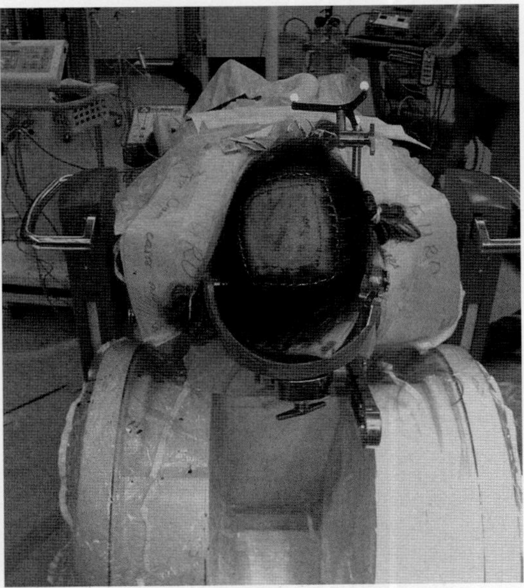

Fig. 2. Patient positioned for surgery with the PoleStar N-10.

shoulder pressure is minimized during imaging (Fig. 2). Some experience is needed to learn the nuances required to achieve this result.

With the MRF attached to the magnet and the infrared cameras positioned (typically at the foot of the table), the magnet is automatically registered. The navigation probe is placed on the scalp over the approximate area of interest; this now becomes the scan position to which the magnet can be moved. Imaging sessions should be as brief as possible and no longer than necessary. We start with an 8-second sequence labeled "esteady" by OMT (the generic name is a "true fast imaging steady state processing"). This sequence combines characteristics of T1 weighting (for tissue) and T2 weighting (for fluids) and has a high signal-to-noise ratio (SNR). Adjustments to the magnet position are made as needed using these short sequences. We then acquire a 1-minute T1-weighted image without contrast, followed by a 3.5-minute image enhanced with intravenous gadolinium. This sequence, with 4-mm thick slices, usually provides excellent views of the lesion (Fig. 3). Longer scanning sequences are used on occasion for thinner slices and hence greater stereotactic accuracy, a higher SNR, or more detailed reconstructed views. We use the PoleStar mainly for surgery on patients with tumors that enhance with contrast on T1-weighted imaging, but esteady or T2-weighted sequences are preferable in some cases (eg, for a low-grade astrocytoma).

When imaging is completed, the navigation probe is placed on standard landmarks to confirm accuracy and the magnet is lowered below the table. The probe is held in one place to ensure that navigation is not affected by magnet movement (as occurs if there is relative movement between the patient's head and the PRF). After standard preparation and draping, surgery is begun. When possible, the preoperative imaging coil is kept beneath the drapes, obviating the need for coil replacement before intraoperative scanning. Standard instruments are used, including drills, an operating microscope, and ultrasonic aspirators. The initial placement of MRI-compatible

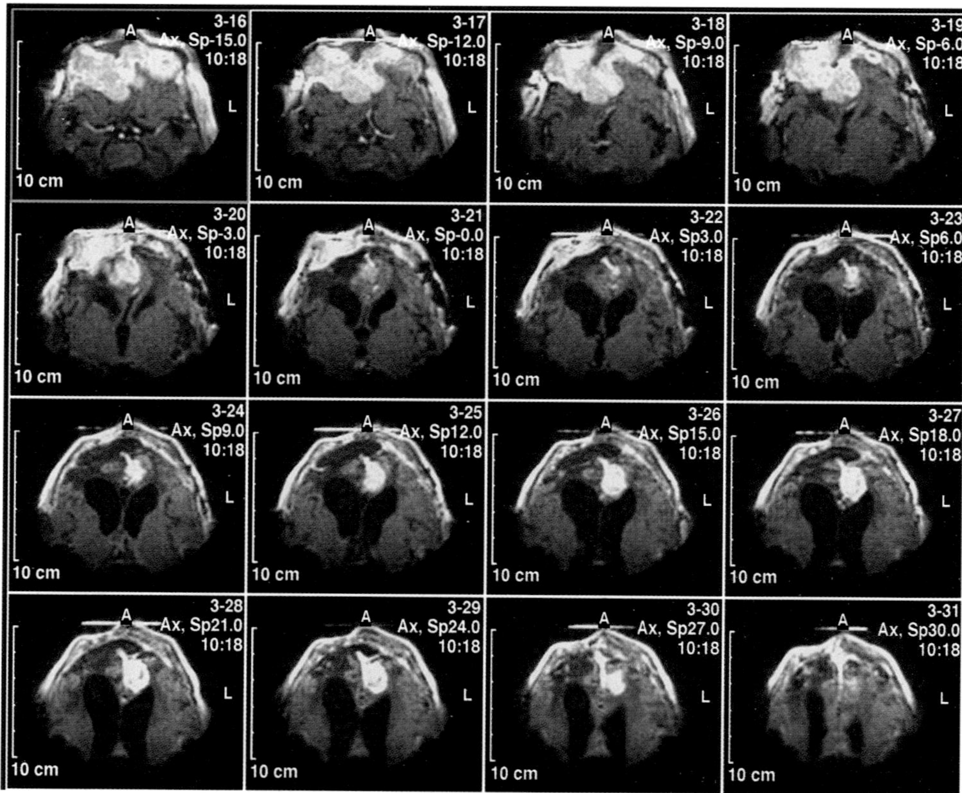

Fig. 3. Preoperative 3.5-minute image in patient with a recurrent meningioma.

retractors facilitates scanning later on. Surgery is continued until a new image is needed to rule out a residual lesion or to confirm that the surgical goals have been reached. To scan, the magnet is returned to the scan position without the need for new draping. The same imaging sequence as described previously is repeated. When appropriate, surgery can proceed with the magnet in the imaging position and successive scans can be performed (eg, for glioma resection; see case illustration of patient 1). Surgery is completed with the magnet lowered, and a final scan is obtained before the patient is awakened from anesthesia.

Patient data

Most surgery in the PoleStar N-10 was done for patients with intracranial tumors but not exclusively. These data are summarized in Table 3.

iMRI could not be obtained in 6 patients because of equipment failure. In 3 patients, planned iMRI was aborted because the patient's large body habitus made imaging in the PoleStar N-10 impossible. Neither problem has been noted to date after surgery on 12 patients in the PoleStar N-20.

Effect on surgery

In 61 of 184 patients undergoing surgery with the PoleStar N-10, iMRI revealed an additional lesion that warranted resection. Diagnoses in these cases were mainly glioma, pituitary adenoma, and skull base meningioma. In 24 patients, imaging demonstrated that the surgical goals had been reached and therefore prevented unnecessary and potentially harmful dissection from being performed. Diagnoses were similar in these patients, although the most common lesion was pituitary adenoma.

Table 3
Patient data: iMRI experience with the PoleStar N-10

Diagnoses			No.
Tumor			153
Seizures			9
Inflammatory			12
Hematoma			3
Cavernoma			1
Hydrocephalus			3
Infarction			1
Cerebrospinal fluid leak			2
Total			184
Procedure	**No.**	**Position**	**No.**
Craniotomy	118	Supine	157
Transsphenoidal	43	Prone	11
Biopsy and other	20	Lateral	13
Additional time (h)			**No. scans**
Range 0.25–4.0			Range 1–9
Mean 1.4			Mean 3.1
First 10 procedures 2.6			
Last 50 procedures 1.1			

Case illustrations

Patient 1

A 28-year-old man complained of headaches. He was grossly neurologically intact, but neuropsychologic testing revealed significant cognitive deficits. dMRI revealed a nonenhancing mass growing from the left centrum semiovale to the left lateral ventricle, and this was demonstrated on the preoperative image in the OR (Fig. 4A). A left frontal transcortical approach was made, with bipolar stimulation to identify and avoid the primary motor cortex and corticospinal tract. After initial resection, with the frozen section consistent with oligodendroglioma and intraoperative imaging showing residual tumor (see Fig. 4B), microsurgical removal was continued with the magnet raised (see Fig. 4C). The "Compare" function shows progressive resection over time, from left to right, until gross imaging removal was achieved (see Fig. 4D). The patient was neurologically intact after surgery.

Patient 2

This 64-year-old woman had undergone two previous craniotomies for craniopharyngioma 14 and 10 years earlier. She now presented with an inferior visual field deficit, and dMRI showed a recurrent retrosuprachiasmatic cyst (Fig. 5A). Now, with iMRI guidance, a right coronal burr hole was made. Using a skull-mounted Navigus guide (Image-Guided Neurologics, Melbourne, FL), the navigational probe was used to plan a trajectory and distance to the cyst. A catheter was passed, and 6 mL of murky fluid was aspirated. The catheter was left in place and secured to a reservoir. iMRI showed the cyst before and after drainage and confirmed catheter placement (see Fig. 5B).

Patient 3

A 25-year-old man with intractable seizures was found to have an enhancing right temporal mass. The PoleStar N-20 was positioned for

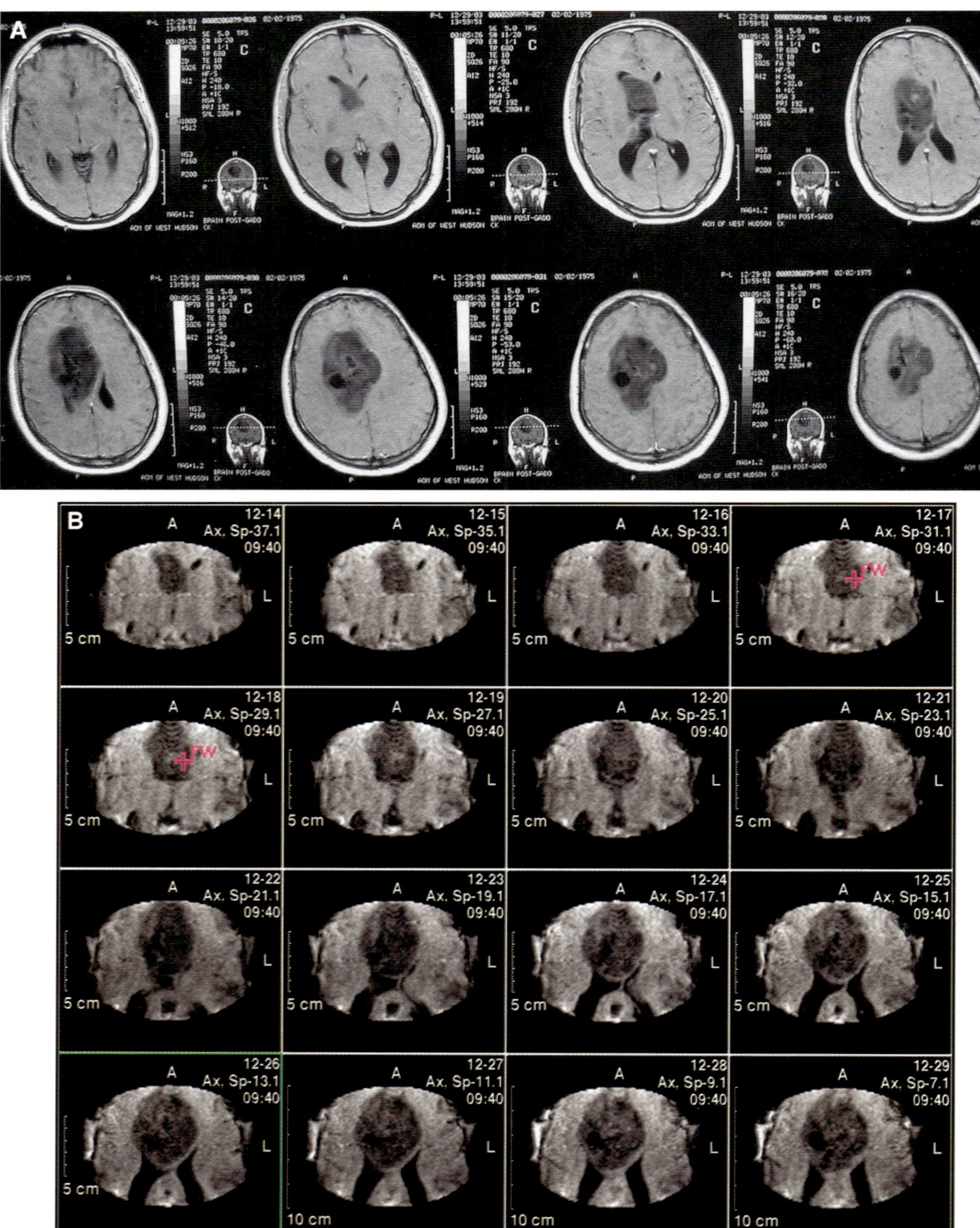

Fig. 4. (*A*) Diagnostic MRI in 28-year-old man with headache. (*B*) Preoperative image obtained with the PoleStar N-10. (*C*) Operating with the microscope through the magnet poles. (*D*) Compare function shows progressive removal at the midlevel of the tumor from left to right.

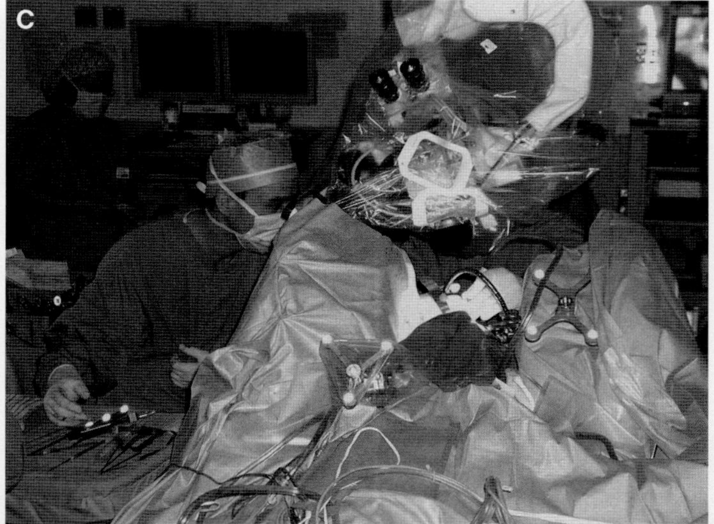

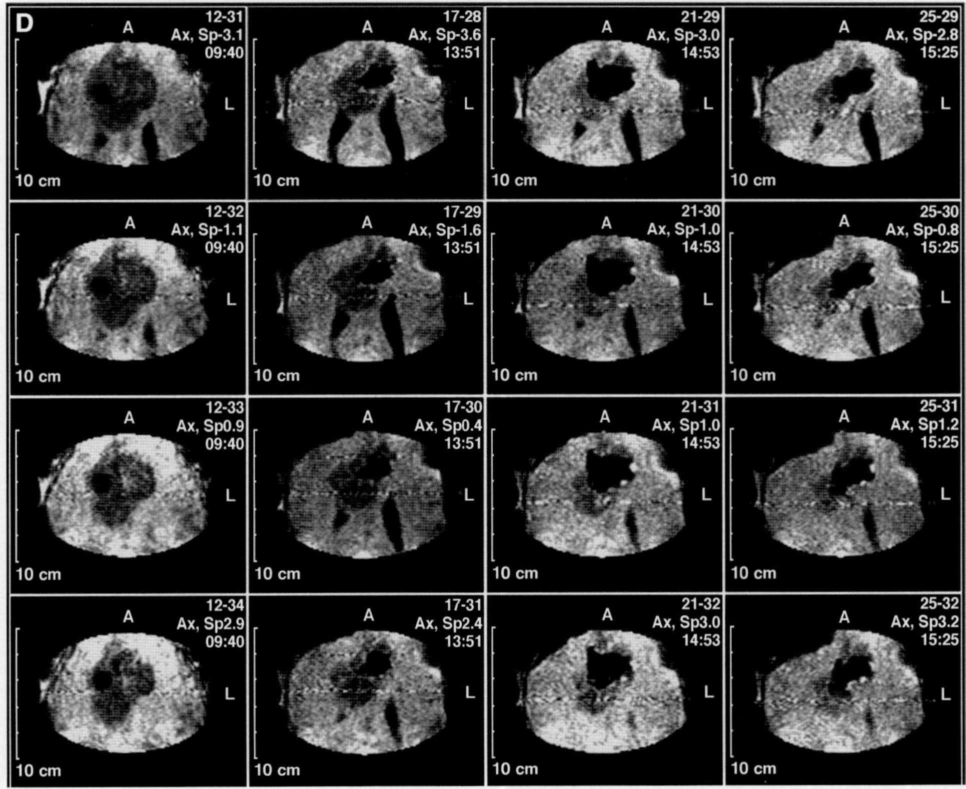

Fig. 4 (*continued*)

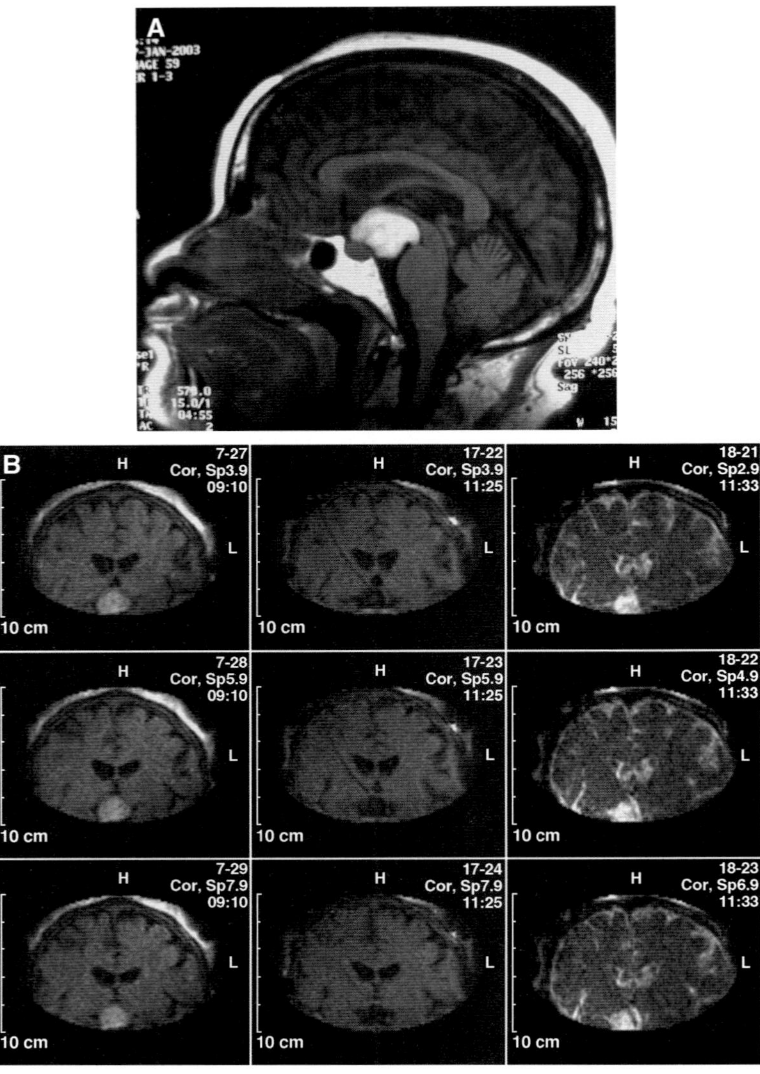

Fig. 5. (*A*) Diagnostic MRI showing recurrent craniopharyngioma cyst. (*B*) Compare display demonstrates cyst on T1-weighted coronal images before (*left*) and after (*center*) drainage; esteady scan (*right*) shows catheter in place.

surgery, and a preoperative image was obtained (Fig. 6A, B). The patient's large body habitus would have made imaging in the PoleStar N-10 impossible. After resection, the Compare function demonstrated no further enhancement (see Fig. 6C). Pathologic examination revealed a pilocytic astrocytoma.

Discussion

Is brain imaging in the OR necessary? It is fair to say that it is not required for the preoperative image, because any patient coming for elective surgery will have had such a study done before. Surgical navigation for the purpose of planning operative exposures and biopsy trajectory can likewise be done with images acquired, analyzed, and processed before the patient arrives in the OR [7]. This "decoupling" of imaging from surgery is, in fact, cited as an advantage of frameless stereotaxy over the frame-based approach [13]. What intraoperative imaging offers are two main advantages. First, and perhaps most dramatic, is the reduction in guesswork resulting from images

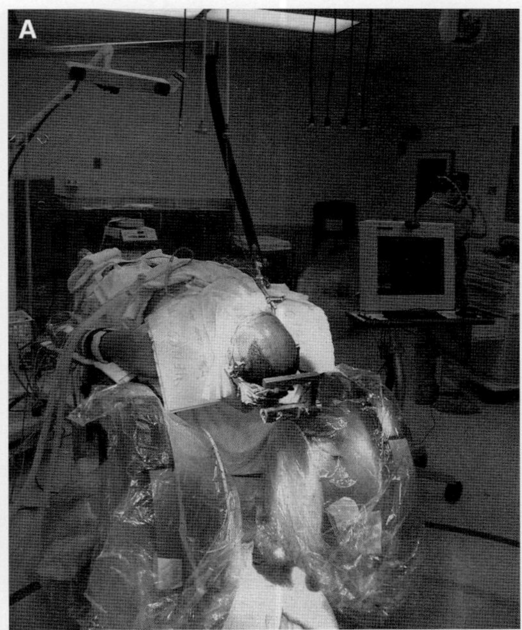

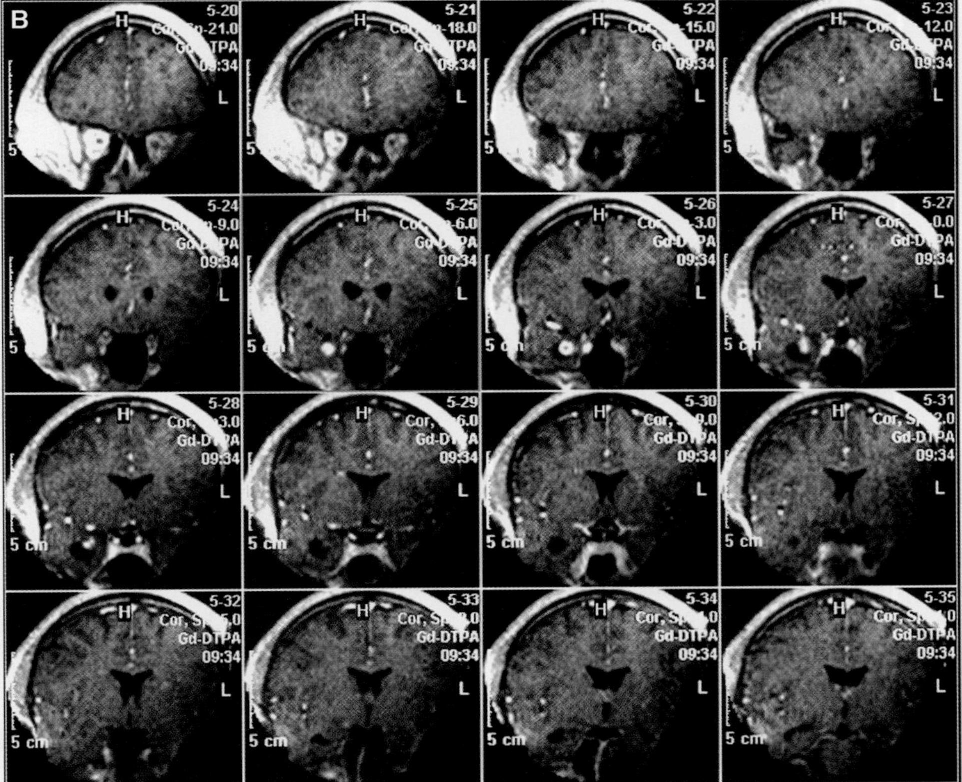

Fig. 6. (*A*) Patient positioned for right temporal surgery in the PoleStar N-20. (*B*) Preoperative coronal T1-weighted image with contrast. (*C*) Compare function before (*left*) and after (*right*) resection.

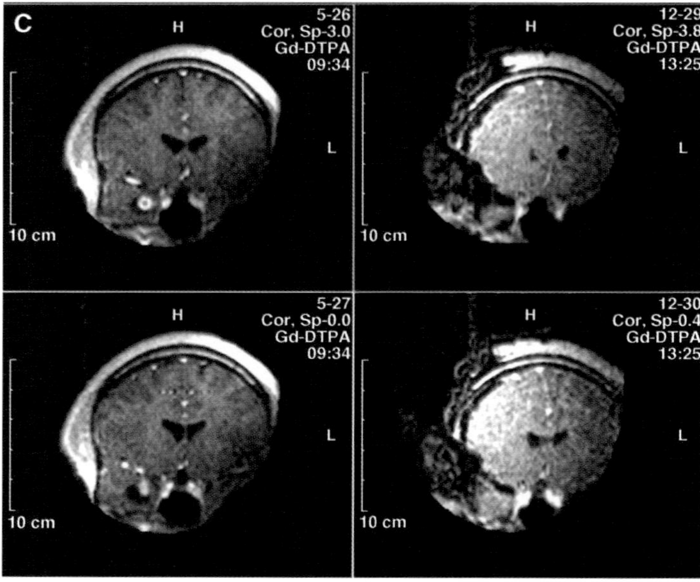

Fig. 6 (*continued*)

obtained during surgery. With the right kind of image, surgeons should no longer face surprises on postoperative scans, wishing that they had removed a large amount of residual tumor or that they had avoided the temptation to "go a little further," with consequent morbidity. After all, does any neurosurgeon who has the technology available not obtain an MRI or CT scan after surgery? How much better it would be to be able to do so during an operation. Second, by accounting for brain shift, surgical navigation can be updated rather than rendered useless or even harmful almost as soon as the dura is open [14,15].

For the foreseeable future, intraoperative imaging means iMRI. Intraoperative CT scanning, introduced 20 years ago [16] and recently refined [17], has certain advantages, including lower cost, lack of need for radiofrequency or magnetic shielding, and speed of image acquisition. It does involve the use of ionizing radiation and, perhaps more importantly, does not provide the soft tissue contrast needed for much brain imaging. Ultrasonography has been used in the neurosurgical OR and continues to be developed [18,19] but is unlikely to approach the imaging capability of iMRI. It does have the advantages of lower cost and easier integration into the OR, however.

So what kind of iMRI is necessary? As noted in the introductory section, various systems have been described and made commercially available. These have been categorized by magnet field strength [10] or by the ergonomics of patient versus magnet movement [20]. A more practical approach may to be ask how much iMRI we need. Is the ideal unit one that provides all the functions of dMRI or one that is the easiest to implement in a variety of ways? There are only so many patients with low-grade gliomas or pituitary adenomas, the indications often cited (for good reason) as being best served by iMRI. It is not possible to define a new standard for intracranial surgery for a relatively infrequent indication, nor can the issue of cost be completely ignored. Although some studies have shown early results suggesting the cost-efficiency of iMRI [9,21], much more work needs to be done in this area.

Innovative and exciting investigation of iMRI applications continues to be done at certain centers, where "full function" iMRI systems have been implemented [22–24]. These units provide not only images that are of diagnostic quality, or nearly so, but the possibility of "advanced" techniques, such as diffusion tensor imaging, functional MRI, or magnetic resonance angiography. In addition to their high capital costs, however, these units may require special personnel for their operation, mandate the surgeon to move out of the familiar OR environment, or have constraints on patient positioning—all for progressively fewer returns on increasing investment and effort. We would suggest that iMRI will become a routine part of the neurosurgical OR only when many, if not most, neurosurgeons can use it as they would any other "high tech" instrument, such as an operating microscope or "conventional" surgical navigation system. At present, and we expect in the future, it is low magnetic field strength systems that provide this unique combination of usable information and ease of use. We have shown as well that advanced applications may be possible at a low magnetic field strength, with the demonstration of motor functional MRI acquired in the PoleStar N-10 [25].

The data and images provided in this article demonstrate that for most patients who need elective intracranial surgery, and for most neurosurgeons, iMRI with a low field strength magnet and integrated navigation is an excellent adjunct that more than meets the requirements for intraoperative imaging.

Summary

Low magnetic field strength MRI provides the anatomic information needed for intracranial procedures in which intraoperative imaging is needed. Stereotactic accuracy is proven. The distinct advantage of this technologic approach is that it allows the neurosurgical team to operate an iMRI system with minimal disruption to the OR routine. Technical improvements are likely to increase the power and versatility of low field strength iMRI. Logic dictates that ergonomics and economics will make this the iMRI technique desired by most neurosurgeons.

References

[1] Black P, Moriarty T, Alexander E III, et al. Development and implementation of intraoperative magnetic resonance imaging and its neurosurgical applications. Neurosurgery 1997;41(4):831–42 discussion 842–45.

[2] Sutherland G, Kaibara T, Louw D, Hoult D, Tomanek B, Saunders J. A mobile high-field magnetic resonance system for neurosurgery. J Neurosurg 1999;91(5):804–13.

[3] Fahlbusch R, Ganslandt O, Buchfelder M, Schott W, Nimsky C. Intraoperative magnetic resonance imaging during transsphenoidal surgery. J Neurosurg 2001;95(3):381–90.

[4] Hall WA, Martin AJ, Liu H, et al. High-field strength interventional magnetic resonance imaging for pediatric neurosurgery. Pediatr Neurosurg 1998; 29(5):253–9.

[5] Bohinski RJ, Kokkino AK, Warnick RE, et al. Glioma resection in a shared-resource magnetic resonance operating room after optimal image-guided frameless stereotactic resection. Neurosurgery 2001;48(4):731–42 discussion 742–44.

[6] Hadani M, Spiegelman R, Feldman Z, Berkenstadt H, Ram Z. Novel, compact, intraoperative magnetic resonance imaging-guided system for conventional neurosurgical operating rooms. Neurosurgery 2001;48(4):799–807 discussion 807–9.

[7] Germano I. The NeuroStation System for image-guided frameless stereotaxy. Neurosurgery 1995;37: 348–50.

[8] Levivier M, Wikler D, De Witte O, Van de Steene A, Baleriaux D, Brotchi J. PoleStar N-10 low-field compact intraoperative magnetic resonance imaging system with mobile radiofrequency shielding. Neurosurgery 2003;53(4):1001–6 discussion 1007.

[9] Schulder M, Sernas TJ, Carmel PW. Cranial surgery and navigation with a compact intraoperative MRI system. Acta Neurochir Suppl (Wien) 2003; 85:79–86.

[10] Schulder M, Liang D, Carmel PW. Cranial surgery navigation aided by a compact intraoperative magnetic resonance imager. J Neurosurg 2001;94(6): 936–45.

[11] Dorward NL, Alberti O, Palmer JD, Kitchen ND, Thomas DG. Accuracy of true frameless stereotaxy: in vivo measurement and laboratory phantom studies. Technical note. J Neurosurg 1999;90(1):160–8.

[12] Schulder M, Fontana P, Lavenhar MA, Carmel PW. The relationship of imaging techniques to the accuracy of frameless stereotaxy. Stereotact Funct Neurosurg 1999;72(2–4):136–41.

[13] Dorward NL, Paleologos TS, Alberti O, Thomas DG. The advantages of frameless stereotactic biopsy over frame-based biopsy. Br J Neurosurg 2002;16(2):110–8.

[14] Dorward N, Alberti O, Velani B, et al. Postimaging brain distortion: magnitude, correlates, and impact on neuronavigation. J Neurosurg 1998; 88(4):656–62.

[15] Nimsky C, Ganslandt O, Hastreiter P, Fahlbusch R. Intraoperative compensation for brain shift. Surg Neurol 2001;56(6):357–64; discussion 364–5.

[16] Lunsford L, Parrish R, Albright L. Intraoperative imaging with a therapeutic computed tomographic scanner. Neurosurgery 1984;15(4):559–61.

[17] Hum B, Feigenbaum F, Cleary K, Henderson F. Intraoperative computed tomography for complex craniocervical operations and spinal tumor resections. Neurosurgery 2000;47:374–81.

[18] Unsgaard G, Gronningsaeter A, Ommedal S, Nagelhus Hernes TA. Brain operations guided by

real-time two-dimensional ultrasound: new possibilities as a result of improved image quality. Neurosurgery 2003;51(2):411–2.

[19] Hernes TA, Ommedal S, Lie T, Lindseth F, Lango T, Unsgaard G. Stereoscopic navigation-controlled display of preoperative MRI and intraoperative 3D ultrasound in planning and guidance of neurosurgery: new technology for minimally invasive image-guided surgery approaches. Minim Invasive Neurosurg 2003;46(3):129–37.

[20] Kanner AA, Vogelbaum MA, Mayberg MR, Weisenberger JP, Barnett GH. Intracranial navigation by using low-field intraoperative magnetic resonance imaging: preliminary experience. J Neurosurg 2002; 97(5):1115–24.

[21] Hall WA, Kowalik K, Liu H, Truwit CL, Kucharezyk J. Costs and benefits of intraoperative MR-guided brain tumor resection. Acta Neurochir Suppl (Wien) 2003;85:137–42.

[22] Black P, Jaaskelainen J, Chabrerie A, Golby A, Gugino L. Minimalist approach: functional mapping. Clin Neurosurg 2002;49:90–102.

[23] Hall W, Liu H, Martin A, Pozza C, Maxwell R, Truwit C. Safety, efficacy, and functionality of high-field strength interventional magnetic resonance imaging for neurosurgery. Neurosurgery 2000;46(3):632–41; discussion 641–2.

[24] Nimsky C, Ganslandt O, Fahlbusch R. Functional neuronavigation and intraoperative MRI. Adv Tech Stand Neurosurg 2004;29:229–63.

[25] Schulder M, Azmi H, Biswal B. Functional magnetic resonance imaging in a low-field intraoperative scanner. Stereotact Funct Neurosurg 2003;80(1–4): 125–31.

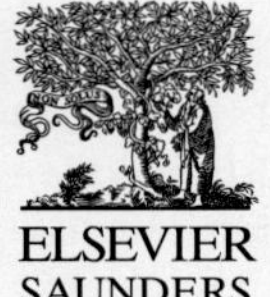

ELSEVIER
SAUNDERS

Neurosurg Clin N Am 16 (2005) 155–164

NEUROSURGERY
CLINICS
OF NORTH AMERICA

Adaptation of a standard low-field (0.3-T) system to the operating room: focus on pituitary adenomas

Borimir J. Darakchiev, MD[a], John M. Tew Jr, MD[a,b], Robert J. Bohinski, MD, PhD[a,b], Ronald E. Warnick, MD[a,b,*]

[a]*Department of Neurosurgery, The Neuroscience Institute, University of Cincinnati College of Medicine, ML 0515, 231 Albert Sabin Way, Cincinnati, OH 45267–0515, USA*

[b]*Mayfield Clinic, ML 0515, 231 Albert Sabin Way, Cincinnati, OH 45267-0515, USA*

Tumors of the pituitary gland were of interest to surgeons even before the establishment of neurosurgery as a separate specialty. Surgical treatment of the pituitary gland via the transsphenoidal approach evolved through many stages, from its ingenious introduction that was later abandoned and subsequently rediscovered decades later. In 1907, Schloffer pioneered its introduction, using the transsphenoidal approach to the gland via a superolateral nasoethmoidal route to remove a large intra- and suprasellar mass [1]. Two years later, Hirsch [2], who, like Schloffer, was from Austria, used the inferolateral endonasal transsphenoidal approach. In 1910, Harvey Cushing further refined the transsphenoidal approach by not only combining the best of the previous routes to the sphenoid sinus but by introducing the oronasal midline rhinoseptal transsphenoidal approach. This approach, with minor modifications, remains the standard surgical corridor used today by most neurosurgeons. In his remarkable Weir Mitchell lecture published in a 1914 issue of the *Journal of the American Medical Association* [3], Cushing described his experience using the transsphenoidal route for 247 pituitary adenoma cases.

Cushing noted two major drawbacks with this approach: first, the visualization of the field was suboptimal, and, second, the intraoperative assessment and removal of larger tumors with suprasellar extension were difficult. These difficulties were apparently major considerations in his decision to abandon the transsphenoidal approach and to adopt the transcranial approach. In the 1920s, Norman Dott of Edinburgh, a scholar of Cushing's in Boston, revived the use of the transsphenoidal route and introduced the approach in Europe [1]. In the early 1950s, Gerard Guiot of Paris studied this technique with Dott and further improved it with the introduction of intraoperative radiologic control [1].

With the innovative work and vision of Jules Hardy [1,4,5] in Montreal, interest in the transsphenoidal approach in North America was reborn. After training in transsphenoidal surgery with Guiot in France, Hardy made significant contributions to the neurosurgical field throughout his career, most importantly by the introduction of televised intraoperative fluoroscopy, operative microsurgical techniques, and the concept of pituitary microadenomas.

Neurosurgeons still face suboptimal intraoperative visualization of the pathoanatomic relations of the parasellar and suprasellar structures despite advances in magnification, illumination, microsurgical instrumentation, and technique during the last century. Limitations in visualization are especially pronounced in the surgical treatment of macroadenomas, which invade the cavernous sinuses or the suprasellar space. Implications of better visualization aimed at optimal tumor resection can be critical in the determination of the need for a second surgery or adjuvant therapy (eg, radiotherapy) and in patients in whom

* Corresponding author. c/o Editorial Office, Department of Neurosurgery, ML 0515, 231 Albert Sabin Way, Cincinnati, OH, 45267–0515.

E-mail address: www.mayfieldclinic.com (R.E. Warnick).

doi:10.1016/j.nec.2004.07.003

neurosurgery.theclinics.com

a potentially resectable residual tumor is found on postoperative imaging. Several intraoperative imaging tools have been used to optimize the extent of resection and achieve the operative goals of transsphenoidal surgery since Hardy introduced fluoroscopic guidance as the first intraoperative imaging modality [4]. More sophisticated technologies have included frameless image guidance [6,7], ultrasonography [8–10], endoscopy [11], and intraoperative MRI (iMRI) [12–17].

The use of iMRI, particularly low-field units, during transsphenoidal pituitary adenoma surgery has been a subject of special interest in recent years. The University of Cincinnati Medical Center has developed substantial experience with its use in intracranial procedures, including transsphenoidal surgery. In 2001, we reported our initial results with the Hitachi AIRIS II 0.3-T vertical-field, open-magnet scanner (Hitachi Medical Systems America, Twinsburg, Ohio) for pituitary surgery [15]. In this article, we analyze the literature and review the current status of intraoperative low-field magnets used in the surgical treatment of pituitary adenomas. We describe the evolution of this technology in our practice and provide additional follow-up on our initial patients.

Intraoperative MRI in transsphenoidal neurosurgery: background

Literature review

In the late 1990s, Black et al [18] and Tronnier et al [19] reported the first use of iMRI scanners in neurosurgery. Their efforts rapidly triggered interest in this technology, predominantly for brain tumors, within the neurosurgical community as evidenced by an increasing number of publications, [20–26]. Several centers published their experience with iMRI during transsphenoidal procedures for pituitary macroadenomas [12–17]. The objectives of these studies were assessment of the safety and reliability of iMRI and the effectiveness of this imaging on completeness of tumor resection.

One of the first publications on the use of iMRI in transsphenoidal surgery was a preliminary report by Steinmeier et al [25] on a mixed group of patients. Eighteen patients underwent transsphenoidal procedures for two craniopharyngiomas, 15 nonsecreting macroadenomas, and one cystic macroprolactinoma. Based on the iMRI information, 3 of 5 patients underwent a second resection for residual tumor. Testing the reliability of iMRI by comparison with follow-up MRI scans (2–3 months), the authors established a high correlation between the two modes of imaging, thus concluding that iMRI was a reliable imaging diagnostic tool.

In a second more extensive study from the same institution, Fahlbusch et al [13] used the same open magnetic resonance imager (0.2-T Magnetom Open, Siemens AG, Erlangen, Germany) for 44 patients who had similar characteristics, that is, nonsecreting intra- and suprasellar pituitary macroadenomas. With suspicion of a residual tumor in 54% of patients based on the iMRI scans, repeat exploration was performed. However, only 34% of these patients had residual tumors that were found and resected. Although these false-positive iMRI interpretations occurred in 16% of patients, use of this technique led to an increased rate of complete tumor removal (from an initial 43% to 70% after additional resection). In the authors' experience, the major advantages of iMRI were the ability to maximize the extent of tumor removal, avoidance of artifact interference with the postoperative MRI scans, and early planning for any additional treatments needed. Two other smaller retrospective reports by Martin et al [12] and Pergolizzi et al [17] confirmed the benefits of iMRI. We later discuss our institutional experience with low-field iMRI in pituitary macroadenomas.

Current intraoperative MRI technologies for magnetic resonance operating rooms in neurosurgical applications

The iMRI evolved around three basic magnet configurations: the high-field strength, 1.5-T, cylindric, superconducting short-bore magnet [26–28]; the 0.5-T "double-doughnut" configuration [29,30]; and the biplanar, open, low-field, 0.12- to 0.3-T design [15,19,20,25,31–34]. These systems differ with respect to magnet field strength, distribution of the magnetic fringe field, image quality, speed of image acquisition, imaging capabilities (eg, functional MRI, magnetic resonance angiography, magnetic resonance spectroscopy), ability to use real-time MRI, operative position relative to the magnet isocenter, and cost-effectiveness.

In practical terms, the performance of surgery in a strong magnetic field is a complex task that relates to the strength and design of the MRI unit. Major limitations of such an environment prohibit the use of ferromagnetic surgical instruments, anesthesia equipment, and conventional operating microscopes. The strength of the magnetic fringe fields in the iMRI unit is a function of the distance from the magnet isocenter. Therefore, the field strength decays as the distance increases.

As described by Rubino et al [33], three magnetic fringe zones have been characterized that define the usability of ferromagnetic medical and surgical equipment. Zone I involves the area between the magnet isocenter and the 10-mT fringe field or 20-G line. Only MRI-compatible instruments, patient monitoring devices, and anesthesia equipment may be brought into this area. Zone II extends between the 10-mT and the 0.5-mT fringe fields (20-G to 5-G field lines). Zone II allows the use of most standard neurosurgical instruments by trained personnel but requires an MRI-compatible operating microscope. Zone III, which lies beyond the 0.5-mT fringe field (5-G line), is safe for the use of all standard instruments, operating microscopes, and frameless stereotaxy platforms.

The ability to perform surgery in any of these three zones essentially defined the design and organization of the contemporary iMRI operating rooms (ORs). Of the three approaches described, each offers its own advantages and disadvantages. The first iMRI scanner developed at Brigham and Women's Hospital in Boston by Peter McLaren. Black and Ferenc Jolesz [18] was based on the 0.5-T double-doughnut system that placed the surgical field within the MRI isocenter (zone I). Thus, iMRI scans could be obtained in real time during surgery without transporting the patient. This set up was costly, however, requiring the use of MRI-compatible surgical instrumentation.

In contrast to operations performed within the magnet, Tronnier et al [19] and Steinmeier et al [25] described the development of an alternative approach in Germany, known as the "twin operating theater." This concept consisted of two components. First, a conventional operating theater within the zone III field allowed surgery to be performed with the use of ferromagnetic instruments and an operating microscope. Second, a radiofrequency-shielded OR was designed for use with a low-field (0.2-T) MRI scanner. With the ORs located next to each other, patients can be transported from one room to another during surgery, thus permitting the goal of intraoperative imaging. Obvious disadvantages associated with this system were the inconvenience of transporting the patients, increased OR time, and risk of contamination.

A third approach described by the same authors [19,25] was initially used in small series for patients undergoing brain biopsies and transsphenoidal procedures. Rubino et al [33], Fahlbusch et al [13], Bohinski et al [15,31], and others further developed and used this approach. In a specially designed iMRI sterile OR, surgeons could operate within the weak magnetic fringe fields (beyond the 5-G line, zone III) and in close proximity to the magnet. Rotation of the table into the magnet volume allowed intraoperative images to be obtained quickly. This third concept combined the best of the first two approaches, namely, the ease of performing intraoperative imaging and the use of standard ferromagnetic equipment, and avoided patient transportation, time delays, and contamination to a sterile field.

Intraoperative MRI Center at the University of Cincinnati

Most experience with the use of iMRI in transsphenoidal surgery in the treatment of pituitary adenomas was acquired with low-field magnet scanners [12–17]. At our center, we developed an iMRI facility that includes a low-field magnet (Hitachi AIRIS II, 0.3-T, vertical-field, open-magnet imaging system).

Organization and intraoperative MRI setup

Our setup is based on the twin operating theater concept [19,25] in which one OR, which houses the Hitachi AIRIS II imaging magnet, links to a separate but adjacent conventional OR (Fig. 1). Our iMRI OR functions as a shared resource that provides services for diagnostic and intraoperative imaging. The addition of convenient access to the iMRI OR for outpatients undergoing diagnostic imaging distinguishes our facility from other previously described OR designs. This access permits the facility to be used not only for surgical procedures but for diagnostic imaging. With a location at a site close to but distinct from the main hospital OR suites, the iMRI center was also designed to incorporate scrub sinks and a self-sufficient material storage room.

The unit undergoes sterile cleansing between each diagnostic and intraoperative imaging session according to the requirements of the Joint Commission on accreditation of Health Care Organizations for OR environments. The facility was strategically built in the basement of the

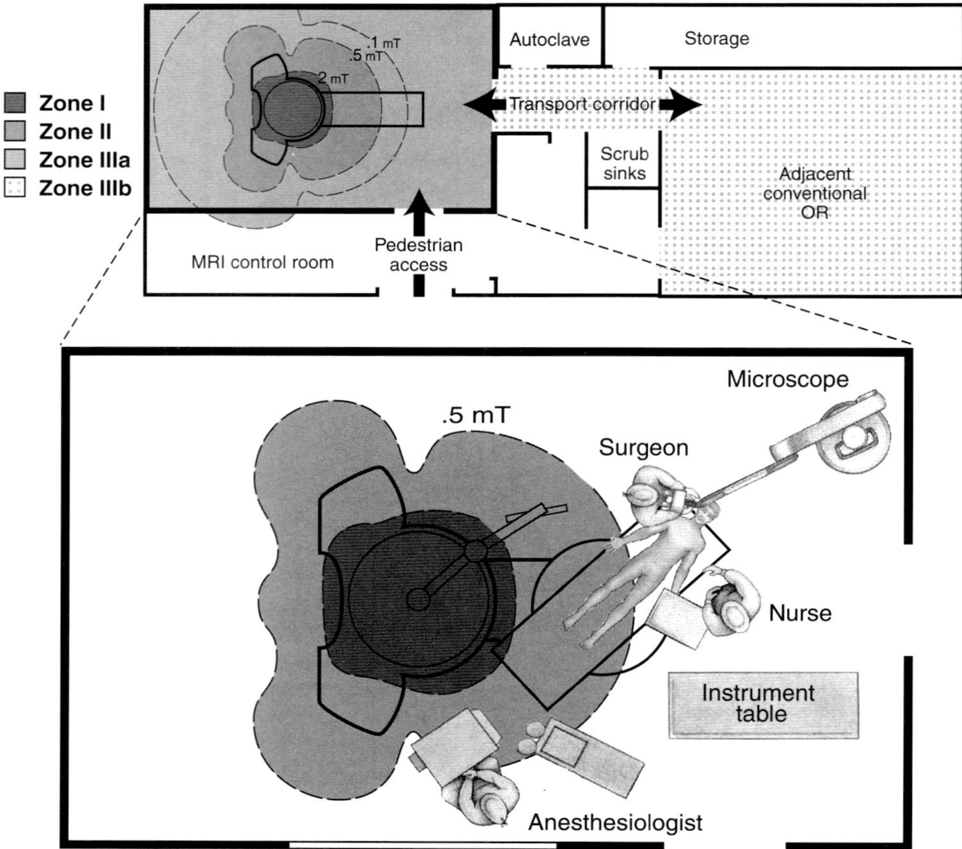

Fig. 1. Floor plan and layout of our twin operating theater design at the University of Cincinnati Medical Center. Transsphenoidal procedures are performed in the intraoperative MRI operating room. Patient positioning in magnetic fringe field zone III with the tabletop rotated to 120° (operative position). (*Courtesy of* the Mayfield Clinic, Cincinnati, OH.)

university hospital close to key departments (ie, radiology and emergency), the intensive care unit, and the main OR complex. This proximity facilitates patient transportation, pre- and postanesthesia care, and radiology interpretation of the scans.

Description of the low-field Hitachi magnet

The imaging device is a commercially available Hitachi AIRIS II, 0.3-T, vertical-field, open MRI unit that is used at many centers solely for diagnostic imaging purposes. The system has two horizontally oriented magnets that are separated by a distance of 17 in. The magnet has a vertical-field dual-column design that is common to the open MRI concept (Fig. 2). The magnet generates a horizontal spatial distribution of the static magnetic field (see Fig. 1B). The installation of this magnet in a fully functional OR environment at the University of Cincinnati Medical Center represents the first instillation of its kind in the United States.

Additional features of this scanner include a variable-position, radiofrequency-shielded, liquid crystal display (LCD) monitor; open-design radiofrequency receiver coils; a gantry illumination system; and custom-designed sterile gantry drapes. Two radiofrequency receiver coils were developed specifically for this setting. First, a nonsterile double-loop solenoid coil is sterile draped within the operative field. Second, a sterilizable single-loop solenoid coil can be placed directly in the operative field. Both coils must be placed vertically within the magnetic field for optimal image quality. The Hitachi AIRIS II table has

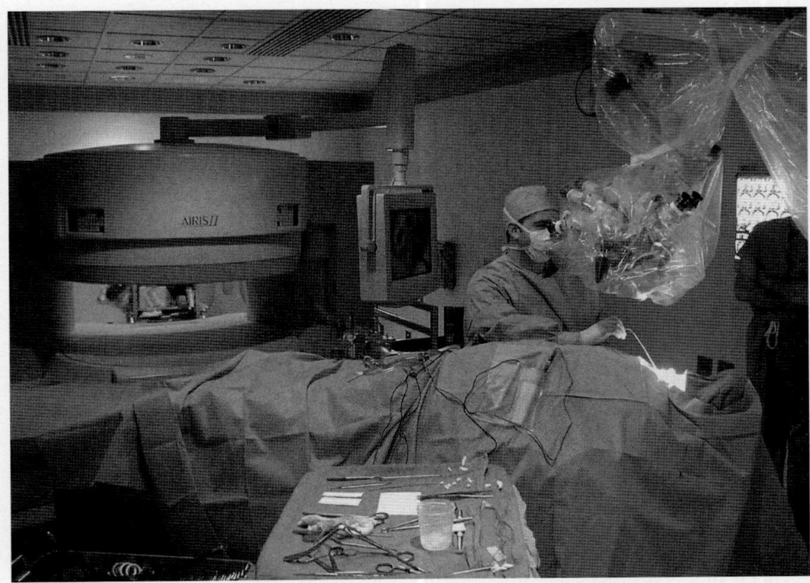

Fig. 2. Hitachi AIRIS II 0.3-T, vertical-field, open MRI system within its own operating room at the University of Cincinnati Medical Center during a transsphenoidal tumor resection. (*Courtesy of* the Mayfield Clinic, Cincinnati, OH.)

motorized controls that permit not only horizontal and vertical movement but rotation from 0° to 120° (0° corresponds to the patient's head located at the isocenter of the magnet, and 120° lies beyond the 5-G field line). The addition of this table to the system brought increased maneuverability during the patient positioning part of the process.

Practical aspects of transsphenoidal procedures in the intraoperative MRI environment: anesthesia, patient positioning, surgery, and imaging

Induction of anesthesia and intubation with a nonferromagnetic endotracheal tube is typically performed with the patient lying on a stretcher positioned next to the Hitachi AIRIS II tabletop. The gas exchange circuit is passed through the magnet and connected to an MRI-compatible anesthesia machine (Narcomed MRI; North American Drager, Telford, Pennsylvania), which is located opposite the scanner table. Vital signs are monitored with an MRI-compatible monitor (Omni-Trak 3150; In Vivo Research, Orlando, Florida). After intubation, the patient is transferred onto the tabletop, which is rotated to 120° (see Fig. 2) [35]. This rotation (as described previously) positions the patient's head in zone III, thus allowing the safe use of standard surgical instruments and the operating microscope. When positioning is completed, a double-loop solenoid coil is placed around the patient's head, centered at the level of the sella. Sterile draping of the operative field is performed in a standard manner.

A standard transsphenoidal sublabial-transseptal approach [36] is performed by an otolaryngologist, with exposure facilitated by an MRI-compatible titanium speculum. It can be left in place during imaging because it does not cause MRI artifacts in the sellar region. Confirmation of the surgical trajectory to the sella at the completion of the otolaryngologist's part of the exposure is occasionally obtained by imaging before opening the sellar floor. The MRI-compatible titanium speculum or a syringe filled with gadolinium contrast is used as guidance (Fig. 3). X-ray fluoroscopy was not used for localization in any procedure.

The microneurosurgical part of the procedure is also performed in a standard manner with the use of typical surgical instruments and a neurosurgical operating microscope (OPMI NC-4; Carl Zeiss, Thornwood, New York). All procedures are performed by four senior neurosurgeons whose combined experience exceeds 1500 transsphenoidal surgeries. A variable-position radiofrequency-shielded LCD monitor displays the microscope's field of view for the scrub nurse and observers in

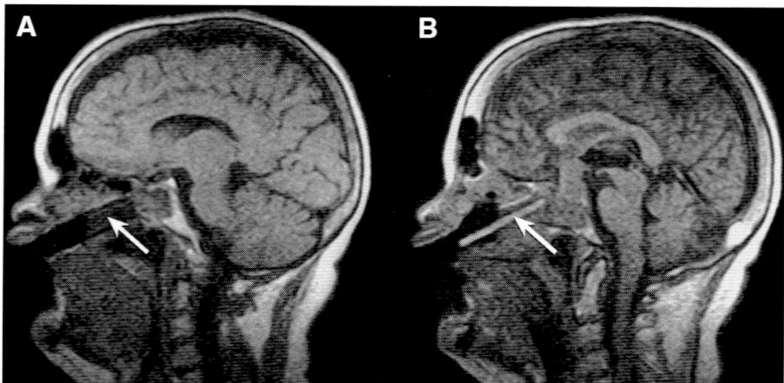

Fig. 3. Intraoperative MRI was occasionally used to verify the trajectory to the floor of the sella before its exposure. (*A*) Sagittal midline image with a cylinder-shaped signal void from the titanium speculum pointing at the sella (*arrow*). (*B*) An alternative localization technique using a tuberculin syringe filled with gadolinium (*arrow*). (*Courtesy of* the Mayfield Clinic, Cincinnati, OH.)

the room. During the surgical part of the procedure, the rotating tabletop remains angled at 120° (operative position). The procedure continues until the surgeon believes that all the accessible neoplasm has been removed. The table with the MRI-compatible speculum in place is swiveled back into the magnet to 0° for image acquisition. These steps, which can be completed within seconds, require neither additional manpower nor excessive OR time for repositioning. At the completion of iMRI, the patient is returned to operating position for closure or re-exploration. Second and, occasionally, third intraoperative imaging procedures can be performed to verify the completeness of tumor removal.

At the completion of the initial tumor resection, intraoperative imaging consisted of a T1-weighted, localizing, precontrast scout sequence in the sagittal plane (repetition time [TR] = 340 milliseconds, echo time [TE] = 20 milliseconds, 240-mm field of view [FOV], 4-mm slice thickness, 0.5-mm slice gap, acquisition time = 1 minutes 27 seconds), followed by precontrast sequences in the coronal plane (TR = 450 milliseconds, TE = 20 milliseconds, 220-mm FOV, 3-mm slice thickness, 0.5-mm slice gap, acquisition time = 5 minutes 46 seconds). If a satisfactory resection was established, postcontrast coronal sequences were performed for confirmation purposes. In cases in which additional resection was needed, the contrast imaging was delayed until the repeat precontrast sequences demonstrated that the goal of the surgery was achieved. Our practice is to obtain postcontrast images after the completion of surgical removal so as to avoid artifacts from a contrast leak in the surgical field, which can confuse interpretation of the images. The contrast agent used was Omniscan (gadodiamide, 287 mg/mL; Nycomed, Princeton, New Jersey). A standard single dose (0.2 mL/kg [0.1 mmol/kg]) of Omniscan was administered in all patients. The time for the intraoperative imaging session, including review of the images and patient positioning adjustments, averaged 30 minutes. Typically, the surgical team remained scrubbed during this first imaging process. The surgeon was then able to review the images inside the iMRI OR with the in-suite MRI-compatible monitor. A final intraoperative imaging procedure was not performed routinely after closure to conserve operative time and resources. We obtain postoperative imaging within 1 to 3 months after surgery, particularly in patients who require additional treatment (eg, stereotactic radiosurgery).

Results

Between 1998 and 2004 at the University of Cincinnati Medical Center, 115 patients with pituitary macroadenomas underwent iMRI-assisted transsphenoidal surgery. The first 30 of these patients were included in a prospective study protocol previously reported [15]. We summarize our experience with this group of patients and discuss their additional follow-up.

Patient characteristics

Patients included 18 men and 12 women who ranged in age from 24 to 74 years (mean = 51 years). Twenty-six patients had newly diagnosed tumors, and 4 patients presented with recurrent disease after previous surgical resection. The clinical presentation included visual field deficits in 16 patients, endocrine disturbances (acromegaly in 6 patients, hypopituitarism in 3 patients, and Cushing's disease in 2 patients), and headaches in 3 patients. All hormone-secreting tumors were confirmed with immunostaining. Tumor size was consistent with macroadenomas in all cases and averaged 27 mm in maximal diameter. All patients had suprasellar extension of the tumor, including grade 1 (5 patients), grade 2 (16 patients), and grade 3 (9 patients) according to the scale of Knosp et al [37]. Patient information was collected prospectively and analyzed in a standardized computer database.

Surgical results and clinical follow-up

Of the first 30 iMRI surgical procedures, 29 were completed uneventfully; one patient had an unsuspected intraventricular hemorrhage that was detected by intraoperative scans and treated successfully with an emergent craniotomy. Second and third re-explorations were performed for resection of residual tumors demonstrated on iMRI in 19 patients and 3 patients, respectively. The goals of surgery varied based on the extent of tumor growth into the cavernous sinuses and suprasellar space. Although we strive for optimal tumor removal, the planned surgical goal in some cases was clearly subtotal resection (STR). For example, for 13 patients with macroadenomas of grade 2 or greater, the surgical goal was decompression of the optic chiasm, followed by radiation treatment to the residual tumor that invaded the cavernous sinuses. The criteria for optimal STR based on the MRI scans included the absence of residual resectable tumor 3 mm or greater from the optic apparatus and the presence of a noninvasive plane along the cavernous sinuses. In the remaining 17 patients, who had no imaging evidence of invasive disease, gross total resection (GTR) was planned. iMRI successfully demonstrated residual resectable tumor in 56% of patients after GTR and in 77% of patients after STR. GTR was typically accomplished after a second exploration when imaging indicated the presence of residual tumor (Fig. 4). The intraoperative images were of diagnostic quality and comparable to postoperative 1.5-T localization MRI scans performed in patients who also underwent radiosurgical treatment. Compared with the postoperative images, the presence of residual tumor was more effectively detected on the iMRI scans because of the absence of signal interference from the fat graft and sellar reconstruction.

At the clinical follow-up, 15 of 16 patients with visual field deficits had improvement that was documented by formal visual testing. One patient developed a delayed postoperative hematoma that caused acute visual decline and necessitated emergent reoperation. Endocrine function improved in most of the patients. The 3 patients with hypopituitarism continued on long-term hormonal replacement therapy. All 6 patients with acromegaly showed gradual postoperative normalization of growth hormone levels and insulin-like growth factor 1. As part of a planned STR, 3 of the 6 patients underwent postoperative adjuvant stereotactic radiosurgical treatment for nonresectable tumors that invaded the cavernous sinuses; their hormonal levels also normalized after treatment with octreotide (sandostatin). Although the signs of hypercortisolism in the 2 patients with Cushing's disease resolved after surgery, these patients developed panhypopituitarism that required medical management as a result of the total hypophysectomies performed. All patients with less specific symptoms (eg, headache) reported symptomatic improvement. No complications were attributed to interaction between the magnet and anesthesia equipment or surgical instrumentation.

Drawbacks of intraoperative MRI

In our experience, two factors that can potentially interfere with intraoperative imaging interpretation in transsphenoidal procedures are blood products and contrast media. Blood products, which accumulated in the surgical field, including the sphenoid sinus and sella, need to be distinguished from residual tumor. Clotted blood had isointense signal on pre- and postcontrast sequences. Tumor and normal gland enhance after contrast administration, which is typically more pronounced in the gland. Leaking of contrast mixed with blood products in the surgical cavity can be another confusing element that makes differentiation from residual tumor more difficult. Therefore, we abandoned our initial approach of contrast administration immediately after the first surgical attempt. We now reserve contrast imaging for the final preclosure stage of the procedure, only after the precontrast sequences demonstrate that the planned extent of resection has been achieved. With this practice, we have successfully avoided the issue of confusing imaging artifacts

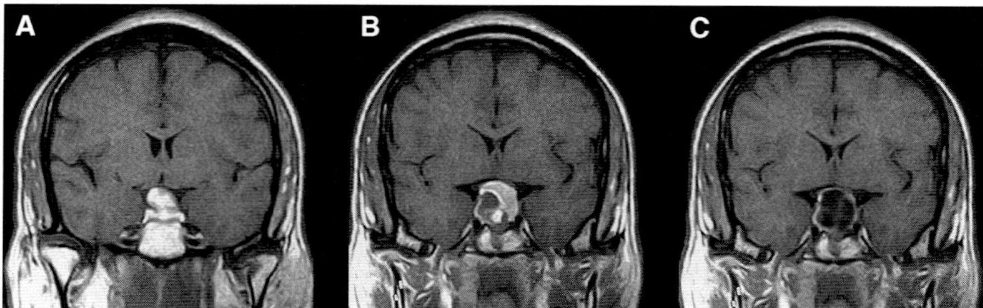

Fig. 4. Intraoperative MRI (iMRI) coronal, T1-weighted, contrast-enhanced serial views. (*A*) iMRI scan before a planned gross total resection (GTR) in a patient with a pituitary macroadenoma with suprasellar extension. (*B*) First iMRI scan after the initial resection demonstrated residual tumor. (*C*) During a repeat surgical exploration, GTR was confirmed with this second intraoperative imaging. (*Courtesy of* the Mayfield Clinic, Cincinnati, OH.)

from contrast in the surgical field and thus can accomplish the surgical goals.

Discussion

At our iMRI center at the University of Cincinnati Medical Center (1998–2004), we have successfully operated on more than 100 patients with pituitary macroadenomas via the transsphenoidal approach. In our experience, the Hitachi AIRIS II 0.3-T shared-resource MRI scanner was especially valuable in providing intraoperative images of diagnostic quality and detecting residual tumor amenable to further resection. With use of the iMRI scanner, we eventually accomplished our planned surgical goals in all patients; without this scanner, we would have accomplished these goals in only 34% of the patients. As described in the previous section, iMRI demonstrated residual resectable tumor in 56% of patients for whom GTR was the goal of surgery and in 77% of patients for whom STR was the goal. This difference indicates that the likelihood of incomplete resection is greater in larger invading tumors, for which iMRI becomes especially valuable. Our experience generally showed a higher incidence of residual disease found with iMRI when compared with other reports [13]. Possible factors that may have contributed to this incidence included reliance on the immediate availability of a "second iMRI look," a learning curve with this new technology, and inclusion of patients with extremely large difficult-to-resect tumors referred to our center.

Some characteristics in our setup are unique and allow for significant flexibility in terms of practicality and convenience. Our facility is based on the twin operating theater concept and offers a significant advantage in ease of use that is facilitated by the rotating tabletop. The surgeon can operate within magnetic-fringe field zone III with conventional surgical instruments and a microscope, thus saving significant resources and time. The use of the second "conventional" OR is reserved exclusively for cranial cases that require lateral or "park-bench" patient positioning, which the MRI tabletop cannot accommodate. The location of our unit is close to strategic facilities, such as the main OR complex; intensive care unit; and radiology, anesthesia, and emergency departments. This location facilitates patient care and transportation as well as communication among specialists during image interpretation.

One of the most important features of our iMR-OR design is the shared resource capability that allows for out- or inpatient diagnostic use when the unit is not in use as an intraoperative imager. This aspect of the unit makes it cost-effective when compared with other available designs. Our approximate costs included $1 million for the Hitachi AIRIS MRI scanner, $1.5 million for the twin operating theater construction, and $250,000 for annual operating expenses. In our cost analysis, we determined that our iMRI facility covers its expenses by performing 1000 diagnostic scans per year (20 per week). During a 2-year period (2002–2003), we performed almost 1200 diagnostic scans annually and thus surpassed our "break even" point.

Although use of iMRI increases operative time, this drawback is common in other similar systems. Each intraoperative imaging session in our patients added an average of 30 minutes to the OR time. However, this additional OR time was justified by a more precise tumor resection, which could potentially prevent or delay a second procedure or adjuvant treatment for patients.

In our experience, iMRI provides the surgeon with the unique capability to maximally accomplish the planned goal of surgery. Such accuracy is especially important in nonsecreting pituitary macroadenomas in which resection is the only means to minimize the chance of recurrence. iMRI allows the surgeon to assess the extent of tumor resection immediately and to detect any surgical complications. The potential benefits of iMRI are a decrease in the rates of a second surgical resection because of undetected residual tumor (at least during the immediate and intermediate postoperative periods) and a greater opportunity for detection of smaller targets when additional treatment (eg, stereotactic radiosurgery) is needed. A clear measure of the effectiveness of iMRI on tumor recurrence and survival rates has not yet been demonstrated because of the slow growth rate of these tumors. Such a potentially beneficial relation needs to be demonstrated in a prospective, controlled, long-term follow-up trial.

Summary

iMRI is a reliable and safe tool to monitor the extent of resection and to avoid complications in the transsphenoidal surgical approach for pituitary tumors. The best indication for its application in transsphenoidal surgery is for patients with pituitary macroadenomas with suprasellar extension. The low-field 0.3-T magnet has a diagnostic imaging quality that provides surgeons with good intraoperative detail of the anatomic relations in the sellar region. In our experience, iMRI provided a distinct benefit in planned STR for invasive macroadenomas that compress the optic chiasm and in planned GTR for noninvasive tumors. The iMRI design adopted at our center includes important features, such as the use of ferromagnetic surgical instruments, elimination of patient transportation, and capability as a shared resource, that allow multipurpose diagnostic use and increased cost-effectiveness.

References

[1] Lanzino G, Laws ER. Key personalities in the development and popularization of the transsphenoidal approach to pituitary tumors: an historical overview. Neurosurg Clin N Am 2003;14:1–10.

[2] Hirsch O. Endonasal method of removal of hypophyseal tumors. JAMA 1910;55:772–4.

[3] Cushing H. Surgical experiences with pituitary disorders. JAMA 1914;63:1515–25.

[4] Hardy J, Wigser SM. Trans-sphenoidal surgery of pituitary fossa tumors with televised radiofluoroscopic control. J Neurosurg 1965;23(6):612–9.

[5] Hardy J. Transsphenoidal microsurgery of the normal and pathological pituitary. Clin Neurosurg 1969; 16:185–217.

[6] Elias WJ, Chadduck JB, Alden TD, Laws ER Jr. Frameless stereotaxy for transsphenoidal surgery. Neurosurgery 1999;45(2):271–7.

[7] Hardy J. Frameless stereotaxy for transsphenoidal surgery. Neurosurgery 2000;46(5):1269–70.

[8] Ram Z, Shawker TH, Bradford MH, Doppman JL, Oldfield EH. Intraoperative ultrasound-directed resection of pituitary tumors. J Neurosurg 1995; 83(2):225–30.

[9] Ram Z, Bruck B, Hadani M. Ultrasound in pituitary tumor surgery. Pituitary 1999;2(2):133–8.

[10] Suzuki R, Asai J, Nagashima G, et al. Transcranial echo-guided transsphenoidal surgical approach for the removal of large macroadenomas. J Neurosurg 2004;100(1):68–72.

[11] Jho HD, Carrau RL. Endoscopic endonasal transsphenoidal surgery: experience with 50 patients. J Neurosurg 1997;87(1):44–51.

[12] Martin CH, Schwartz R, Jolesz F, Black PM. Transsphenoidal resection of pituitary adenomas in an intraoperative MRI unit. Pituitary 1999;2(2): 155–62.

[13] Fahlbusch R, Ganslandt O, Buchfelder M, Schott W, Nimsky C. Intraoperative magnetic resonance imaging during transsphenoidal surgery. J Neurosurg 2001;95(3):381–90.

[14] McPherson CM, Bohinski RJ, Dagnew E, Warnick RE, Tew JM. Tumor resection in a shared-resource magnetic resonance operating room: experience at the University of Cincinnati. Acta Neurochir Suppl (Wien) 2003;85:39–44.

[15] Bohinski RJ, Warnick RE, Gaskill-Shipley MF, et al. Intraoperative magnetic resonance imaging to determine the extent of resection of pituitary macroadenomas during transsphenoidal microsurgery. Neurosurgery 2001;49(5):1133–43.

[16] Hlavin ML, Lewin JS, Arafah BM. Intraoperative magnetic resonance imaging for assessment of chiasmatic decompression and tumor resection during transsphenoidal pituitary surgery. Tech Neurosurg 2000;6:282–8.

[17] Pergolizzi RS Jr, Nabavi A, Schwartz RB, et al. Intra-operative MR guidance during trans-sphenoidal pituitary resection: preliminary results. J Magn Reson Imaging 2001;13(1):136–41.

[18] Black PM, Moriarty T, Alexander E III, et al. Development and implementation of intraoperative magnetic resonance imaging and its neurosurgical applications. Neurosurgery 1997;41(4):831–42.

[19] Tronnier VM, Wirtz CR, Knauth M, et al. Intraoperative diagnostic and interventional magnetic resonance imaging in neurosurgery. Neurosurgery 1997;40(5):891–900.
[20] Bernstein M, Al-Anazi AR, Kucharczyk W, Manninen P, Bronskill M, Henkelman M. Brain tumor surgery with the Toronto open magnetic resonance imaging system: preliminary results for 36 patients and analysis of advantages, disadvantages, and future prospects. Neurosurgery 2000;46(4): 900–9.
[21] Kaibara T, Saunders JK, Sutherland GR. Advances in mobile intraoperative magnetic resonance imaging. Neurosurgery 2000;47(1):131–8.
[22] Lewin JS. Interventional MR imaging: concepts, systems, and applications in neuroradiology. AJNR Am J Neuroradiol 1999;20(5):735–48.
[23] Schwartz RB, Hsu L, Wong TZ, et al. Intraoperative MR imaging guidance for intracranial neurosurgery: experience with the first 200 cases. Radiology 1999; 211(2):477–88.
[24] Seifert V, Zimmermann M, Trantakis C, et al. Open MRI-guided neurosurgery. Acta Neurochir (Wien) 1999;141(5):455–64.
[25] Steinmeier R, Fahlbusch R, Ganslandt O, et al. Intraoperative magnetic resonance imaging with the Magnetom open scanner: concepts, neurosurgical indications, and procedures: a preliminary report. Neurosurgery 1998;43(4):739–48.
[26] Sutherland GR, Kaibara T, Louw D, Hoult DI, Tomanek B, Saunders J. A mobile high-field magnetic resonance system for neurosurgery. J Neurosurg 1999;91(5):804–13.
[27] Hoult DI, Saunders JK, Sutherland GR, et al. The engineering of an interventional MRI with a movable 1.5 tesla magnet. J Magn Reson Imaging 2001;13(1): 78–86.
[28] Martin AJ, Hall WA, Liu H, et al. Brain tumor resection: intraoperative monitoring with high-field-strength MR imaging-initial results. Radiology 2000; 215(1):221–8.
[29] Black PM, Alexander E III, Martin C, et al. Craniotomy for tumor treatment in an intraoperative magnetic resonance imaging unit. Neurosurgery 1999; 45(3):423–31.
[30] Zimmermann M, Seifert V, Trantakis C, Raabe A. Open MRI-guided microsurgery of intracranial tumours in or near eloquent brain areas. Acta Neurochir (Wien) 2001;143(4):327–37.
[31] Bohinski RJ, Kokkino AK, Warnick RE, et al. Glioma resection in a shared-resource magnetic resonance operating room after optimal image-guided frameless stereotactic resection. Neurosurgery 2001;48(4):731–42.
[32] Hadani M, Spiegelman R, Feldman Z, Berkenstadt H, Ram Z. Novel, compact, intraoperative magnetic resonance imaging-guided system for conventional neurosurgical operating rooms. Neurosurgery 2001;48(4):799–807.
[33] Rubino GJ, Farahani K, McGill D, Van De Wiele B, Villablanca JP, Wang-Mathieson A. Magnetic resonance imaging-guided neurosurgery in the magnetic fringe fields: the next step in neuronavigation. Neurosurgery 2000;46(3):643–53.
[34] Schulder M, Sernas TJ, Carmel PW. Cranial surgery and navigation with a compact intraoperative MRI system. Acta Neurochir Suppl (Wien) 2003; 85:79–86.
[35] McPherson CM, Bohinski RJ, Dagnew E, Warnick RE, Tew JM Jr. Clinical experience with a shared-resource, intraoperative magnetic resonance imaging center for resection of intracranial neoplasms. Tech Neurosurg 2002;7(4):274–84.
[36] Chandler W. Surgical approaches to the pituitary fossa. In: Robertson JT, Coakham HB, Robertson JH, editors. Cranial base surgery. New York: Churchill Livingstone; 2000. p. 163–9.
[37] Knosp E, Steiner E, Kitz K, Matula C. Pituitary adenomas with invasion of the cavernous sinus space: a magnetic resonance imaging classification compared with surgical findings. Neurosurgery 1993; 33(4):610–8.

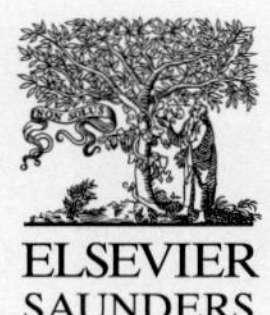

ELSEVIER
SAUNDERS

Neurosurg Clin N Am 16 (2005) 165–172

NEUROSURGERY
CLINICS
OF NORTH AMERICA

1.5 T: spectroscopy-supported brain biopsy

Walter A. Hall, MD[a,b,c,*], Charles L. Truwit, MD[c,d,e]

[a]*Department of Neurosurgery, University of Minnesota Medical School, MMC #96, 420 Delaware Street SE, Minneapolis, MN 55455, USA*

[b]*Department of Radiation Oncology, University of Minnesota Medical School, 420 Delaware Street SE, Minneapolis, MN 55455, USA*

[c]*Department of Radiology, University of Minnesota Medical School, 420 Delaware Street SE, Minneapolis, MN 55455, USA*

[d]*Department of Pediatrics, University of Minnesota Medical School, 420 Delaware Street SE, Minneapolis, MN 55455, USA*

[e]*Department of Neurology, University of Minnesota Medical School, 420 Delaware Street SE, Minneapolis, MN 55455, USA*

Since the 1970s, the technique for performing brain biopsy has changed significantly as the ability of the neurosurgeon to visualize the target site has improved [1–9]. Initially, CT allowed clinicians to obtain images of the brain in the axial plane using x-rays. The first brain biopsies were performed in the CT scanner in a freehand manner [1]. Stereotactic head frames were introduced in the early 1980s and were first combined with CT guidance until MRI became available by the end of the decade. MRI represents one of the most important technologic advances for neurosurgeons developed over the last 20 years. This radiologic tool can demonstrate the brain in axial, coronal, and sagittal projections with excellent soft tissue discrimination.

After stereotaxis and MRI, the next significant advancement in neurosurgery was frameless neuronavigation systems. These systems rely on acquiring preoperative images immediately or several days before a planned surgical procedure. With neuronavigation, the imaging is oriented to a constant set of fiducial markers that are fastened to the head of the patient. Optical, ultrasound, or radiofrequency sensors are used to detect the movement of surgical instruments, such as a brain biopsy needle during surgery, with respect to these reference points. Neuronavigation, however, is limited by two distinct disadvantages: the potential for movement of the fiducial markers during the procedure, resulting in registration inaccuracy, and the ability of the brain to shift once the cranium is opened and cerebrospinal fluid is drained.

In the mid-1990s, MRI was adapted for use in a surgical environment in which intraoperative imaging could provide near–real-time updates of the operative site without concern for brain shift [10–16]. Lesions within the brain could now be accessed or resected without fear of displacement, and neurosurgeons would have the ability to alter their surgical approach dynamically to compensate for brain shift [5,7]. The capability to alter the surgical approach during surgery is not possible with framed or frameless stereotaxy unless it is combined with intraoperative CT or MRI. The ability to visualize the biopsy needle directly within the target tissue during surgery has resulted in an increase in the diagnostic yield for brain biopsy when it is performed with intraoperative MRI guidance compared with conventional stereotaxis [2,5].

The first intraoperative MRI-guided brain biopsies were performed in a freehand fashion as was initially done with the advent of CT, largely because there was no way to direct the passage of the needle through the brain or to stabilize the needle once it had reached the intended target [3].

Drs. Hall and Truwit each have a financial interest in Image-Guided Neurologics.

* Corresponding author.

E-mail address: hallx003@umn.edu (W.A. Hall).

doi:10.1016/j.nec.2004.07.002

Such concerns led to the development of various trajectory guides that facilitated tissue sampling [4,17]. To further enhance the diagnostic yield of intraoperative MRI-guided brain biopsy, particularly for patients thought to harbor a neoplastic process, magnetic resonance spectroscopy (MRS) was performed during the procedure to identify areas in the brain having increased levels of certain metabolites believed to represent tumor, which were then sampled in near–real time [6,8,18,19].

MRI-guided brain biopsy technique

MRI-guided brain biopsy can be performed under local or general anesthesia. We have tended to use general anesthesia more commonly, because it is difficult for a patient to remain calm for extended periods. The noise associated with MRI scanning could startle the patient during the procedure, which may lead to displacement of the head and the biopsy needle while it is within the brain. Many of the lesions that are biopsied are in locations where it would be difficult for the patient to maintain the proper position for the entire duration of the procedure.

Patients are placed under general anesthesia before or after transport to the intraoperative MRI suite. An MRI-visible marker is placed on the scalp at the location where the skull will undergo perforation. By defining a safe and accurate trajectory for the brain biopsy, the neurosurgeon can ensure that critical structures are avoided and that a diagnostic sample is obtained. At the University of Minnesota, two flexible radiofrequency coils are placed around the surgical site to perform high-resolution scanning. The scalp is shaved and then prepared in a sterile manner. The skin is incised, and a twist drill craniostomy or a burr hole is made through the skull. The dura mater is incised, and the base of the trajectory guide (Navigus; Image-Guided Neurologics, Melbourne, Florida) is secured in place with three self-tapping titanium screws (Fig. 1). A variable-diameter guide tube is then snapped into the base and secured in place with a plastic locking nut. The alignment stem is inserted into the guide tube to determine an appropriate trajectory in multiple MRI planes for the biopsy using prospective stereotaxy [5,20]. To visualize the alignment stem, it is filled with saline or contrast, depending on which MRI sequences best demonstrate the target lesion. After a trajectory has been chosen that encounters the target in at least two projections, the guide tube is locked in place and the alignment stem is removed. In a stepwise fashion with periodic "snap-shot" MRI updates, the titanium brain biopsy needle is gradually advanced toward the target in near–real time.

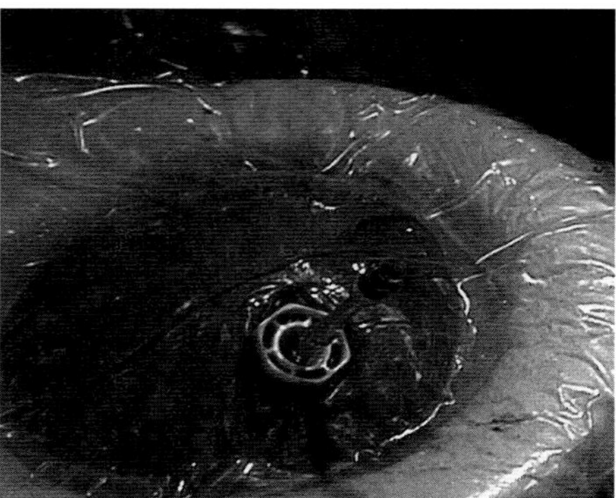

Fig. 1. Navigus trajectory guide (Image-Guided Neurologics, Melbourne, Florida) enables the neurosurgeon to choose a safe and accurate surgical pathway for brain biopsy while securing the needle in place at the time when the tissue samples are obtained. The biopsy is being performed through a radiofrequency coil, and the alignment stem has been inserted into the guide tube.

For most lesions, T2-weighted, orthogonal, half-Fourier acquisition single-shot turbo spin echo (HASTE) imaging is used to determine the surgical trajectory to the target because of its rapid scan acquisition time. Once the biopsy needle reaches the target, imaging is performed in two orthogonal planes along the entire length of the biopsy needle to document the location of the biopsy and to confirm the accuracy of the procedure (Fig. 2). Multiple samples are usually obtained from the target tissue at different depths and in different directions for frozen section and permanent pathologic analysis. At present, we still confirm the presence of pathologic tissue before leaving the operating room; however, in the future, we will probably forego this practice because of the accuracy of the sampling technique. While the pathologist is analyzing the tissue samples, the biopsy needle is removed and the sample site is evaluated for intraoperative hemorrhage. Because the presence of hyperacute blood (before conversion of intracellular oxyhemoglobin to deoxyhemoglobin) can be difficult to detect on MRI, a combination of HASTE, gradient echo (GE)-T2*, and turbo fluid-attenuated inversion recovery sequences has proved

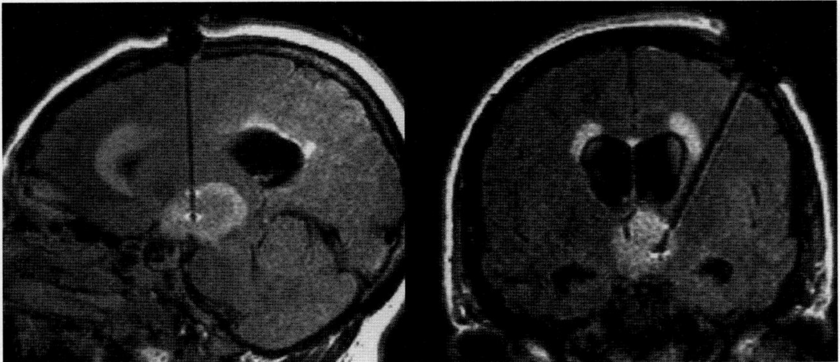

Fig. 2. Orthogonal sagittal (left) and coronal (right) turbo fluid-attenuated inversion recovery MRI along the entire length of the titanium brain biopsy needle once it has reached the target in the left thalamus found to be an astrocytoma.

sensitive to detect intraoperative hemorrhage accurately (Fig. 3). After the presence of diagnostic tissue has been confirmed, the trajectory guide is removed and the scalp is sutured closed. The patient is then transported to the recovery room for extubation. Usually, the patient is discharged home the following morning, although some patients have been discharged home the same day at their own request after several hours of observation. Performing outpatient brain biopsies should clearly help to curtail rising medical costs.

Prospective stereotaxy

Prospective stereotaxy represents a novel way to determine the surgical path for the brain biopsy needle using the trajectory guide that starts at the target and moves from the target to the distal end of the alignment stem. After the neurosurgeon has chosen the biopsy location (target point), it is necessary to determine two additional points in space to align the trajectory guide with the target. The second point is the pivot point, which is located at the tip of the alignment stem. The third point is a point in space that represents the desired location of the alignment stem, which can be oriented until all three points are collinear, thereby ensuring that the passage of the biopsy needle through the trajectory guide will encounter the target.

The alignment stem is filled with an appropriate fluid for visualization on MRI and then inserted into the guide tube before performing prospective stereotaxy. The alignment stem can be

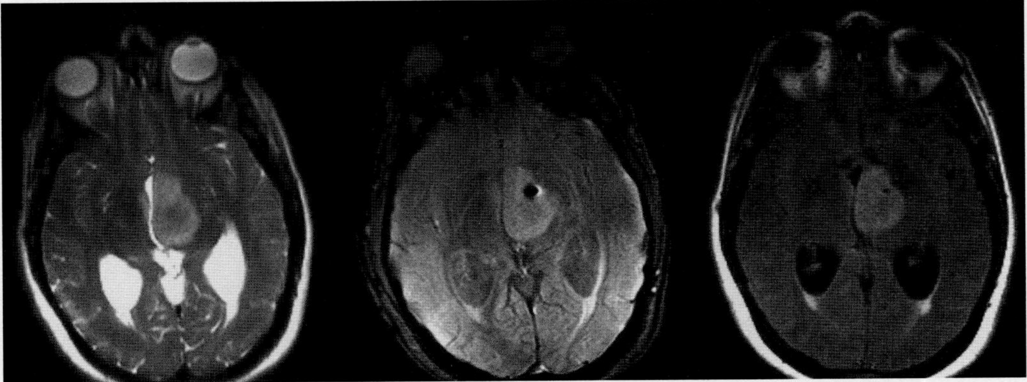

Fig. 3. A combination of half-Fourier acquisition single-shot turbo spin echo (left), gradient echo (GE)-T2* (middle), and turbo fluid-attenuated inversion recovery (right) sequences has proved sensitive to detect accurately the presence or absence of intraoperative hemorrhage after brain biopsy. The prominent signal void seen within the left thalamus on the GE-T2* image is thought to represent air because of its sharp border.

rotated freely in space because of a ball joint until all three points are aligned, which can be completed in less than 5 minutes. After the points are aligned, scanning along the entire length of the alignment stem is performed to confirm that the trajectory guide is pointed toward the target and that the biopsy needle will access the tissue of interest once it is passed through the brain. If the surgical path is considered satisfactory, the locking nut is tightened to prevent redirection or displacement of the trajectory guide while the biopsy is being performed.

Magnetic resonance spectroscopy–guided brain biopsy

Since April 1998, we have used MRS to guide brain biopsy in the intraoperative MRI unit [6,18,19]. Successfully combining the trajectory guide with MRS to guide brain biopsy was first accomplished in January 1999 [6]. The MRS techniques that we have used during brain biopsy include single-voxel spectroscopy (SVS) or turbo spectroscopic imaging (TSI) obtained under general anesthesia individually or in combination. General anesthesia is used to prevent movement of the head during the examination, which would invalidate the MRS data. A phased-array head coil was used to acquire the MRS data initially in the ACS-NT 1.5-T, high-field, short-bore, interventional MRI system (Philips Medical Systems; Best, The Netherlands) and, more recently, using the 1.5-T Intera I/T system (Philips Medical Systems) (Fig. 4). SVS (1.5-cm^3 $\times$ 1.5-cm^3 $\times$ 1/5-cm^3 voxel, 1-Hz spectral resolution, echo time (TE)/repetition time (TR) = 136/2000 milliseconds, 4.5-minute acquisition) was obtained on a region of interest in the brain to be biopsied and on a control area in a comparable location in the contralateral hemisphere [7]. TSI (32-mm $\times$ 32-mm grid of spectra in a single plane, 0.66-cm^3 $\times$ 0.66-cm^3 $\times$ 2.0-cm^3 spatial resolution, 4.4-Hz spectral resolution, TE/TR = 272/2000 milliseconds, turbo factor = 3, 11-minute acquisition) was performed on a single axial slice to measure brain metabolites [7]. Intravenous contrast was not used during MRS to prevent alteration of the spectral data by those agents. Regions of elevated phosphocholine on SVS and TSI, which are believed to represent areas of rapid membrane turnover and increased cellular density suspicious for tumor tissue, were selected for biopsy during the procedure (Fig. 5). If elevated phosphocholine was not identified on MRS, areas of contrast enhancement were chosen for biopsy.

MRI- and magnetic resonance spectroscopy–guided brain biopsy results

The first 35 MRI-guided brain biopsies performed between January 1997 and June 1998 were freehand, because the trajectory guide had not yet been developed for clinical use [3]. At that time, the brain biopsy needle was stabilized in the burr hole using bone wax after it had reached the target. All 35 brain biopsies yielded diagnostic tissue, and the

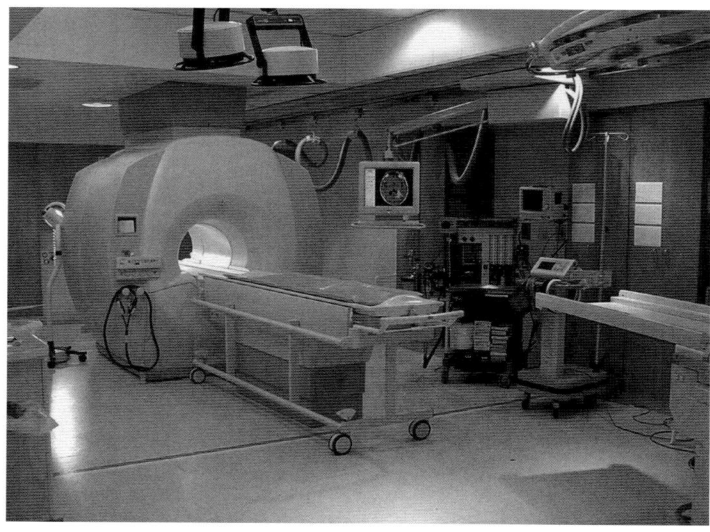

Fig. 4. Intera I/T intraoperative MRI system (Philips Medical Systems, Best, The Netherlands).

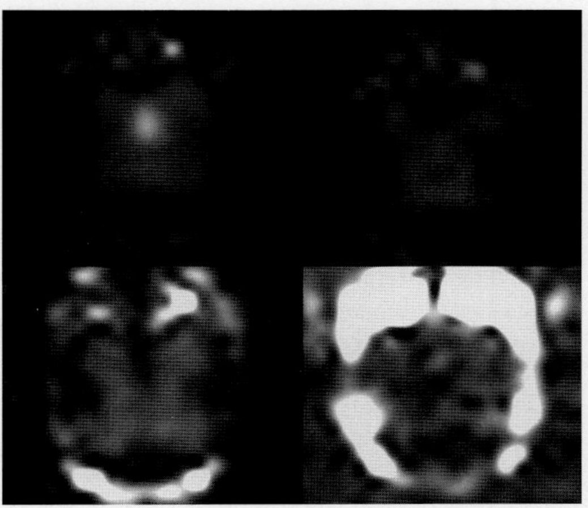

Fig. 5. Turbo spectroscopic imaging (TSI) metabolite map of the left thalamic astrocytoma. The upper left panel represents the TSI phosphocholine map, and the creatine map is in the upper right panel. The *N*-acetylaspartate map is in the lower left panel, and the lactate/lipid map is in the lower right panel. The tumor clearly demonstrates an elevated phosphocholine level representative of rapid membrane turnover and increased cellular density.

diagnoses obtained included 28 primary brain tumors, 1 metastatic tumor, one meningioma, one cerebral infarct, one demyelinating process, and three cases of radiation necrosis. One patient with a pontine glioma had a temporary hemiparesis after the biopsy that improved with physical therapy, and another patient who experienced scalp cellulitis was successfully treated with antibiotics. No patient sustained a clinically or radiographically significant hemorrhage during the procedure. Six of these patients had SVS at the time of their biopsies. The results of the SVS in five of the patients demonstrated elevated phosphocholine levels in comparison to the creatine levels, with a decrease in the *N*-acetylaspartate levels. The diagnoses found in these five patients were astrocytoma, anaplastic astrocytoma, and three glioblastomas multiforme. In the single patient in whom the phosphocholine level was not elevated, radiation necrosis was found. The results of the SVS correlated well with the pathologic findings in each case.

After the advent of the trajectory guide, the results of the first 40 brain biopsies that were performed in 38 patients between January 1999 and March 2000 were reviewed for safety and accuracy [5]. All biopsies were diagnostic, and there were no clinically or radiographically significant hemorrhages detected. Thirty-three (83%) lesions were primary brain tumors, 5 were radiation necrosis, 1 was vasculitis, and 1 was a demyelinating process. One patient with a lesion adjacent to the motor cortex sustained a temporary hemiparesis related to edema that occurred with the passage of the biopsy needle, and another elderly patient experienced a fatal myocardial infarction after the biopsy despite preoperative cardiac clearance. The accuracy of the device was measured to be 2 mm at a depth of 70 mm within the brain [5].

Over a concurrent 12-month period, we coupled MRS with the use of the trajectory guide in an attempt to improve the diagnostic yield in 17 patients [6]. Before the procedure, 10 patients had TSI and 7 patients had TSI and SVS. All tissue samples were diagnostic, and the diagnoses obtained included six glioblastomas multiforme, three anaplastic astrocytomas, three anaplastic oligodendrogliomas, germinoma, ganglioglioma, astrocytoma, and two cases of radiation necrosis. No clinically or radiographically significant hemorrhage was visible on postbiopsy imaging. In all 7 patients who had SVS, there was a 100% spectral correlation with the pathologic results. In the 17 patients who had TSI, the correlation was similar in only 13 (76%), however. In those patients who had SVS and TSI, the results correlated in 6 (86%) of 7 patients. Overall, it was thought that the MRS data enhanced the diagnostic yield of brain biopsy [6].

To determine the utility of TSI, a group of 26 patients underwent brain biopsy using this imaging technique [19]. An area of elevated phosphocholine was seen on TSI in 17 of 21 patients who had a confirmed neoplasm on pathologic examination of the biopsy sample. Radiation necrosis was found in 5 patients in whom the phosphocholine level was low and consistent with that diagnosis. Four patients with tumors had low phosphocholine levels that were indistinguishable from the levels present in radiation necrosis. Of the 10 patients who had SVS in addition to TSI, the results were qualitatively similar for both techniques, although more spectral contamination was seen with TSI than with SVS. Quantitative analysis of TSI was limited by the low spatial resolution for that technique. The diagnostic yield for TSI-guided brain biopsy was 100%.

In our first 140 brain biopsies performed under MRI guidance, we sought to determine what influence the imaging had on surgical decision making [21]. In 42 (30%) brain biopsies, we used

MRS to guide the brain biopsy. Twenty-nine (71%) patients had TSI and 21 (48%) patients had SVS. Twenty-one (48%) patients had TSI alone, 13 (31%) patients had SVS alone, and 8 (19%) patients had TSI and SVS. In the patients who were thought to have tumor, the areas of elevated phosphocholine on SVS, TSI, or both were targeted during the biopsy. In those 8 patients who had SVS and TSI, there was excellent correlation between the phosphocholine levels. Radiation necrosis was diagnosed in 10 (20%) patients, glioblastoma multiforme in 12 (24%), anaplastic oligodendroglioma in 6 (12%), anaplastic astrocytoma in 6 (12%), astrocytoma in 2 (4%), oligodendroglioma in 4 (8%), germinoma in 1 (2%), and lymphoma in 1 (2%). SVS was performed in 5 patients with radiation necrosis, 1 with anaplastic oligodendroglioma, 3 with glioblastoma multiforme, 2 with anaplastic astrocytoma, and 2 with astrocytoma. TSI was obtained in 6 patients with glioblastoma multiforme, 4 with radiation necrosis, 4 with oligodendroglioma, 3 with anaplastic astrocytoma, 2 with anaplastic oligodendroglioma, 1 with lymphoma, and 1 with germinoma. The diagnoses that were found in those patients who had TSI and SVS were three glioblastomas multiforme, three anaplastic oligodendrogliomas, one anaplastic astrocytoma, and one case of radiation necrosis.

Review of brain biopsy results

The first CT-guided brain biopsies were performed freehand [1]. The diagnostic yield was 90% and ranged from 79% to 97% in 344 patients having this type of biopsy [1]. The morbidity rate was 7.8% and ranged from 2% to 14%, and the mortality rate was 2.5% and ranged from 0.5% to 4.7%. Stereotactic head frames were used shortly after the development of CT to guide the performance of brain biopsy. A review of 17 stereotactic brain biopsy series that included nearly 7500 patients demonstrated that the diagnostic rate was 91% and ranged from 80% to 99%, the morbidity rate was 3.5% and ranged from 0% to 13%, and the mortality rate was 0.7% and ranged from 0.5% to 2.6%. Diagnostic failure in stereotactic brain biopsy patients was attributed to small sample size, small target size, displacement of the lesion away from the biopsy needle, inability to penetrate the lesion with the biopsy needle, inaccurate tissue targeting resulting in sampling error, poor target choice in areas of high T2-weighted signal on MRI, and lesion proximity adjacent to the ventricular system resulting in the aspiration of cerebrospinal fluid [2].

Intraoperative MRI-guided brain biopsy results

The presence of MRI in the operating room allows for intracranial tissue to be sampled in near–real time [3]. Compared with conventional frame-based brain biopsy, intraoperative MRI-guided brain biopsy has a diagnostic yield of 100% in some reports and allows for the confirmation that a clinically or radiographically detected hemorrhage has not been sustained during the procedure [5]. Of the first 140 cases that were performed using 0.5-T midfield intraoperative MRI at the Brigham and Women's Hospital, 63 were brain biopsies [12]. The lesions were located in various areas throughout the brain, including the thalamus, basal ganglia, brain stem, cerebellum, deep white matter, and cerebral hemispheres. One patient sustained an intraoperative hemorrhage that was detected on intraoperative scanning and was emergently evacuated. The authors concluded that the intraoperative MRI enabled them to evaluate the surgical site rapidly and to intervene dynamically if necessary [12].

Using a low-field 0.2-T MRI scanner, 10 brain biopsies were performed in a series of 27 patients [14]. All brain biopsies yielded diagnostic tissue, and the authors concluded that they could adjust for brain shift during the operative procedure by obtaining updated image sets. Another group performed 16 brain biopsies in the magnetic fringe fields using the same low-field intraoperative MRI system [15]. Fifteen (94%) of the 16 brain biopsies were diagnostic, and the single nondiagnostic biopsy attempt was aborted because the brain stem tumor could not be safely accessed through the cerebellum. No hemorrhages were detected that required surgical evacuation, and the only morbidity that was experienced was a temporary hemiparesis that resulted after a lesion near the motor cortex was biopsied. Using a low-field 0.2-T vertical gap system, 36 neurosurgical procedures were performed over a 1-year period, of which 12 cases were brain biopsies [16]. One patient had postoperative hand weakness after a brain biopsy that demonstrated a lymphoma, and all biopsies yielded diagnostic tissue. There were several technical issues raised by the authors concerning brain biopsy using their intraoperative MRI system, including poor image quality in five cases, instrumentation concerns in two cases, and the probe not being visualized in three cases. The two most useful features of intraoperative MRI-guided surgery that were noted by the authors were the ability to visualize the brain biopsy needle within the region of interest and to confirm the absence of intra-operative hemorrhage.

Technical advances in intraoperative MRI-guided brain biopsy

Neurosurgeons operating in the intraoperative MRI environment realized rapidly the need to guide biopsy needles through the brain and then to secure the needle in place once it had reached the target tissue. Frameless stereotaxy has been combined with an optical triangulation system to localize the burr hole, to plan the surgical pathway, and to guide the needle to the target at some intraoperative MRI sites [17]. In the first 20 procedures that were performed in this manner, there were 15 brain biopsies, three abscess drainages, one cyst aspiration, and one fenestration for multiloculated hydrocephalus. The positional accuracy of this system was believed to be comparable to that of conventional stereotaxy, with a mean error of 1.5 mm [17].

Prospective stereotaxy represents another advancement in the evolution of intraoperative MRI-guided brain biopsy [5,20]. Although framed or frameless stereotaxy and prospective stereotaxy require preoperative images to locate the target and to plan the surgical approach, the two techniques are quite different during the performance of the biopsy. Frameless stereotaxy requires that fiducial markers be placed on the scalp before the preoperative imaging is obtained to register or localize the markers with respect to the position of the target. An external probe is used to register the fiducial markers, which will generate an image on a computer monitor, which is then viewed by the neurosurgeon. Once the fiducial markers have been registered, the target can then be displayed on the monitor by changing the position of the probe in space. The most concerning issue that is associated with frameless stereotaxy is the potential for brain shift with subsequent displacement of the target once the dura mater is opened and cerebrospinal fluid is lost. Prospective stereotaxy does not require fiducial markers, because the imaging will demonstrate the target and the trajectory that the biopsy needle will traverse to reach the target. After aligning the trajectory guide, the biopsy needle can be passed in a stepwise fashion in near–real time until the target is encountered. The techniques are diametrically opposed. Frameless stereotaxy demonstrates the target lesion on a computer screen as it is related to an external probe in contrast to prospective stereotaxy, which displays the desired trajectory on a computer monitor as it is determined. By rotating the alignment stem that is within the guide tube like a joy stick, the surgical channel can be directed toward the target. Concerns about brain shift are minimized with prospective stereotaxy.

The trajectory guide can be used with frameless and prospective stereotaxy, and two other MRI-compatible needle stabilization devices are also currently available (MRI Devices Corporation, Waukesha, Wisconsin; Snapper-Stereo-Guide, MagneticVision, Zurich, Switzerland) [17]. Since the introduction of the trajectory guide at our institution, our diagnostic rate for brain biopsy has been 100%. Biopsies have been safe and accurate, with the alignment of the device being rapid and efficient without extending the length of the operative procedure. MRS measures specific metabolites noninvasively within the brain, which may help to distinguish tumor recurrence from radiation necrosis in patients with brain tumors who have received radiation therapy, much like positron emission tomography. By combining the use of the trajectory guide with MRS, we hope to enhance our diagnostic yield for patients who have intraoperative MRI-guided brain biopsies.

References

[1] Wen DY, Hall WA, Miller DA, Seljeskog EL, Maxwell RE. Targeted brain biopsy: a comparison of freehand computed tomography-guided and stereotactic techniques. Neurosurgery 1993;32:407–13.

[2] Hall WA. The safety and efficacy of stereotactic biopsy for intracranial lesions. Cancer 1998;82: 1749–55.

[3] Hall WA, Martin AJ, Liu H, Nussbaum ES, Maxwell RE, Truwit CL. Brain biopsy using high-field strength interventional MR imaging. Neurosurgery 1999;44:807–14.

[4] Hall WA, Liu H, Truwit CL. Navigus trajectory guide. Neurosurgery 2000;46:502–4.

[5] Hall WA, Liu H, Martin AJ, Maxwell RE, Truwit CL. Brain biopsy using prospective stereotaxis and a trajectory guide. J Neurosurg 2001;91: 67–71.

[6] Hall WA, Martin AJ, Liu H, Truwit CL. Improving diagnostic yield in brain biopsy: coupling spectroscopic targeting with real time needle placement. J Magn Reson Imaging 2001;13:12–5.

[7] Hall WA, Liu H, Martin AJ, Truwit CL. Minimally invasive procedures: interventional MR image-guided neurobiopsy. Neuroimaging Clin N Am 2001;11:705–13.

[8] Hall WA, Liu H, Truwit CL. MR spectroscopy-guided biopsy of intracranial neoplasms. Tech Neurosurg 2002;7:291–8.

[9] Liu H, Hall WA, Truwit CL. Remotely-controlled approach to stereotactic neurobiopsy. Comput Aided Surg 2002;7:237–47.

[10] Hall WA, Liu H, Martin AJ, Pozza CH, Maxwell RE, Truwit CL. Safety, efficacy, and functionality of high-field strength interventional magnetic resonance imaging for neurosurgery. Neurosurgery 2000;46:632–42.

[11] Sutherland GR, Kaibara T, Louw D, Hoult DI, Tomanek B, Saunders J. A mobile high-field magnetic resonance system for neurosurgery. J Neurosurg 1999;91:804–13.

[12] Black PMcL, Moriarty T, Alexander E III, Steig P, Woodard EJ, Gleason L, et al. Development and implementation of intraoperative magnetic resonance imaging and its neurosurgical implications. Neurosurgery 1997;41:831–45.

[13] Steinmeier R, Fahlbusch R, Ganslandt O, Nimsky C, Buchfelder M, Kaus M, et al. Intraoperative magnetic resonance imaging with the Magnetom open scanner: concepts, neurosurgical indications, and procedures: a preliminary report. Neurosurgery 1998;43:739–47.

[14] Tronnier VM, Wirtz CR, Knauth M, Lenz G, Pastyr O, Bonsanto MM, et al. Intraoperative diagnostic and interventional magnetic resonance imaging in neurosurgery. Neurosurgery 1997;40:891–900.

[15] Rubino GJ, Farahani K, McGill D, Van de Wiele B, Villablanca JP, Wang-Mathieson A. Magnetic resonance imaging-guided neurosurgery in the magnetic fringe fields: the next step in neuronavigation. Neurosurgery 2000;46:643–54.

[16] Bernstein M, Al-Anazi AR, Kucharczyk W, Manninen P, Bronskill M, Henkelman M. Brain tumor surgery with the Toronto open magnetic resonance imaging system: preliminary results for 36 patients and analysis of advantages, disadvantages, and future prospects. Neurosurgery 2000;46:900–9.

[17] Bernays RL, Kollias SS, Khan N, Romanowski B, Yonekawa Y. A new artifact-free device for frameless, magnetic resonance imaging guided-stereotactic procedures. Neurosurgery 2000;46:112–7.

[18] Liu H, Hall WA, Martin AJ, Truwit CL. An efficient chemical shift imaging scheme for magnetic resonance-guided neurosurgery. J Magn Reson Imaging 2001;14:1–7.

[19] Martin AJ, Liu H, Hall WA, Truwit CL. Preliminary assessment of turbo spectroscopic imaging for targeting in brain biopsy. AJNR Am J Neuroradiol 2001;22:959–68.

[20] Liu H, Hall WA, Truwit CL. Neuronavigation in interventional MR imaging: prospective stereotaxy. Neuroimaging Clin N Am 2001;11:697–706.

[21] Hall WA, Liu H, Maxwell RE, Truwit CL. Influence of 1.5-tesla intraoperative MR imaging on surgical decision making. Acta Neurochir (Wien) 2002;85: 29–37.

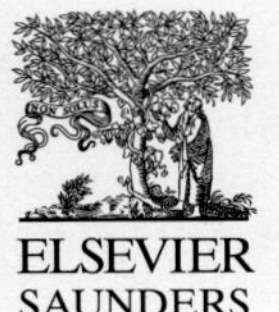

ELSEVIER
SAUNDERS

Neurosurg Clin N Am 16 (2005) 173–183

NEUROSURGERY
CLINICS
OF NORTH AMERICA

Epilepsy surgery with intraoperative MRI at 1.5 T

John J. Kelly, MD, Walter J. Hader, MD, S. Terry Myles, MD, Garnette R. Sutherland, MD*

Division of Neurosurgery, Department of Clinical Neurosciences, University of Calgary, Foothills Medical Centre, 1403 29th Street NW, Calgary, T2N 2T9 Alberta, Canada

Epilepsy and its treatment

Epilepsy is a term that represents a heterogeneous group of syndromes with different etiologies, severities, clinical impact, and treatment options. The cardinal feature of epilepsy is a predisposition to recurrent unprovoked seizures that are classified as partial or generalized [1]. Epileptic seizures occur when a population of hyperexcitable neurons discharge excessively [2]. Current understanding of epileptogenesis, the cellular and molecular mechanisms by which epilepsy develops, remains incomplete [1].

As knowledge of the natural history and pathophysiology of epilepsy syndromes increases, the approach to treatment changes. An important conceptual advance has resulted—the view that surgical therapy should not be considered a last resort but rather the treatment of choice for defined surgically remediable syndromes [3]. Contemporary surgical procedures for the treatment of epilepsy include resection, disconnection, and neural modulation. Advances in diagnosis, neuroimaging, and microsurgery are contributing to improvements in the safety and efficacy of epilepsy surgery.

Surgical management of epilepsy is based on a number of variables, including the type of epilepsy, localization of the epileptogenic focus, patient's wishes, and surgeon's expertise. Before proceeding with surgery, it is imperative that reasonable evidence indicates a structural abnormality of the brain or that clinical and electrographic analysis localizes the epileptogenic focus. The immediate goal of surgery is maximal safe resection of epileptogenic tissue or anatomic and functional disconnection to eliminate or reduce the number of clinically significant seizures without causing significant deficit. Other goals include decreasing medication dependence and improving quality of life together with global brain function.

Efficacy of epilepsy surgery

Surgical treatment of focal epilepsy has a reported success rate, with respect to seizure control, ranging from 33% to 90% [4–13]. Surgical outcome has improved in recent trials and case series [5,6,9,10,13]. Factors predicting this include patient selection based on the presence of a single unilateral MRI abnormality, unilateral hippocampal sclerosis, and localized ipsilateral ictal and interictal epileptiform activity [5,14]. Factors associated with poor outcome include nonlocalizing electroencephalographic (EEG) results, absence of an MRI abnormality, bilateral atrophy, suspected cortical dysplasia, and multiple cortical MRI abnormalities [5].

When the preoperative electrophysiologic workup, clinical history, and adjunctive test results are considered and a single abnormality is identified on MRI, the surgical success rate (Engel class I or II) ranges from 80% to 90% [15]. Surgical cure of epilepsy is more likely with complete resection of the MRI abnormality or, in nonlesional cases with EEG localization only, complete resection of the appropriate anatomic structures [16]. As imaging techniques improve

This work was supported by a grant from the Canadian Foundation for Innovation.

* Corresponding author. Seaman Family Magnetic Resonance Research Centre, Foothills Hospital, 1403 29th Street NW, Calgary, Alberta, Canada T2N 2T9.

E-mail address: garnette@ucalgary.ca (G.R. Sutherland).

doi:10.1016/j.nec.2004.07.006

neurosurgery.theclinics.com

and the results of studies evaluating failed surgical procedures become available, it is evident that persisting epileptogenic foci often correlate with residual imaging and pathologic abnormalities [5].

Epilepsy surgery: a brief history

Two main factors have contributed to the advancement of epilepsy surgery: scientific knowledge and technology. Understanding the natural history and pathophysiology of epilepsy allowed classification of the epilepsies and identification of surgically remediable syndromes. Over the past century, evaluation and treatment of epilepsy were refined, in large part, as a result of the development of diagnostic and localization technologies, including EEG, electrocorticography (ECoG), CT, MRI, frameless stereotaxy/neuronavigation, and intraoperative imaging.

In 1886, Horsley [17], working with Jackson and Ferrier, surgically removed posttraumatic scar and surrounding brain parenchyma successfully while treating a patient with focal epilepsy. In 1929, Berger [18] published the first work describing human scalp EEG recordings. Fischer and Lowenbach [19] were the first to demonstrate epileptiform spikes on EEG in 1934. Shortly thereafter, the application of ECoG for detection of the epileptogenic focus during surgery was reported by Foerster and Altenburger [20]. The hallmark of epilepsy, the interictal spike, was described in 1936 by Jasper [21] and Gibbs et al [22].

In 1934, Wilder Penfield and colleagues established the Montreal Neurological Institute (MNI). The MNI opened its laboratory of EEG and neurophysiology in 1939, the first of its kind dedicated to selecting epilepsy patients for surgery and providing the technology for intraoperative recordings. EEG was established as the primary modality for seizure localization in the pre- and intraoperative evaluation of epilepsy surgery patients. Penfield and Jasper [23] further advanced invasive EEG monitoring in 1954 through the use of chronically implanted epidural electrodes. This unique group established the multidisciplinary approach to the investigation, treatment, and follow-up of patients with epilepsy.

Microsurgical technique significantly improves surgical treatment of epilepsy. The operating microscope, introduced to neurosurgery in the early 1960s, provides magnification and superior illumination. This is of particular importance today, an era of minimalism, when operations to remove only MRI-defined abnormalities take place through restricted surgical corridors. Microsurgical dissection allows removal of a target through anatomic cisterns with minimal injury to adjacent structures.

The introduction of CT brain imaging by Hounsfield in 1973 advanced the preoperative evaluation and localization of neurosurgical pathologic findings. Patient evaluation improved further when Lauterbur and Mansfield developed MRI, which permits multiplanar imaging with superior soft tissue resolution. MRI allows detection of subtle cortical abnormalities and excludes neoplastic, vascular, and infectious causes of seizures. Imaging resolution has improved localization of epileptogenic foci, reducing the need for invasive monitoring and allowing tailored surgical resections. Frameless stereotaxy, developed during the past decade, allows precise craniotomy placement and optimizes the surgical trajectory, thereby avoiding critical structures during dissection. Unfortunately, tissue dissection, cerebrospinal fluid loss, brain retraction, and gravity result in brain shift, invalidating localization coordinates based on preoperative images [24,25]. This problem, to some extent, fueled the development of intraoperative imaging systems that could not only correct for brain shift but provide a method of resection control during surgery.

Intraoperative MRI (iMRI) permits near–real-time updating of intracranial anatomy and surgical progress. iMRI, coupled with neuronavigation, optimizes each technology's complementary features. The utility of iMRI was recognized quickly, and the technique has been successfully applied to the full spectrum of neurosurgical disorders, including epilepsy. Through the introduction of high-resolution MRI systems, improved electrophysiologic monitoring, and iMRI, the concept of tailored resections targeting the epileptogenic focus has evolved.

Since 1999, all surgical procedures performed for treatment of epilepsy at the University of Calgary have used iMRI as an adjunct. This report focuses on the development of the iMRI system, together with the experience gained from 70 patients with intractable epilepsy.

Methods and materials

Technology

The iMRI system consists of a mobile, ceiling-mounted, 1.5-T magnet. The current system, introduced in 1997, has been successfully used during 485 neurosurgical procedures, of which 70 (14%) were performed for intractable epilepsy.

The operating suite containing the iMRI system consists of two parts. The main operating room is 7.6 m × 10.4 m. Attached is a small alcove measuring 2.4 m × 3.8 m that houses the 5-tonne magnet. The magnet tracks along beams attached to the ceiling, allowing movement into the operating room to the anesthetized patient for imaging. The magnet returns to the alcove when imaging is complete, allowing a return to full operating room capacity (Fig. 1).

Lines on the operating room floor indicate areas of 5-G and 50-G, with the magnet in docked and imaging positions. These lines permit the operating suite to function like a typical neurosurgical operating room. The anesthesiologist is positioned opposite the alcove at the far end of the room, outside the 5-G line. The operating microscope, neuronavigation system, ultrasonic aspirator, and electrophysiologic monitoring or ECoG equipment are also moved outside the 5-G line during imaging.

The cantilevered operating table was designed specifically for this iMRI system. It is composed of MRI-compatible materials and is secured to the floor. Movements occur in six axes using hydraulics, optimizing patient positioning. The stationary table eliminates risk associated with patient movement and aids with accuracy of the neuronavigation system. The radiofrequency (RF) coil consists of two parts. The bottom half is built into a Sugita type four-pin head holder that provides rigid immobilization (Fig. 2).

Images are obtained at different points throughout the procedure. Intraoperative surgical planning images are obtained after induction of anesthesia, patient positioning, and head fixation. Interdissection images are acquired at various stages of the surgical dissection. For imaging, a transparent C-arm drape is placed over the wound and the patient. The upper half of the RF coil is placed over the lower half of the coil, and the magnet is moved into position. On average, imaging and reregistration of the navigation coordinates take 30 minutes. Quality assurance images are acquired after wound closure but before reversal of anesthesia. These sequences confirm completion of the surgical objective, exclude acute complications, and eliminate the need for delayed postoperative imaging.

The 1.5-T magnet provides images that approach diagnostic quality and include T1-weighted, T2-weighted, fluid-attenuated inversion recovery (FLAIR), magnetic resonance angiography, diffusion-weighted imaging, or perfusion sequences. In general, gadolinium was not administered to the epilepsy cohort.

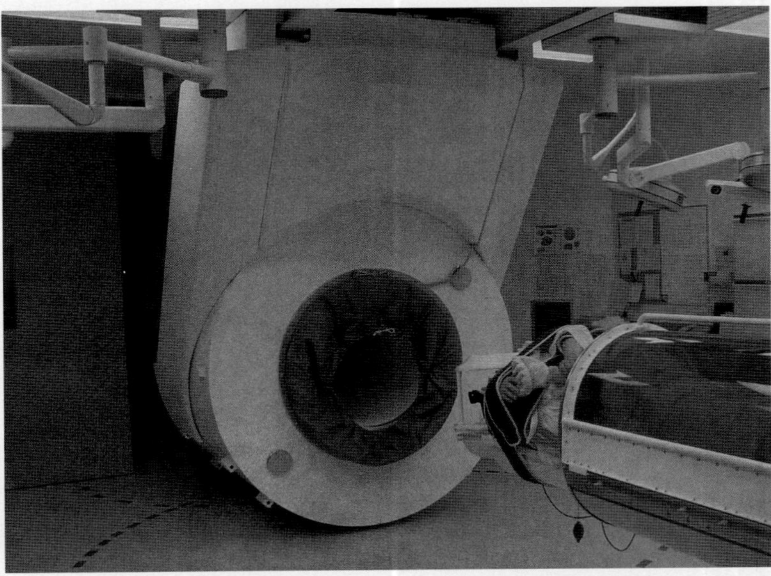

Fig. 1. The 1.5-T, 6-tonne, ceiling-mounted magnet is shown moving out of its alcove into imaging position.

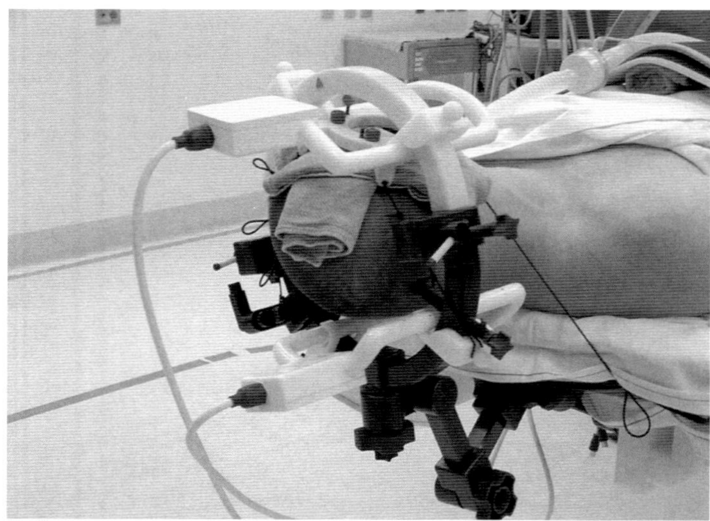

Fig. 2. Patient positioning for a selective amygdalohippocampectomy, with head fixation achieved using a Sugita type four-pin head holder with an integrated radiofrequency coil. The reference array for registration of surgical navigation coordinates is also shown.

Patient selection

The findings in 70 epilepsy patients include cortical dysplasia, ganglioglioma, gangliocytoma, pleomorphic xanthoastrocytoma (PXA), dysembryoplastic neuroepithelial tumor (DNET), and epilepsy without identifiable structural abnormalities on MRI. Patients with neoplastic or vascular lesions as a cause of seizures have not been included.

The patients underwent a complete history, physical examination, and seizure localization using EEG, MRI, and neuropsychologic evaluation. Amytal testing was performed when there was a question as to the functionality of the contralateral temporal lobe and language localization. Selective positron emission tomography, single photon emission computed tomography, and functional MRI (fMRI) were selectively acquired to provide confirmation of the seizure focus and its relation to eloquent cortex. Invasive monitoring using subdural electrode grids or strips was selectively employed before the definitive surgical procedure for confirmation of the epileptogenic focus.

Data, including age at seizure onset; age at surgery; side of surgery; surgical procedure; histopathology; seizure description; pre-, intra-, and postoperative imaging characteristics; and perioperative clinical evaluation results, were prospectively recorded. Patients were classified into four groups: temporal lobe epilepsy (TLE), benign lesions (ganglioglioma, gangliocytoma, DNET, and PXA), cortical dysplasia, and corpus callosotomy. Surgical outcome was based on the Engel classification [26].

Results

Since 1999, 70 patients have undergone 70 surgical procedures for refractory epilepsy at the University of Calgary using iMRI (Table 1). Fifty-nine (84%) patients were adults (age >17 years), and 11 were pediatric patients (age <18 years). Of the 70 procedures performed, 62 (89%) were first operations and 8 were reoperations. TLE predominated in this series. Fifty-one (73%) patients underwent operations for TLE; of these 51 operations, 31 (44%) procedures were selective amygdalohippocampectomies (SelAHs). The 20 remaining procedures for TLE were more extensive temporal lobe resections, including eight (11%) reoperations for residual epileptogenic tissue. Nine (13%) patients underwent resections of benign brain lesions presumed to be the cause of their epilepsy. Resections for cortical dysplasia were performed in 7 (10%) patients. Three (4%) patients underwent corpus callosotomy for generalized epilepsy (Table 2). Eleven pediatric patients, with ages ranging between 12 months and 16 years, were treated for refractory epilepsy.

Table 1
Patient characteristics

	Totals (N = 70)	TLE (N = 51) SelAH [31]	ATL [20]	Benign lesion (N = 9)	Cortical dysplasia (N = 7)	Corpus callosotomy (N = 3)
Age (y)	33 ± 13	35 ± 11	37 ± 13	22 ± 15	23 ± 20	24 ± 13
Gender						
Male	33	15	11	8	3	2
Female	36	16	9	1	4	1
Seizure type		Focal	Focal	Focal	Focal	Generalized
Preoperative evaluation						
MRI						
Normal		0	2 (10%)			
MTS		26 (84%)	13 (65%)			
Benign lesion				9		
Cortical dysplasia		1 (3%)	1 (5%)		7	
Other		4 (13%)	4 (20%)			
EEG telemetry		28	15	9	7	3
Invasive monitoring	18 (26%)	3	9	2	4	0
Previous operation	8 (11%)	0	8	0	0	0

Abbreviations: ATL, anterior temporal lobectomy; MTS, mesial temporal sclerosis; SelAH, selective amygdalohippocampectomy.

Procedures included five resections of benign lesions, three cortical dysplasia resections, two SelAHs, and one corpus callosotomy.

In most patients, surgical planning images were obtained (Table 3). Neuronavigation was registered based on these images in 38 (55%) patients. Sequences included T1-weighted images in all cases and T2-weighted or FLAIR images in select cases. Interdissection images were obtained in 69 (98.6%) patients. T1-weighted sequences were obtained in all cases. Acquisition of other sequences, including T2-weighted and FLAIR images, was individualized to each case. Interdissection imaging revealed residual tissue in 18 (26%) cases, necessitating further resection. Interdissection images were sufficient in 51 (73%) cases demonstrating complete resection of the surgical target. Quality assurance images were obtained after 18 (26%) operations. The need for delayed postoperative imaging was eliminated in all cases. One acute complication, an operative site hematoma, was identified. The patient was redraped, the operative site was reopened, and the hematoma was evacuated.

The duration of imaging studies was approximately 30 minutes, adding, on average, 90 minutes to the procedural time.

Patient seizure outcomes were determined after surgery during the hospital stay and at 3, 6, and 12 months after surgery, followed by yearly clinical assessments thereafter (Table 4). All patients remained on their preoperative antiepileptic medication regimen until 1 year after surgery. At 1 year, tapering of medications was initiated based on each patient's outcome and seizure burden.

Table 2
Pathologic findings

Pathologic finding	Total (N = 70)
TLE	
Normal	8 (11%)
Mesial temporal sclerosis	37 (53%)
Other/gliosis	8 (11%)
Focal cortical dysplasia	7 (10%)
Benign lesions	9 (13%)
Ganglioglioma	4 (6%)
Gangliocytoma	3 (4%)
DNET	2 (3%)
Pleomorphic xanthoastrocytoma	1 (1%)

Table 3
iMRI

	Patients	Surgical planning	Interdissection	Residual tissue	Quality assurance	Neuronavigation
All procedures	70	65 (93%)	69 (99%)	18 (26%)	18 (26%)	39 (56%)
TLE	51 (73%)					
SelAH	31 (61%)	30 (97%)	30 (97%)	10 (32%)	10 (32%)	20 (65%)
ATL	20 (39%)	18 (90%)	20	4 (20%)	4 (20%)	7 (35%)
Cortical dysplasia	7 (10%)	5 (71%)	7	0	0	4 (57%)
Corpus callosotomy	3 (4%)	3	3	1 (33%)	1 (33%)	3
Benign lesion	9 (13%)	9	9	3 (33%)	3 (33%)	5 (56%)

Abbreviations: ATL, anterior temporal lobectomy; SelAH, selective amygdalohippocampectomy.

Of the 70 patients, 61 (87%) have had follow-up of 6 months or longer (mean duration = 21 months, range: 6–51 months). Fifty-nine patients underwent operations for TLE, cortical dysplasia, or benign lesions, with follow-up greater than 6 months. Of these, 41 (70%) remain seizure-free (Engel class I). Outcome for the remaining patients includes 10 (17%) in Engel class II, 4 (7%) in Engel class III, and 4 (7%) in Engel class IV.

Discussion

Epilepsy surgery and intraoperative MRI: current status

The application of iMRI to epilepsy surgery is new, first reported in 1999 [27]. Since that initial publication, only five papers devoted solely to this topic have appeared [28–32]. The reports are small case series documenting and describing the application of iMRI to epilepsy (Table 5).

The University of Calgary's publication was a case series of 14 patients who underwent various operations for TLE and were monitored using the 1.5-T iMRI system. The utility of iMRI during epilepsy surgery was demonstrated by identification of unexpected residual tissue on interdissection imaging in 50% of patients. One acute postoperative hematoma was observed and removed before reversal of anesthesia [30].

Harvard University published a case series of 13 patients who underwent surgery using the General Electric (Waukesha, Wisconsin) Signa SP 0.5-T iMRI system for treatment of benign intracerebral lesions producing seizures. The use of iMRI during lesional epilepsy surgery was demonstrated to be safe and effective, providing guidance throughout the surgical procedure [32].

The University of Erlangen-Nuremberg has made two contributions to the literature. The first publication evaluated whether iMRI using the Magnetom Open 0.2-T iMRI system aided

Table 4
Surgical procedures and patient outcomes

	All patients	Patients (follow-up >6 mo)	Seizure outcome: Engel class (follow-up >6 mo)			
			Class I	Class II	Class III	Class IV
All procedures	70	59 (84%)	41 (70%)	10 (17%)	4 (7%)	4 (7%)
TLE						
SelAH	31 (33%)	30 (51%)	20 (67%)	7 (23%)	1 (3%)	2 (7%)
ATL	20 (29%)	15 (25%)	9 (60%)	1 (7%)	3 (20%)	2 (13%)
Cortical dysplasia	7 (10%)	7 (10%)	5 (71%)	2 (29%)		
Benign lesion	9 (13%)	7 (12%)	7 (100%)			
Reoperations for TLE	8/51 (16%)	8 (14%)	5 (63%)	1 (9%)	1 (9%)	1 (9%)
Corpus callosotomy	3 (3%)	2 (66%)				

Abbreviations: ALT, anterior temporal lobectomy; SelAH, selective amygdalohippocampectomy.

Table 5
iMRI during epilepsy surgery

Description	Year of publication	Authors	Source
Intraoperative MRI in epilepsy surgery	2000	Buchfelder M, et al	J Magn Reson Imaging 12:547–55
Optimizing epilepsy surgery with intraoperative MRI	2002	Kaibara T, et al	Epilepsia 43:425–9
Intraoperative magnetic resonance for the surgical treatment of lesions producing seizures	2002	Walker DG, et al	J Clin Neurosci 9:515–20
Use of iMRI in tailored temporal lobe surgeries for epilepsy	2002	Buchfelder M, et al	Epilepsia 43:864–73
Standardization of amygdalohippocampectomy with iMRI: preliminary experience	2002	Schwartz TH, et al	Epilepsia 43:430–6

surgery individualized to each patient. The series included 61 patients with pharmacoresistant epilepsy. iMRI provided a reliable assessment of the extent of the surgical procedure and a means for identification of residual tissue during surgery [29]. The second publication examined the utility of iMRI for immediate assessment of the extent of resection after operations for TLE. The case series of 58 patients using the same iMRI system provided a reliable evaluation of the extent of resection after temporal lobe procedures when compared with delayed postoperative studies [28].

The Neurological Institute of New Jersey reviewed a series of five patients to determine whether iMRI using the PoleStar 0.12-T system was beneficial for standardization of amygdalohippocampectomy. The authors concluded that iMRI is a useful adjunct for the surgical treatment of mesial TLE and is a reliable method of standardizing complete hippocampectomy [31].

Based on this literature, it can be concluded that iMRI technology is safe and feasible. The benefit of iMRI in epilepsy surgery, however, has not been equivocally established. Further studies, including randomized clinical trials comparing epilepsy procedures performed with and without iMRI guidance, are necessary to provide objective evidence.

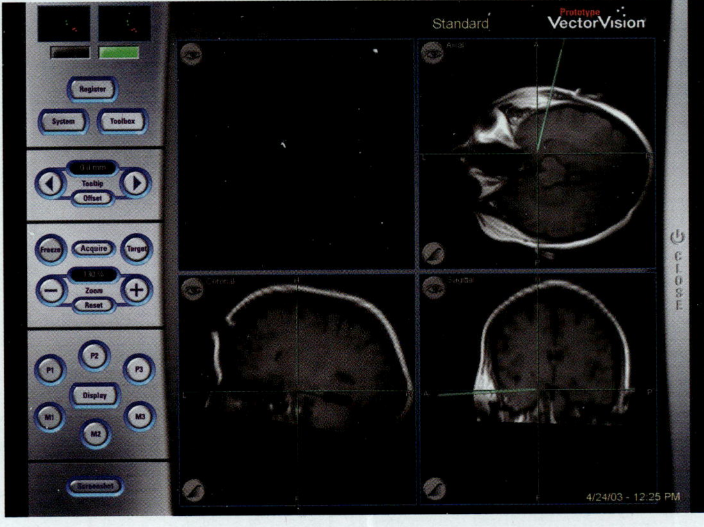

Fig. 3. Intraoperative surgical planning T1-weighted MRI scans registered to a frameless navigation system (BrainLab, Redwood City, California). The screenshot demonstrates the surgical trajectory.

Advantages of intraoperative MRI in epilepsy surgery

Surgical planning images update existing diagnostic studies with the patient anesthetized and positioned for surgery. Neuronavigational setup and coordinate registration occur at this time, thereby eliminating the need for patient transport for repeat diagnostic imaging and its associated cost. This stage optimizes craniotomy placement and target localization (Fig. 3).

Interdissection imaging provides resection control through visualization of intracranial contents, including the surgical target and normal brain parenchyma. The navigational system and the surgeon's anatomic knowledge are updated. Surgeons typically overestimate the amount of resection. In the present series, 18 (26%) cases demonstrated unexpected residual tissue during imaging, necessitating further resection.

The main indication for quality assurance imaging has been acute complication identification and avoidance. This imaging sequence also eliminated the need for delayed postoperative image evaluation of the extent of resection.

Disadvantages of iMRI include economic costs and impact on surgical rhythm. The cost of iMRI technology, including installation cost and service contracts, has limited this technology to a few centers. Imaging during surgery disrupts rhythm and increases procedural time. On average, iMRI added 90 minutes to each case. Disruption of the surgical rhythm is not unlike that encountered during acquisition of traditional ECoG.

Epilepsy surgery and intraoperative MRI at the University of Calgary

Our experience has involved application of a 1.5-T iMRI system to a heterogeneous group of patients with TLE, cortical dysplasia, benign lesions producing seizures, and generalized seizure disorders treated by corpus callosotomy (Figs. 4, 5).

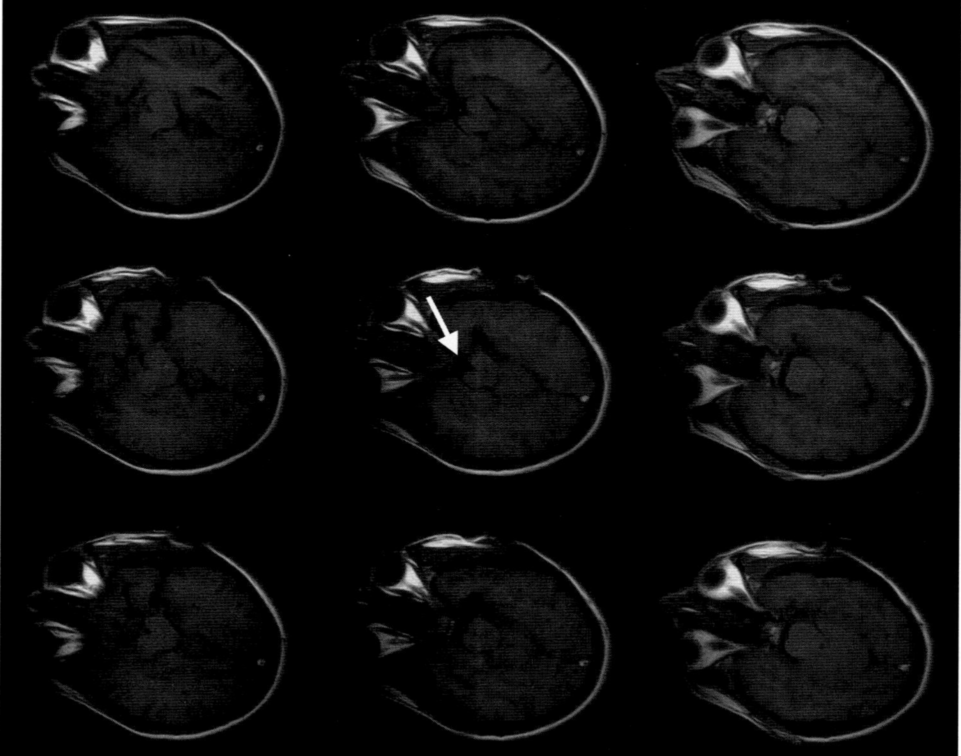

Fig. 4. Surgical planning (*upper row*), interdissection (*middle row*), and quality assurance (*lower row*) T1-weighted MRI scans from a patient with intractable temporal lobe epilepsy. The surgical planning study shows the targeted amygdala and hippocampus. Unsuspected residual amygdala (*arrow*) was present on the interdissection study and was removed before the quality assurance study.

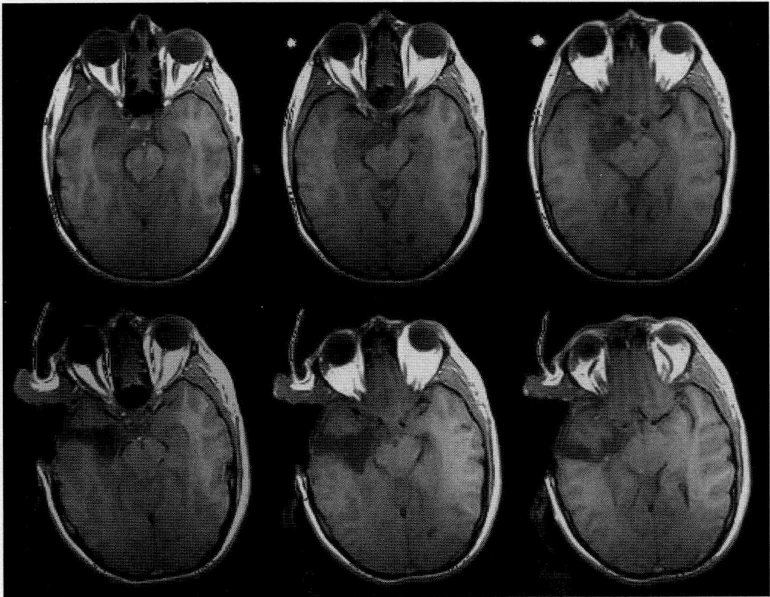

Fig. 5. Surgical planning (*upper row*) and interdissection (*lower row*) T1-weighted MRI scans from a patient with a dysembryoplastic neuroepithelial tumor of the right mesial temporal lobe causing intractable epilepsy. The surgical planning study demonstrates the hypointense lesion. The interdissection study demonstrates complete resection of the lesion.

The iMRI system has been applied to different types of epilepsy operations and is compatible with other technologies routinely used during the surgical management of epilepsy.

After introduction of the iMRI system, anterior temporal lobectomy (ATL) was the most common procedure performed for intractable epilepsy. Over time, the comfort level in performing selective procedures with iMRI guidance increased. Consequently, more selective and less invasive procedures are now performed.

Areas of cortical dysplasia are often subtle and are best identified using 1.5-T or higher iMRI systems. Single to noise, a prerequisite for image quality, is field dependent. Outcome after removal of cortical dysplasia and benign lesions associated with epilepsy is related to the extent of removal of the MRI abnormality. In the present series, dysplastic areas were occasionally visually indistinguishable from normal parenchyma, making iMRI and neuronavigation invaluable. ECoG, when used during these procedures, complemented the iMRI data by providing electrographic localization.

Corpus callosotomy was performed on three patients in an attempt to improve their quality of life. One of the disconnection procedures benefited from interdissection MRI, which showed unexpected incomplete division of the body of the corpus callosum.

Approximately 20% to 50% of patients with TLE develop recurrent seizures after surgery. Reasons for failure include bitemporal EEG abnormalities, incomplete resection of abnormal tissue, and initially unidentified extratemporal lesions. Eight of our patients underwent repeat operations for recurrent seizures after temporal lobectomy. In all these cases, failure was related to incomplete resection of epileptogenic medial temporal lobe structures. It may be concluded that iMRI would decrease the likelihood of such patients.

Neuronavigation was frequently integrated with the iMRI. After interdissection imaging, the neuronavigation system was updated with newly acquired data, thereby restoring navigational accuracy and reducing the problem associated with brain shift. iMRI was particularly beneficial for patients undergoing selective resections of medial temporal structures, where residual tissue was identified in 50% of cases.

We decided to develop an iMRI system based on a moveable magnet for a number of reasons. The operating room looks and functions as a normal surgical theater between imaging studies. MRI-incompatible surgical microscopes, neuronavigation systems, anesthesia and electrophysiologic equipment, and other surgical adjuncts can be accommodated. The potential for moving the magnet to an adjacent diagnostic room permits image acquisition on other patients. Technology sharing is important in a health care system burdened by escalating costs.

Based on the results described, our surgical results are comparable to those reported in the literature with respect to seizure control. We found iMRI of value for target localization and resection control. Given the nature of the disease process and the different factors that influence patient outcome, however, it will be difficult to unequivocally prove the benefit of iMRI during epilepsy surgery without a large randomized control trial.

Advancing epilepsy surgery means improving surgical efficacy. Further advancements in imaging techniques, and their fusion, will improve localization of the epileptogenic focus. Refinements of surgical techniques are necessary to optimize management of the epileptogenic focus with minimal disruption of normal brain parenchyma. Ultimately, surgical intervention in appropriately selected patients will maximally reduce seizure frequency while minimizing neurologic and neuropsychologic deficits. Incorporating surgical robotics into this environment will augment surgical precision and accuracy, allowing precise removal or modulation of abnormal tissue.

Summary

Despite the infancy of iMRI in epilepsy surgery and the paucity of literature on this topic, some conclusions may be reached. Although iMRI is a useful adjunct during epilepsy procedures, a randomized control trial is necessary to determine its true impact.

References

[1] Chang BS, Lowenstein DH. Epilepsy. N Engl J Med 2003;349:1257–66.

[2] Avanzini G, Franceschetti S. Cellular biology of epileptogenesis. Lancet Neurol 2003;2:33–42.

[3] Wiebe S, Blume WT, Girvin JP, Eliasziw M. A randomized, controlled trial of surgery for temporal-lobe epilepsy. N Engl J Med 2001;345:311–8.

[4] Bengzon AR, Rasmussen T, Gloor P, Dussault J, Stephens M. Prognostic factors in the surgical treatment of temporal lobe epileptics. Neurology 1968; 18:717–31.

[5] Clusmann H, Schramm J, Kral T, Helmstaedter C, Ostertun B, Fimmers R, et al. Prognostic factors and outcome after different types of resection for temporal lobe epilepsy. J Neurosurg 2002;97: 1131–41.

[6] Gilliam F, Bowling S, Bilir E, Thomas J, Faught E, Morawetz R, et al. Association of combined MRI, interictal EEG, and ictal EEG results with outcome and pathology after temporal lobectomy. Epilepsia 1997;38:1315–20.

[7] Guldvog B, Loyning Y, Hauglie-Hanssen E, Flood S, Bjornaes H. Predictive factors for success in surgical treatment for partial epilepsy: a multivariate analysis. Epilepsia 1994;35:566–78.

[8] McIntosh AM, Wilson SJ, Berkovic SF. Seizure outcome after temporal lobectomy: current research practice and findings. Epilepsia 2001;42: 1288–307.

[9] Radhakrishnan K, So EL, Silbert PL, Jack CR Jr, Cascino GD, Sharbrough FW, et al. Predictors of outcome of anterior temporal lobectomy for intractable epilepsy: a multivariate study. Neurology 1998; 51:465–71.

[10] Schramm J, Kral T, Grunwald T, Blumcke I. Surgical treatment for neocortical temporal lobe epilepsy: clinical and surgical aspects and seizure outcome. J Neurosurg 2001;94:33–42.

[11] Spencer SS. When should temporal-lobe epilepsy be treated surgically? Lancet Neurol 2002;1:375–82.

[12] Spencer SS, Berg AT, Vickrey BG, Sperling MR, Bazil CW, Shinnar S, et al. Initial outcomes in the Multicenter Study of Epilepsy Surgery. Neurology 2003;61:1680–5.

[13] Zentner J, Hufnagel A, Wolf HK, Ostertun B, Behrens E, Campos MG, et al. Surgical treatment of temporal lobe epilepsy: clinical, radiological, and histopathological findings in 178 patients. J Neurol Neurosurg Psychiatry 1995;58:666–73.

[14] Berkovic SF, McIntosh AM, Kalnins RM, Jackson GD, Fabinyi GC, Brazenor GA, et al. Preoperative MRI predicts outcome of temporal lobectomy: an actuarial analysis. Neurology 1995;45: 1358–63.

[15] Berkovic SF. Surgical treatment of temporal lobe epilepsy. J Neurol Neurosurg Psychiatry 2002;73: 470.

[16] Wyler AR, Hermann BP, Somes G. Extent of medial temporal resection on outcome from anterior temporal lobectomy: a randomized prospective study. Neurosurgery 1995;37:982–90.

[17] Horsley V. Brain-surgery. BMJ 1886;2:670–5.

[18] Berger H. Uber Electrenkephalogramm des Menschen. Arch Psychiatr Nervenkr 1929;87: 527–70.

[19] Fischer M, Lowenbach H. Aktiosstrome des Zentralnerven-systems unter der Einwikung von

Krampfgiften: I. Miteilung Strychnin und Pikrotoxin. Arch Exp Pathol Pharmakol 1934;174:357–82.

[20] Foerster FM, Altenburger H. Elektrobiologische Vorgange an der menslichen Hirnrinde. Dtsch Z Nervenkr 1935;135:277–88.

[21] Jasper H. Localized analyses of the function of the human brain by the electro-encephalogram. Arch Neurol Psychiatry 1936;36:1131–4.

[22] Gibbs F, Lennox W, Gibbs E. The electroencephalogram in diagnosis and localization of epileptic seizures. Arch Neurol Psychiatry 1936;36:1225–35.

[23] Penfield W, Jasper H. Epilepsy and the functional anatomy of the human brain. Boston: Little, Brown; 1954.

[24] Ganslandt O, Behari S, Gralla J, Fahlbusch R, Nimsky C. Neuronavigation: concept, techniques and applications. Neurol India 2002;50:244–55.

[25] Nimsky C, Ganslandt O, Kober H, Buchfelder M, Fahlbusch R. Intraoperative magnetic resonance imaging combined with neuronavigation: a new concept. Neurosurgery 2001;48:1082–9.

[26] Engel JJ. Outcome with respect to epileptic seizures. In: Engel J Jr, editor. Surgical treatment of the epilepsies. New York: Raven Press; 1987. p. 553–71.

[27] Sutherland GR, Kaibara T, Louw D, Hoult DI, Tomanek B, Saunders J. A mobile high-field magnetic resonance system for neurosurgery. J Neurosurg 1999;91:804–13.

[28] Buchfelder M, Fahlbusch R, Ganslandt O, Stefan H, Nimsky C. Use of intraoperative magnetic resonance imaging in tailored temporal lobe surgeries for epilepsy. Epilepsia 2002;43:864–73.

[29] Buchfelder M, Ganslandt O, Fahlbusch R, Nimsky C. Intraoperative magnetic resonance imaging in epilepsy surgery. J Magn Reson Imaging 2000; 12:547–55.

[30] Kaibara T, Myles ST, Lee MA, Sutherland GR. Optimizing epilepsy surgery with intraoperative MR imaging. Epilepsia 2002;43:425–9.

[31] Schwartz TH, Marks D, Pak J, Hill J, Mandelbaum DE, Holodny AI, et al. Standardization of amygdalohippocampectomy with intraoperative magnetic resonance imaging: preliminary experience. Epilepsia 2002;43:430–6.

[32] Walker DG, Talos F, Bromfield EB, Black PM. Intraoperative magnetic resonance for the surgical treatment of lesions producing seizures. J Clin Neurosci 2002;9:515–20.

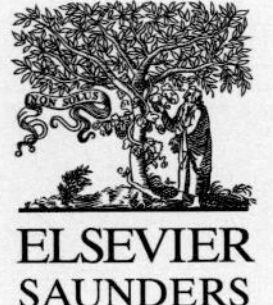
ELSEVIER
SAUNDERS

Neurosurg Clin N Am 16 (2005) 185–200

NEUROSURGERY
CLINICS
OF NORTH AMERICA

1.5 T: intraoperative imaging beyond standard anatomic imaging

Christopher Nimsky, MD*, Oliver Ganslandt, MD, Rudolf Fahlbusch, MD

Department of Neurosurgery, University Erlangen-Nuremberg, Schwabachanlage 6 91054 Erlangen, Germany

In contrast to the subjective estimation of the surgeon about the extent of surgery, intraoperative imaging provides an objective evaluation of surgical effects, thus acting as a measure of quality control during surgery [1]. Because of limited imaging quality, the first attempts in applying ultrasound and CT during neurosurgical procedures in the 1980s were frustrating. Since then, MRI has become the method of choice for the preoperative diagnosis of brain tumors and epilepsy. The closed-bore design and the strong fringe fields of the first MRI scanners prevented their use in the operating room, however. With the development of open MRI systems in the mid-1990s, the concept of intraoperative imaging experienced a renaissance [2–4]. The first designs were based on low-field magnets with magnetic field strengths up to 0.5 T. The use of MRI scanners in the operating environment is safe and reliable as well as applicable to neurosurgical procedures, even if these procedures have to be adapted to the MRI environment to a certain extent. In the meantime, reports on intraoperative MRI for large numbers of patients have been published [5–10].

In contrast to the development of an MRI scanner dedicated to the operating room as pioneered by Black, Jolesz, and General Electric Medical Systems (Milwaukee, Wisconsin) at the Brigham and Women's Hospital in Boston [4], we adapted, in cooperation with the Department of Neurosurgery of the University of Heidelberg and Siemens Medical Solutions (Erlangen, Germany), a low-field MRI scanner for surgical use (0.2-T Magnetom Open) [2,3]. In addition to intraoperative imaging, an integral part of our concept is the possibility of applying neuronavigation simultaneously. We prefer microscope-based neuronavigation, where the extent and localization of a tumor are superimposed on the microscope field of view through contours. Aside from standard neuronavigation based on anatomic information only, which has become a routine tool in many neurosurgical departments, we integrate preoperative functional data from magnetoencephalography (MEG) and functional MRI (fMRI) defining localizations of eloquent brain areas, such as the motor and speech areas, in individual patients, resulting in so-called "functional neuronavigation" [11–15]. Between March 1996 and July 2001, we performed intraoperative low-field MRI in 330 patients [10]. Among these procedures were 240 craniotomies, 59 transsphenoidal approaches, and 31 burr hole procedures. The simultaneous use of intraoperative MRI and functional neuronavigation allowed preservation of neurologic function despite extended resections. The most important indications for intraoperative imaging include gliomas [7–9,16,17], hormonally inactive pituitary tumors [18–21], and pharmacoresistant epilepsy [22–25]. Intraoperative MRI also enables compensation for brain shift by means of an update of the navigation system with intraoperative image data [26–29].

The diagnostic quality of intraoperative low-field MRI systems cannot compete with the image quality of routine neuroradiologic diagnosis,

This work is supported by the Deutsche Forschungsgemeinschaft and the Wilhelm-Sander-Stiftung.

* Corresponding author.

E-mail address: nimsky@nch.imed.uni-erlangen.de (C. Nimsky).

1042-3680/05/$ - see front matter
doi:10.1016/j.nec.2004.07.001

neurosurgery.theclinics.com

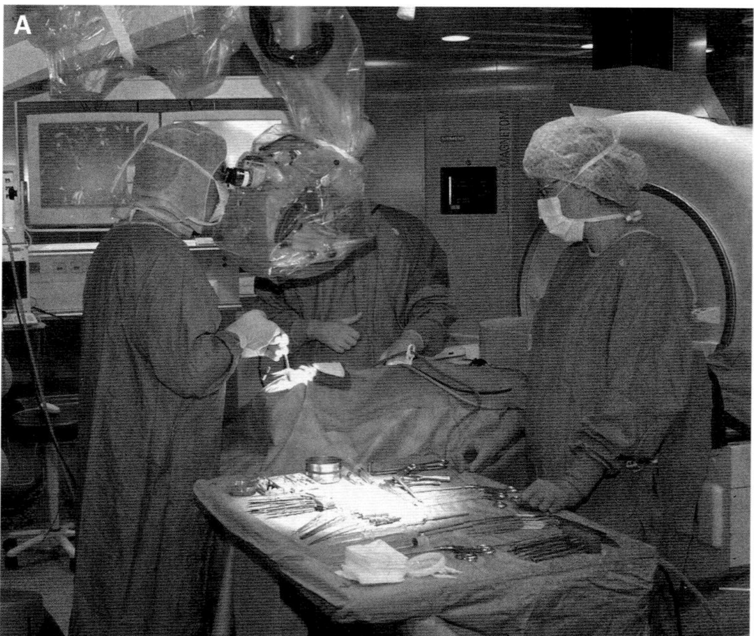

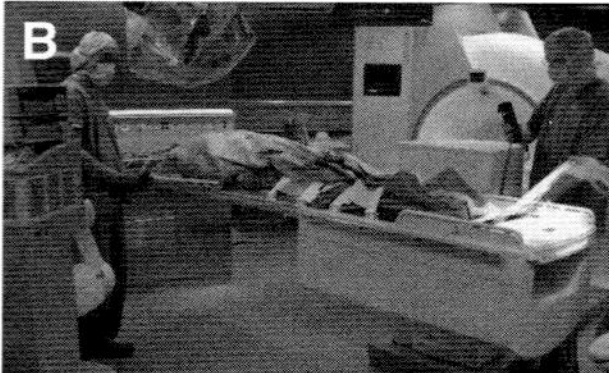

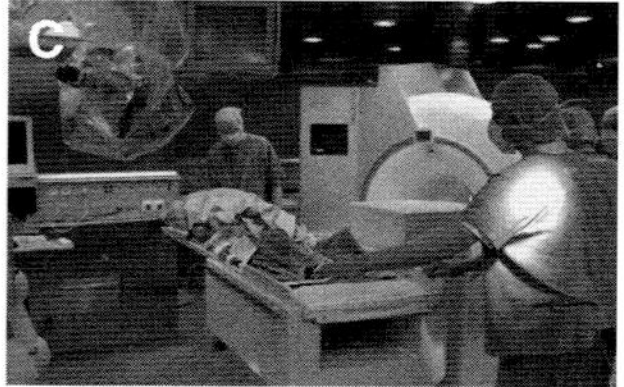

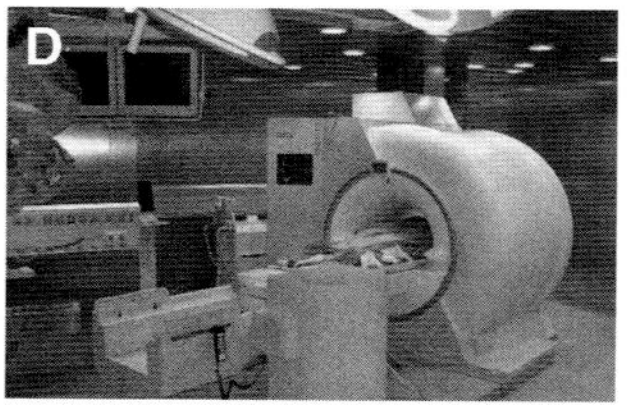

Fig. 1. (*A*) Intraoperative scene in transsphenoidal surgery. (*B–D*) For scanning, the table is rotated 160° and the patient is moved into the center of the scanner.

which is generally performed with high-field magnets. Advances in scanner design, including those resulting from active magnetic shielding, have made it possible to adapt modern high-field scanners to the surgical environment. So far, two different high-field concepts have been realized [30,31]. Basically, as in the intraoperative low-field magnet concepts, there are two possibilities: taking a standard diagnostic scanner and adapting it to the operating environment, as was done in Minneapolis with a Philips scanner (Best, The Netherlands) [31,32], or designing a high-field scanner specifically dedicated for the requirements of an operating room, as was implemented in Calgary with a ceiling-mounted magnet that is moved into the appropriate imaging position during surgery [30,33]. Our approach to realize intraoperative high-field MRI scanning combined with microscope-based neuronavigation resembles the Minneapolis setup, necessitating some kind of intraoperative patient transport for intraoperative imaging. The active magnetic shielding of the high-field magnet results in the 5-G zone being relatively close to the scanner such that the adaptation of a rotating operating table enables combining intraoperative high-field MRI with microscope-based neuronavigation [34]. The main operating position where navigation can be applied is located in the fringe field of the scanner; use of all standard neurosurgical equipment is possible there. In this way, our concept of intraoperative MRI with integration of microscope-based neuronavigation in the low magnetic fringe field [35] can now be applied for high-field magnets. Our operating room was appropriately reconstructed between August 2001 and March 2002. We have been able to operate on patients using intraoperative high-field MRI and integrated microscope-based neuronavigation since the end of April 2002.

Operating room setup

Intraoperative high-field MRI

A rotating surgical table (Trumpf, Saalfeld, Germany) is adapted to a 1.5-T Magnetom Sonata Maestro Class scanner (Siemens Medical Solutions), which is placed in an operating room with radiofrequency (RF) shielding (Figs. 1, 2). The scanner consists of a superconductive 1.5-T magnet with a length of 160 cm and an inner bore diameter of 60 cm equipped with a gradient system with an effective field strength of up to

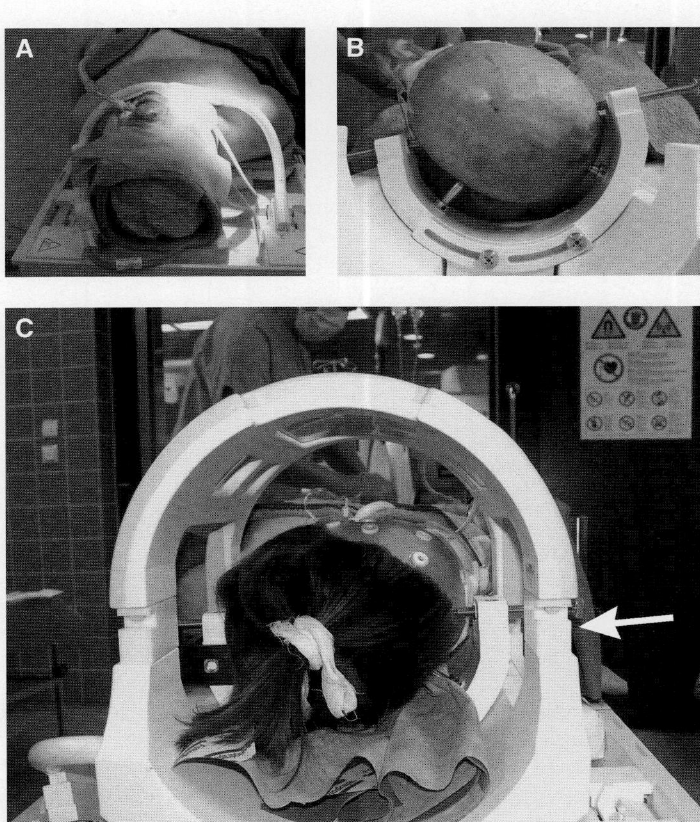

Fig. 2. Different possibilities of coil placement. (*A*) In transsphenoidal surgery, a flexible coil is attached to the head and surgical access is not impeded. (*B*) In craniotomy procedures, the head is fixed in an MRI-compatible head holder, which is placed in the lower part of the standard head coil. (*C*) Sterile adapters (*white arrow*) are placed on the lower part of the head coil, allowing sterile placement of the upper part of the head coil during surgery (image depicts situation before surgery to show the details without draping).

69 mT/m and an effective slew rate of up to 346 T/m/s. The rotating surgical table can be locked into various positions. The principal surgical position is at 160°, with the patient's head at the 5-G line (4-m distance to the center of the scanner). The height of the table, the angle of tilt, and the lateral tilt can be remotely controlled. For imaging, the table is rotated manually for safety reasons so that the table is turned into the axis of the scanner (see Fig. 1).

The ceiling outlet for laminar airflow (Luwa, Frankfurt, Germany) is located above the main operating position. The laminar airflow output is surrounded by a band of fluorescent lamps for optimal illumination. For scanning, the illumination can be turned off from the control room. The entire operating theater has MRI-compatible spot-room lighting. Two ceiling-mounted surgical lamps (Heraeus Med, Hanau, Germany) are installed at the main surgical position. Movable MRI-compatible surgical lamps (Heraeus Med) can be used at the second surgical position in the high magnetic field at the dorsal opening of the scanner. MRI-compatible ventilation (Servo 900C; Siemens Medical Solutions) and MRI-compatible monitoring (Invivo Research, Orlando, Florida) are available for anesthesia. Vital parameters are transferred outside the RF cabin by wireless 2.4-GHz data transfer. The perfusors and infusion pumps are shielded for MRI compatibility (MRI-Caddy; MIPM, Mammendorf, Germany) [36]. All standard gas lines are available on service outlets

Table 1
Sequences used in intraoperative high-field MRI

Sequence	Slice thickness (mm)	TR (ms)	TE (ms)	FOV (mm)	In-plane resolution (mm)	No. acquisitions	Total scan time
Localizer	10	20	50	280	1.1 × 1.1	1	9 s
Pituitary tumors							
T2-HASTE	5	1000	89	230	0.89 × 0.89	5	25 s
T1-SE	3	450	12	270	0.52 × 0.87	4	4 min 57 s
T2-TSE	3	3850	111	210	0.41 × 0.58	4	7 min 17 s
Gliomas/epilepsy surgery							
T2-TSE	4	6490	98	230	0.44 × 0.74	3	5 min 39 s
FLAIR	4	10,000	103	230	0.44 × 0.74	1	6 min 2 s
T1-SE	4	525	17	230	0.89 × 0.89	2	3 min 59 s
EPI	5	30,000	85	230	1.79 × 1.79	2	3 min
MPRAGE	1	2020	4.38	250	0.49 × 0.49i	1	8 min 39 s
Metabolic and functional imaging							
MRS-CSI	10	1600	135	160	6.7 × 6.7	2	12 min 45 s
fMRI	3	1580	60	192	3 × 3	1	3 min 13
DTI	1.9	9200	86	240	1.87 × 1.87	5	5 min 31 s

Abbreviations: CSI, chemical shift imaging; DTI, diffusion tensor imaging; EPI, echo planar imaging; FLAIR, fluid-attenuated inversion recovery; FOV, field of view; HASTE, half-Fourier single-shot turbo spin echo; i, interpolated; min, minutes; MPRAGE, magnetization prepared rapid acquisition gradient echo sequence; MRS, magnetic resonance spectroscopy; s, seconds; SE, spin echo; TE, echo time; TR, repetition time; TSE, turbo spin echo.

at different places in the RF cabin. Compressed air is integrated to operate drills. The service outlets include sockets connected to different electrical circuits so that selected sockets can be switched off from a switchboard in the MRI control room to prevent artifacts generated by individual devices.

The NC4 Multivision microscope (Zeiss, Oberkochen, Germany) is installed at the left side of the head outside the 5-G line. The microscope and other potentially interfering devices are automatically switched off for the MRI measurements. The microscope videotape is documented using Medimage software (Vepro, Pfungstadt, Germany) and in parallel as a recording on commercial S-VHS tapes. Both systems are installed in the MRI control room. Two flat-monitor screens (17.4 in, AS4431ID; Iyamo, Nagano-Shi, Japan) mounted on a ceiling arm (Ondal, Hünfeld, Germany) display the microscope image, the image from the MRI console, or various personal computer (PC) applications. There is also a wall-mounted PC console using Autoview200 (Avocent, Munich, Germany), with which the various PC systems, such as the videotape documentation and the navigation system, can be operated from inside the RF cabin. There is an identical console in the MRI control room. A mobile in-room MRI console is available in the RF room for operating the scanner. The 5-G and 200-G lines are marked on the floor. The 200-G line is also marked by a raised stainless steel strip as a mechanical threshold. All equipment not completely MRI-compatible, such as the navigation microscope and the height-adjustable surgeon's chair, are mechanically secured to the wall of the RF room. The instrument table and the various rotating stools are fully MRI-compatible (Trumpf).

An MRI-compatible four-point head holder made of fiberglass-reinforced plastic was used for head fixation during the craniotomy and burr hole procedures. It is integrated into the common system circular polarized head coil (see Fig. 2B) [37]. The upper part of the head coil may be sterilized using plasma sterilization. Sterile adapters placed onto the lower part of the head coil ensure the possibility of sterile draping (see Fig. 2C). In transsphenoidal surgery that does not require head fixation, imaging is performed using a U-shaped flexible coil adapted to the head (see Fig. 2A). After the patient is moved into the center of the scanner, certain circuits are switched off, including the fluorescent lamps, the operating microscope, and the part of the navigation system that is located in the RF cabin. Imaging then starts with a localizer sequence (all sequence parameters are listed in Table 1).

In transsphenoidal surgery, T2-weighted half-Fourier single-shot turbo spin echo (HASTE) sequences in coronal and sagittal orientations are measured next to give a quick overview. HASTE imaging allows one to obtain a rough estimation of the extent of the resection, allowing nearly immediate continuation of surgery if a tumor remnant is depicted. Afterward, T1-weighted coronal and sagittal spin echo sequences are applied. Additionally, high-resolution, T2-weighted, turbo spin echo sequences are measured. The protocol in transsphenoidal pituitary surgery was modified after having acquired increased experience. Measuring of the T1-weighted images was abandoned, because T2-weighted imaging provided sufficient and even more reliable information than the T1-weighted images, especially regarding better delineation of the intrasellar and parasellar structures.

In glioma surgery, the imaging protocol includes the following axial sequences: T2-weighted turbo spin echo, fluid-attenuated inversion recovery (FLAIR), T1-weighted spin echo, and echo planar imaging dark fluid. In case the tumor showed contrast enhancement in the preoperative images, the T1-weighted axial spin echo sequence was repeated after intravenous application of gadolinium-diethylenetriamine pentaacetic acid at a rate of 0.2-mL/kg of body weight. Afterward, the 1.0-mm, isotropic, three-dimensional (3-D) magnetization prepared rapid acquisition gradient echo sequence (MPRAGE) data set, which is used for navigation, was measured, allowing free-slice reformatting and intraoperative updating of the navigation system [27,28]. In epilepsy surgery and other applications (eg, biopsies), a reduced scanning protocol was applied. If intraoperative imaging resulted in further tumor removal, imaging was repeated after completion of the resection before wound closure. Contrast medium was not applied repeatedly. If preoperative scanning was performed after head fixation and anesthesia induction, identical sequence parameters were used so that the identical pre- and intraoperative slices could be displayed side by side, facilitating image interpretation greatly.

Neuronavigation

Neuronavigation support is provided by the VectorVision Sky Navigation System (BrainLab, Heimstetten, Germany). A fiberoptic connection ensures MRI-compatible integration into the RF room. The camera used to monitor the positions of the microscope and other instruments is ceiling mounted, as is the touch screen that is used to operate the navigation system. A 1.0-mm, isotropic, 3-D MPRAGE data set was acquired before surgery as a navigational reference data set in which functional data could be integrated. For registration, five adhesive skin fiducials were placed in a scattered pattern on the head surface before imaging and registered with a pointer after their position was defined in the 3-D data set, or a LASER scanning device (z-touch; BrainLab) [38] was used for referencing. Functional data from MEG and fMRI, which were acquired before surgery, were integrated into the 3-D data set [11–15]. Furthermore, data from diffusion tensor imaging (DTI) depicting the course of major white matter tracts were integrated, and metabolic maps from magnetic resonance spectroscopy (chemical shift imaging [CSI]) were coregistered to the navigation data set in selected cases [39]. Repeated landmark checks were performed to ensure overall ongoing clinical application accuracy. In case intraoperative imaging depicted some remaining tumor that should be removed, intraoperative image data were used for updating the navigation system. After a rigid registration of pre- and intraoperative images (ImageFusion software; BrainLAB), all data were transferred to the navigation computer, and the initial patient registration file was then restored such that no repeated patient registration procedure was needed.

Clinical experience

Three hundred thirteen patients have been examined with intraoperative high-field MRI through the end of February 2004. Among these operations were 118 transsphenoidal procedures, 47 burr hole procedures, and 148 craniotomies (Table 2). The major groups were patients with gliomas and pituitary adenomas. Intraoperative high-field MRI is a safe and reliable procedure, we did not encounter any adverse events as a result of the high magnetic field, and there were no ferromagnetic accidents as a result of the use of standard instruments in the fringe field at the 5-G zone. With respect to intraoperative work flow, we found a distinct improvement over our previous designs [2,10,35]. The time necessary for intraoperative imaging has been greatly reduced. In general, it took less than 2 minutes from the time the neurosurgeon decided to use intraoperative imaging until the imaging was actually started. With all the anesthesia lines to and from the patient passing through the surgical table's center of rotation, there were no delays, because

Table 2
Histopathologic findings and types of procedures in 313 patients investigated with intraoperative high-field MRI

Histopathologic finding	cr	ts	bh	Total
Pituitary adenoma	3	95	—	98
Glioma	75	—	22	97
Gliosis/hippocampal sclerosis (epilepsy surgery)	29	—	—	29
Craniopharyngioma	4	13	—	17
Meningioma	9	—	—	9
Lymphoma	4	—	5	9
Cavernoma	9	—	—	9
Dysembryoplastic neuroepithelial tumor	5	—	—	5
Gliomatosis	2	—	2	4
Rathke cleft cyst	—	4	—	4
Metastasis	2	—	1	3
Chordoma	—	2	—	2
Others	6	4	3	13
No histology obtained:				
Craniopharyngioma cyst puncture	—	—	9	9
Other cystic lesions	—	—	5	5
Total	148	118	47	313

Abbreviations: bh, burr hole procedure; cr, craniotomy; ts, transsphenoidal surgery.

no rearrangement of the anesthesia equipment was necessary. Also, the preoperative handling, including patient positioning and navigation registration, was less time-consuming. We expect that the possibility of automatic registration of images, which is under development, will result not only in further time saving but in further improved accuracy during clinical applications.

Intraoperative imaging was technically possible in all cases. We encountered technical difficulties in only one case. In one of the first transsphenoidal procedures, a coil cable broke during use of the flexible coil such that the coil had to be replaced. No major artifacts related to the operating room environment were observed. The ability to turn off the fluorescent lamps and specific power outlets from the MRI control room proved helpful. We did not encounter increased problems with artifacts because of the high-field setup but rather fewer artifacts than with the previous system. This may be mainly a result of the improved operating room design, including better flexibility to eliminate artifacts from devices located in the operating room itself as well as an improved coil design for intraoperative imaging, which was one of the major problems with the initial low-field setup.

The flexibility of the rotating surgical MRI table during surgery is similar to that of a standard surgical table. The head holder integrated into the head coil allows some variability of access; the patient can be placed in the supine and prone position or the head can be turned up to a horizontal position. Full lateral placement of the whole patient is only possible in young patients because of the inner core size of the scanner (60 cm). Access to the craniotomy site is limited to a certain extent. The coil adapters sometimes handicapped access to the craniotomy site. A new head holder with a dedicated eight-channel MRI coil is just being developed. We expect that this new device will improve the ergonomics for the neurosurgeon without decreasing image quality.

The intraoperative image quality obtained is clearly superior to that of our previous intraoperative low-field (0.2-T) system. Even the comparison of pre- and intraoperative images did not indicate any significant limitation. Fig. 3 gives an impression of the enhanced image quality of the intraoperative high-field system in comparison to our previous low-field system in two similar cases of frontal low-grade gliomas. We think that the clearly improved image quality will result in more reliable information regarding the extent of resection (ie, presence of residual tumor tissue and its exact location). Aside from improved image quality, the high-field scanner allows significantly shorter examination times such that a more detailed sequence protocol can be measured within the same time frame.

In 92 (29.4%) of all 313 patients, intraoperative MRI resulted in a modification of the surgical strategy (ie, an extension of the resection or a correction of the placement of a biopsy needle or a catheter). Concerning the major application of intraoperative imaging, which is resection control in pituitary adenomas and gliomas, these numbers are even higher (30 [40%] of 74 patients and 31 [43%] of 72 patients, respectively). Comparing these rates with our previous low-field experience (34% and 26%, respectively) [21,40] supports the impression that the clearly improved image quality of the high-field system may also result in increased rates of extended resections.

Transsphenoidal pituitary surgery

Among the 95 patients with pituitary adenomas who were operated on via the transsphenoidal approach, 74 had an intra- and suprasellar extension that seemed accessible and removable

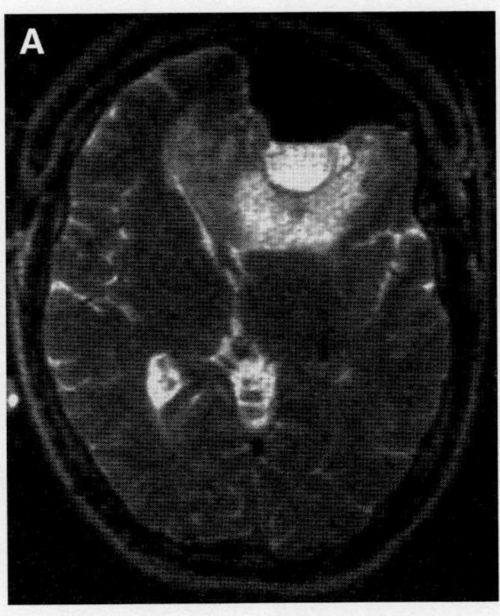

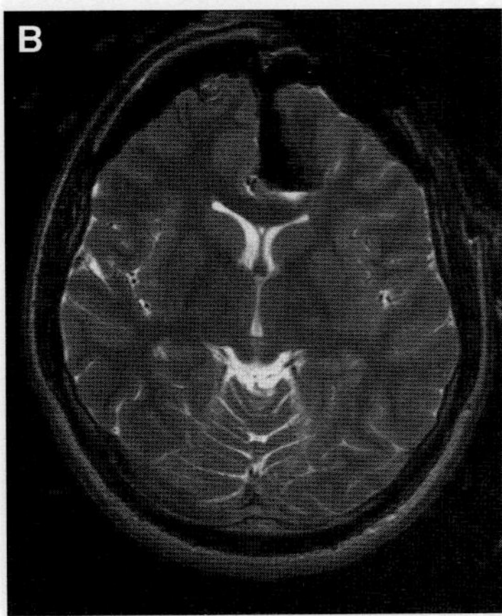

Fig. 3. Comparison of intraoperative image quality in similar clinical cases of left frontal low-grade gliomas examined with T2-weighted imaging. (*A*) Low-field MRI with a 0.2-T Magnetom Open scanner (Siemens Medical Solutions, Erlangen, Germany). (*B*) High-field MRI with a 1.5-T Magentom Sonata scanner.

by the transsphenoidal approach. Repeated inspection of the surgical field during intraoperative MRI revealed some remaining tumor that could be at least partially removed in 30 patients. In 20 of these patients, the resection could be completed, resulting in an increase in the rate of complete removal from 56.7% (42 of 74 patients) to 83.8% (62 of 74 patients). Reliable imaging of suprasellar tumor removal was possible in all cases. Fig. 4 illustrates a typical example of a pituitary adenoma with a distinct suprasellar extension, which could be removed completely. In contrast to the low-field systems, where evaluation of the intrasellar space was rarely possible [21], even the structures of the cavernous sinus could now be evaluated reliably in most patients. Ultra-early (ie, intraoperative) visualization of tumor remnants that are not removable allows the immediate planning of further postoperative treatment options, such as surveillance, radiation therapy, or transcranial surgery. Otherwise, further planning would only be possible some 2 to 3 months after surgery because of early postoperative imaging artifacts preventing reliable image evaluation after transsphenoidal surgery [21,41].

Transsphenoidal surgery of craniopharyngiomas could also be monitored reliably by intraoperative imaging. High-resolution T2-weighted imaging provided valuable information about the extent of resection (Fig. 5). Despite the clearly improved image quality of high-field MRI compared with low-field MRI with regard to craniopharyngioma removal, it is too early to decide whether high-field MRI is more sensitive in the detecting small tumor islets that may give rise to craniopharyngioma recurrence compared with low-field MRI [42].

Burr hole procedures

Exclusion of intracerebral hemorrhage and confirmation of the biopsy site were the major aspects of intraoperative imaging in burr hole procedures (n = 47). In nine patients with large cystic craniopharyngiomas, the cyst could be punctured with a catheter guided by navigation. In four of these patients, intraoperative MRI revealed that the catheter had not penetrated the cyst wall such that no drainage of the cyst to the lateral ventricle was established, leading to a repeated puncture, which was then successful as proved by repeated intraoperative imaging. In five further patients, cysts originating from other tumors could be punctured without any problems. In all 33 burr hole biopsies, a histologic diagnosis could be obtained. Side-by-side display of corresponding pre- and intraoperative slices enabled direct evaluation of the biopsy site (Fig. 6). During the time of intraoperative imaging, frozen section analysis of parts of the biopsy sample was also performed to confirm that a pathologic specimen was obtained. In three patients, intraoperative imaging resulted in a correction of the biopsy needle path. In one patient who was operated on directly in the high magnetic field, the advancement of the biopsy needle could be

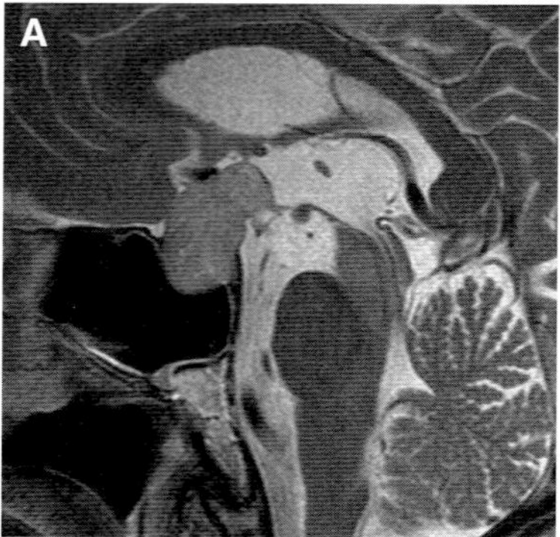

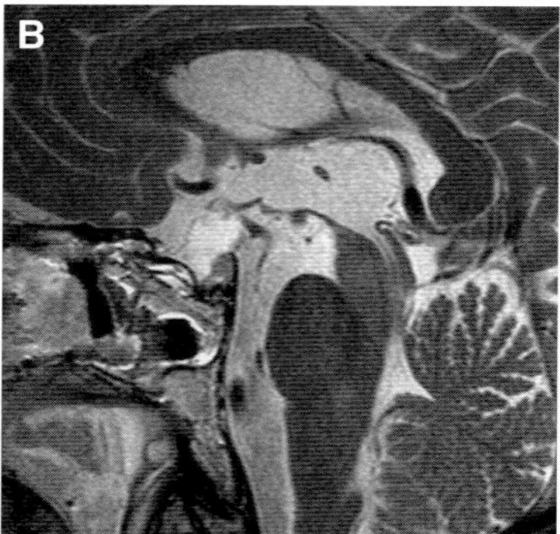

Fig. 4. (*A*) Preoperative T2-weighted imaging in a 53-year-old man with a pituitary adenoma with a distinct suprasellar extension. (*B*) Intraoperative imaging confirms complete removal.

monitored by scanning with a true fast imaging with steady-state precession sequence with a single-slice scan duration of 190 milliseconds.

Glioma surgery

Regarding the treatment of gliomas, at present, the standard treatment is maximum safe resection and, for high-grade gliomas, subsequent adjuvant treatment, such as radio- and chemotherapy [43–45]. With respect to patients undergoing glioma resection (n = 72), intraoperative imaging revealed complete tumor removal initially in 18 (25%) patients. Extension of the resection because of intraoperative imaging resulted in a final gross total removal of 40.3% of gliomas. Of the 29 patients with a finally completed resection, 11 (37.9%) resections were attributable to further tumor removal after intraoperative MRI. In 23 patients with incomplete tumor removal, further resection was abandoned because of the infiltration of eloquent brain cortex or critical anatomic structures despite obvious residual tumor on intraoperative imaging. Additional resection in 31 (43.1%) patients as the result of intraoperative MRI significantly reduced the percentage of final tumor volume compared with first intraoperative MRI. According to a volumetric assessment, the percentages of residual tumor volume were significantly decreased from the first intraoperative scan to the final scan [46]. Even in the subgroup of patients in which no complete resection was intended because of infiltration of eloquent brain areas, intraoperative MRI led to further tumor reduction in 46.5% (20 of 43) of the patients, reducing the tumor volume significantly. In low-grade gliomas, there is little question that complete removal of all tumor tissue is an ideal treatment that may lead to cure. If residual tumor is left

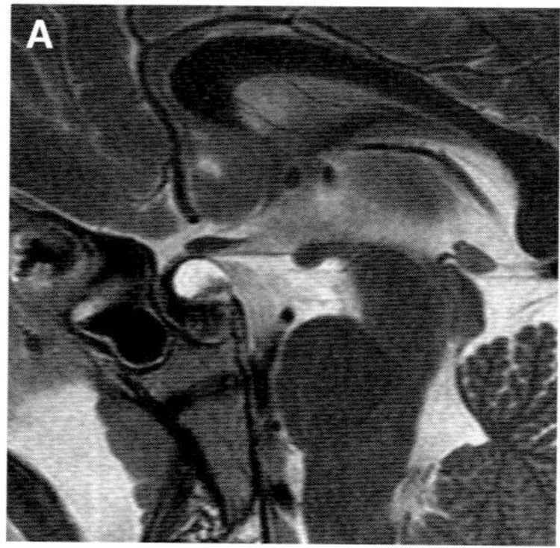

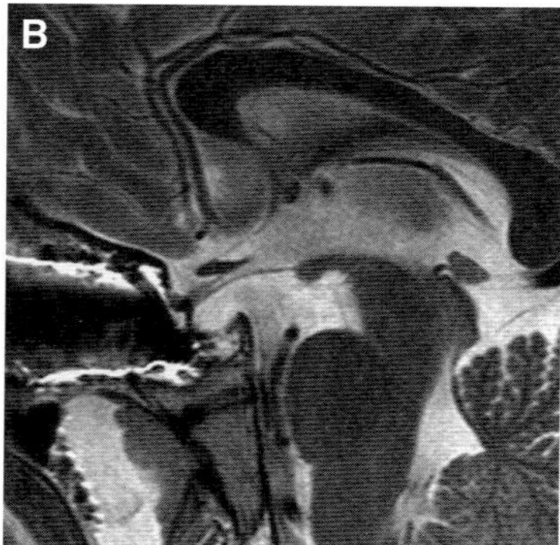

Fig. 5. (*A*) T2-weighted imaging in a 10-year-old girl with a craniopharyngioma that could be removed completely via a transsphenoidal approach. (*B*) Note the high imaging quality with the clear delineation of the pituitary stalk and the infundibulum in the intraoperative images.

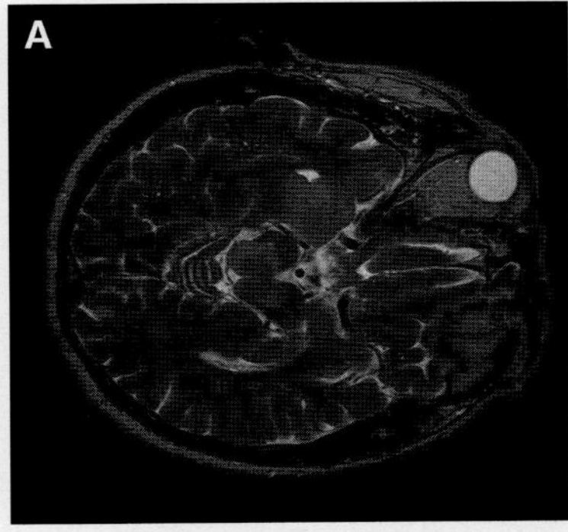

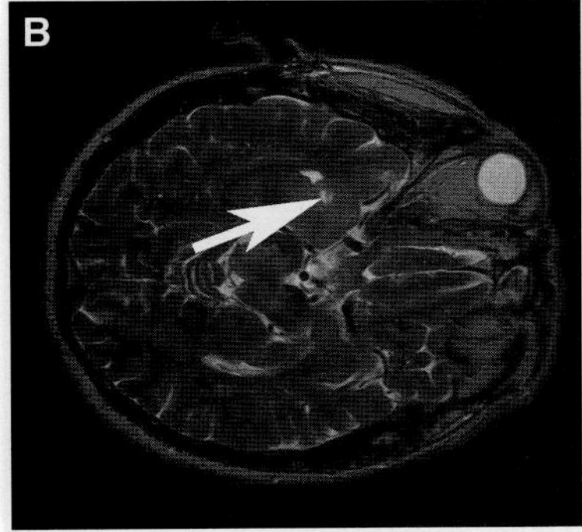

Fig. 6. (*A*) Intraoperative imaging in a biopsy procedure of a diffuse glioma (extending into the internal capsule and into the brain stem) in a 59-year-old man. (*B*) Intraoperative imaging confirms the preplanned navigated biopsy site in the right temporal lobe (*white arrow*). Frozen section analysis confirmed a high-grade glioma, and histologic examination revealed a diffuse astrocytoma, World Health Organization grade III.

behind, it eventually degenerates into a glioblastoma multiforme, limiting the life expectancy of the patient [1]. Even in high-grade gliomas, several reports have supported the benefit of aggressive tumor removal, which was associated with longer survival of patients [47–50]. Fig. 7 depicts an example of resection control in a high-grade glioma. As in transsphenoidal surgery, T2-weighted imaging proved to be most helpful. FLAIR imaging often showed diffuse enhancement at the resection border. Side-by-side and overlay display of corresponding pre- and intraoperative images facilitated imaging interpretation, especially to distinguish between surgically induced changes and tumor remnants.

Other procedures

In all patients, intraoperative MRI provided immediate intraoperative quality control not only in respect to the extent of a resection or the positioning of a catheter or a biopsy needle but with regard to complication avoidance, because we did not encounter any rebleeding. Another interesting indication for intraoperative MRI is epilepsy surgery [22–25]. In epilepsy surgery for nonlesional temporal lobe epilepsy, intraoperative MRI allowed clear delineation of the extent of tailored temporal lobectomies. Furthermore, localization of subdural and hippocampal strip electrodes could be defined by intraoperative imaging.

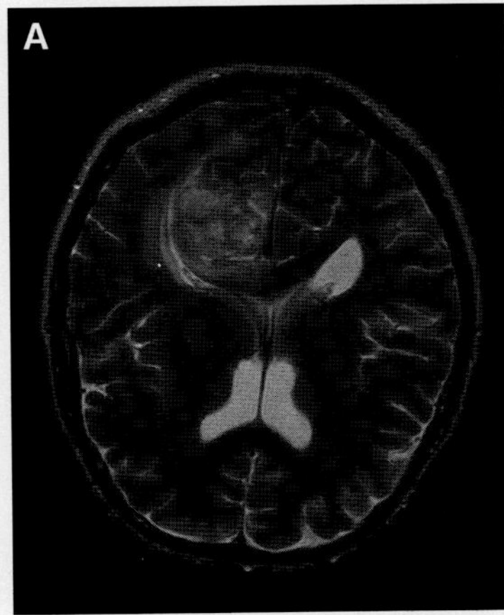

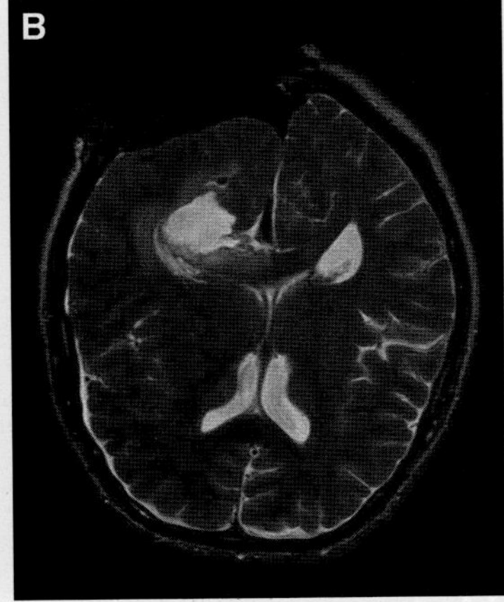

Fig. 7. Right occipital World Health Organization grade IV glioblastoma in a 67-year-old man. T2-weighted imaging reveals complete removal of the main tumor mass and depicts the remaining infiltration zone in the posterior corpus callosum (*A*, preoperative image; *B*, intraoperative image).

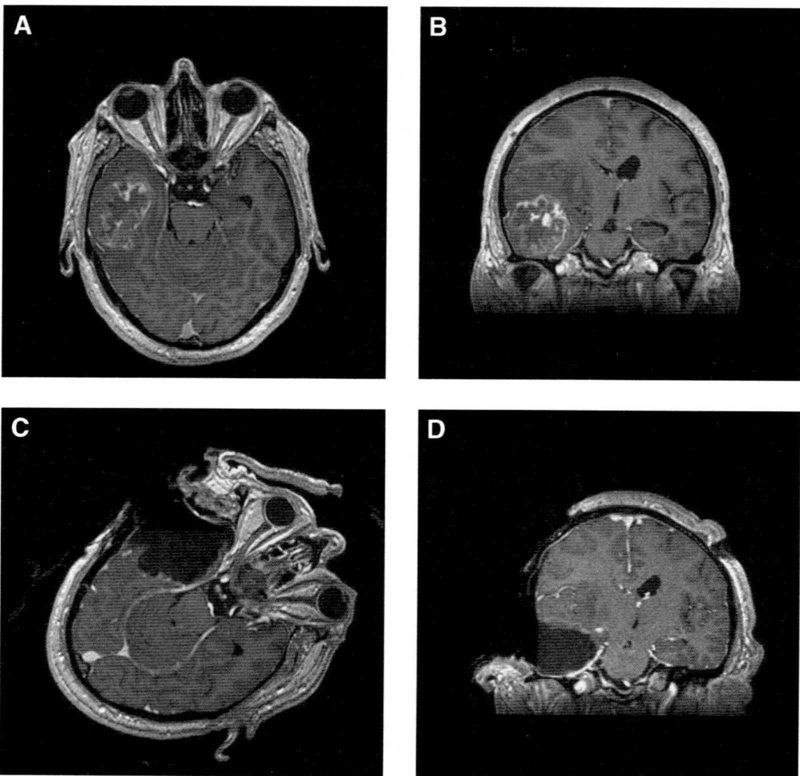

Fig. 8. T1-weighted magnetization prepared rapid acquisition gradient echo sequence images of a right temporal World Health Organization grade IV glioblastoma in a 57-year-old man. Intraoperative imaging confirms the removal of the contrast-enhancing tumor parts (*A, B*: preoperative images; *C, D*: intraoperative images; *A, C*: corresponding axial slices; *B, D*: corresponding coronal slices).

Anatomic neuronavigation guidance

The various other tumor entities that were investigated by intraoperative MRI in smaller numbers included mainly tumors with a difficult location, where navigation guidance was essential, and intraoperative imaging was used to identify tumor remnants and localize them by intraoperative updating of the neuronavigation system, thus compensating for brain shift. The integrated microscope-based neuronavigation was used without problems and with good clinical accuracy. Navigation accuracy was not impeded by the magnetic fringe field. The mean registration error ranged from 0.3 to 2.9 mm. In all navigation cases, the localization error of an additional fiducial, which was not used for the registration, allowed us to document a low target registration error. Only in two cases did the navigation setup fail because of software problems. In total, navigation was applied in 170 patients. The navigation was updated in 42 patients (24.7% of the patients in which navigation was applied) without difficulty. This led to reliable identification of the residual tumor parts and compensated for brain shift. Compared with previous setups that necessitated intraoperative patient reregistration [26–29], which was time-consuming, the implemented update procedure that restores the initial patient registration data facilitated updating. Excluding the patients operated on by a transsphenoidal approach, in which navigation was applied in selected cases only (n = 6), navigation was administered in 84% (164 of 195) of all patients, demonstrating the close integration of imaging and navigation. The remaining 16% of patients who did not undergo navigation were mainly patients with pharmacoresistant epilepsy undergoing tailored temporal lobe resection. In these patients, navigation was not applied routinely, because the various intraoperative anatomic

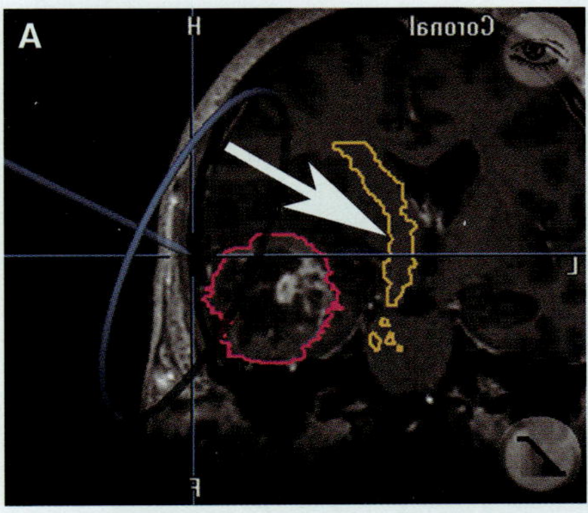

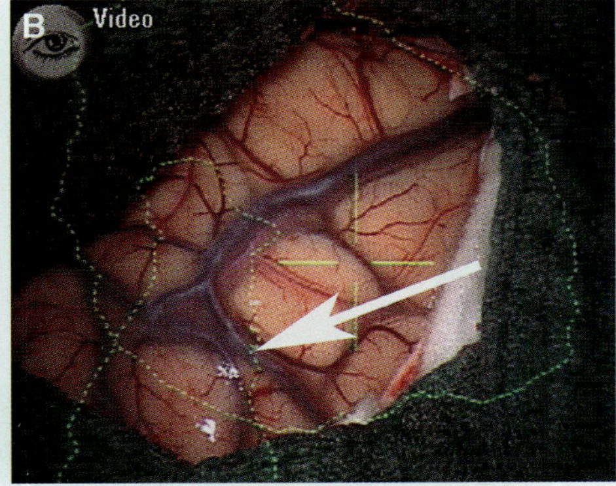

Fig. 9. Navigation screen of the same patient as in Fig. 8. (*A*) The displaced right pyramidal tract is visualized by diffusion tensor imaging and integrated into the navigational data set (*arrow*, coronal T1-weighted image of navigation screen). (*B*) Corresponding microscope view just after dural opening; the tumor contour as well as the contour of the right pyramidal tract is displayed (*arrow*).

landmarks of the temporal lobe were sufficient for reliable guidance. Scanning the 3-D data set, which is used for patient registration, just before surgery after induction of anesthesia and head fixation excluded shifting of registration markers and was a prerequisite for low registration error.

Functional neuronavigation and functional imaging

Functional neuronavigation (ie, integrating functional data into the anatomic navigation data sets) is an important add-on to intraoperative MRI because it prevents resections that are too extensive, which would otherwise result in new neurologic deficits. We had integrated functional or metabolic data in 65 patients and observed prolonged new postoperative neurologic deficits in only 4 of them. To date, data from MEG and fMRI are routinely integrated in functional neuronavigation, allowing identification of eloquent brain areas, such as the motor area and speech-related areas [11,14,15]. This method is open to integrate further modalities, such as magnetic resonance spectroscopy and DTI. Both methods have been used recently as new diagnostic tools in patients with gliomas [51–56]. Magnetic resonance spectroscopy data may provide further information on the diffuse tumor border. Integration of metabolic maps into the neuronavigation data sets enables spatial correlation of metabolic data and histopathologic findings [39].

Functional data from MEG and fMRI only localize function at the brain surface; however, neurologic deficits can occur during tumor resection as a result of damage to deeper structures, such as major white matter tracts. DTI can be used not only to delineate tumor borders but to display the course of white matter tracts, such as the pyramidal tract [57–61]. Knowledge of the course of major white matter tracts in relation to a tumor may help to prevent new postoperative neurologic deficits [62,63]. Registration of these data with the navigation data set [64] should facilitate the intraoperative preservation of these eloquent structures if the intraoperative changes of the brain anatomy, known as brain shift, are taken into account. Fig. 8 illustrates standard anatomic preoperative and corresponding intraoperative imaging in a right temporal glioblastoma. We had integrated DTI data depicting the displaced course of the pyramidal tract into the navigational data set so that these data could be visualized during surgery (Fig. 9). Intraoperative functional imaging (ie, applying intraoperative DTI) revealed a marked shifting of the pyramidal tract because of tumor resection (Fig. 10). As a consequence of this shifting, the preoperative functional data are no longer valid, so the neurosurgeon can no longer rely on the navigation if this shifting is not compensated for. Therefore, it is necessary not only that intraoperative anatomic data be used to compensate for the effects of brain shift [28,29,65] but that functional data be updated [66]. Mathematic models that describe the brain shift phenomenon using finite elements should be helpful in this respect [67,68]. At present, however, only intraoperative functional imaging provides reliable data on the actual intraoperative situation. Whether intraoperative

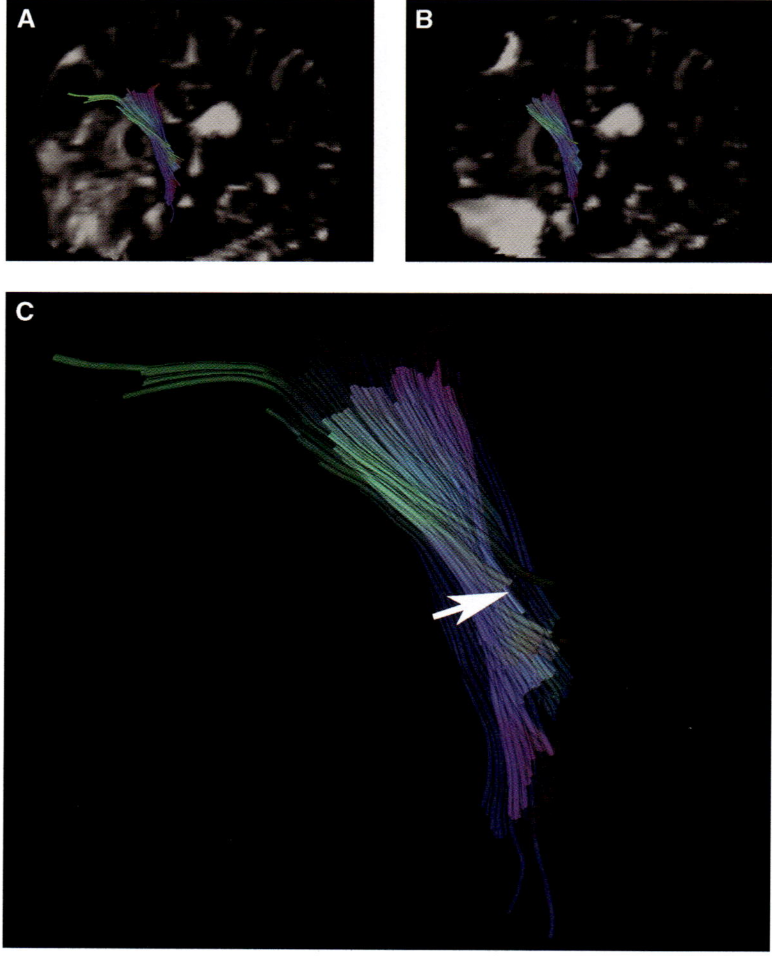

Fig. 10. Comparison between the preoperative (*A*) and intraoperative (*B*) fiber tract visualization of the pyramidal tract with the coregistered B-0 images depicts an inward shifting of the right pyramidal tract after tumor removal. (*C*) The semitransparent overlay of the pre- and intraoperative fiber tracts illustrates the inward shifting, which amounts to approximately 6 mm (*arrow*).

fMRI, despite the open skull, is reliably possible at all is under investigation. Electrical stimulation of the median and tibial nerves as a passive stimulation paradigm may allow identification of the somatosensory cortex [69]. The next steps will be the integration of DTI-based tractography data into the neuronavigation data set along with fMRI, because the combination of fMRI and DTI provides valuable information that cannot be extracted using either method alone [62,70]. Regarding the pyramidal tract, using the fMRI data as seed regions for the DTI fiber-tracking algorithms would be an elegant method.

Other further applications of intraoperative high-field MRI may take place in the field of vascular surgery. Magnetic resonance angiography shows the complete clipping of an aneurysm, and the use of diffusion-weighted imaging should also allow us to evaluate intraoperative blood supply, thus preventing reduced perfusion [71]. Furthermore, intraoperative MRI may also prove useful in spinal surgery, such as for the resection of complex intramedullary tumors or drainage of syringomyelias.

At present, intraoperative high-field MRI with integrated microscope-based neuronavigation is certainly one of the most sophisticated technical methods providing reliable intraoperative quality control. Intraoperative high-field MRI provides intraoperative anatomic images of high quality that are up to the standard of pre- and post-operative neuroradiologic imaging. Compared with the previous low-field MRI systems that were used for intraoperative imaging, not only is the image quality clearly superior but the imaging spectrum is much wider and the intraoperative work flow is improved. Furthermore, high-field MRI offers various modalities beyond standard anatomic imaging, such as magnetic resonance spectroscopy, DTI, and fMRI.

Acknowledgments

The authors thank the entire team of physicists and computer scientists at our neurocenter for their efforts in image processing, namely, P. Grummich, P. Hastreiter, and A. Stadlbauer. They are also grateful to A.G. Sorensen (Department of Radiology/Nuclear Magnetic Resonance Center, Massachusetts General Hospital, Boston, MA) for providing the DTI processing software. Furthermore, they acknowledge the continuing assistance of E. Müller and T. Vetter (Siemens Medical Solutions, Erlangen, Germany).

References

[1] Bradley WG. Achieving gross total resection of brain tumors: intraoperative MR imaging can make a big difference. AJNR Am J Neuroradiol 2002; 23(3):348–9.

[2] Steinmeier R, Fahlbusch R, Ganslandt O, Nimsky C, Buchfelder M, Kaus M, et al. Intraoperative magnetic resonance imaging with the Magnetom open scanner: concepts, neurosurgical indications, and procedures. A preliminary report. Neurosurgery 1998;43(4):739–48.

[3] Tronnier VM, Wirtz CR, Knauth M, Lenz G, Pastyr O, Bonsanto MM, et al. Intraoperative diagnostic and interventional magnetic resonance imaging in neurosurgery. Neurosurgery 1997;40(5): 891–902.

[4] Black PM, Moriarty T, Alexander E III, Stieg P, Woodard EJ, Gleason PL, et al. Development and implementation of intraoperative magnetic resonance imaging and its neurosurgical applications. Neurosurgery 1997;41(4):831–45.

[5] Schwartz RB, Hsu L, Wong TZ, Kacher DF, Zamani AA, Black PM, et al. Intraoperative MR imaging guidance for intracranial neurosurgery: experience with the first 200 cases. Radiology 1999; 211(2):477–88.

[6] Seifert V, Zimmermann M, Trantakis C, Vitzthum HE, Kuhnel K, Raabe A, et al. Open MRI-guided neurosurgery. Acta Neurochir (Wien) 1999;141(5):455–64.

[7] Black PM, Alexander E III, Martin C, Moriarty T, Nabavi A, Wong TZ, et al. Craniotomy for tumor treatment in an intraoperative magnetic resonance imaging unit. Neurosurgery 1999;45(3):423–33.

[8] Schneider JP, Schulz T, Schmidt F, Dietrich J, Lieberenz S, Trantakis C, et al. Gross-total surgery of supratentorial low-grade gliomas under intraoperative MR guidance. AJNR Am J Neuroradiol 2001;22(1):89–98.

[9] Wirtz CR, Knauth M, Staubert A, Bonsanto MM, Sartor K, Kunze S, et al. Clinical evaluation and follow-up results for intraoperative magnetic resonance imaging in neurosurgery. Neurosurgery 2000;46(5): 1112–22.

[10] Nimsky C, Ganslandt O, Tomandl B, Buchfelder M, Fahlbusch R. Low-field magnetic resonance imaging for intraoperative use in neurosurgery: a 5 year experience. Eur Radiol 2002;12(11):2690–703.

[11] Kober H, Möller M, Nimsky C, Vieth J, Fahlbusch R, Ganslandt O. New approach to localize speech relevant brain areas and hemispheric dominance using spatially filtered magnetoencephalography. Hum Brain Mapp 2001;14(4):236–50.

[12] Kober H, Nimsky C, Möller M, Hastreiter P, Fahlbusch R, Ganslandt O. Correlation of sensorimotor activation with functional magnetic resonance imaging and magnetoencephalography in presurgical functional imaging: a spatial analysis. Neuroimage 2001;14(5):1214–28.

[13] Kober H, Nimsky C, Vieth J, Fahlbusch R, Ganslandt O. Co-registration of function and anatomy in frameless stereotaxy by contour fitting. Stereotact Funct Neurosurg 2002;79(3–4):272–83.

[14] Nimsky C, Ganslandt O, Kober H, Möller M, Ulmer S, Tomandl B, et al. Integration of functional magnetic resonance imaging supported by magnetoencephalography in functional neuronavigation. Neurosurgery 1999;44:1249–56.

[15] Ganslandt O, Fahlbusch R, Nimsky C, Kober H, Möller M, Steinmeier R, et al. Functional neuronavigation with magnetoencephalography: outcome in 50 patients with lesions around the motor cortex. J Neurosurg 1999;91:73–9.

[16] Bohinski RJ, Kokkino AK, Warnick RE, Gaskill-Shipley MF, Kormos DW, Lukin RR, et al. Glioma resection in a shared-resource magnetic resonance operating room after optimal image-guided frameless stereotactic resection. Neurosurgery 2001; 48(4):731–44.

[17] Knauth M, Wirtz CR, Tronnier VM, Aras N, Kunze S, Sartor K. Intraoperative MR imaging increases the extent of tumor resection in patients with high-grade gliomas. AJNR Am J Neuroradiol 1999; 20(9):1642–6.

[18] Martin CH, Schwartz R, Jolesz F, Black PM. Transsphenoidal resection of pituitary adenomas in an intraoperative MRI unit. Pituitary 1999;2: 155–62.

[19] Pergolizzi RS, J.,Nabavi A, Schwartz RB, Hsu L, Wong TZ, Martin C, et al. Intra-operative MR guidance during trans-sphenoidal pituitary resection: preliminary results. J Magn Reson Imaging 2001; 13(1):136–41.

[20] Bohinski RJ, Warnick RE, Gaskill-Shipley MF, Zuccarello M, van Loveren HR, Kormos DW, et al. Intraoperative magnetic resonance imaging to determine the extent of resection of pituitary macroadenomas during transsphenoidal microsurgery. Neurosurgery 2001;49(5):1133–44.

[21] Fahlbusch R, Ganslandt O, Buchfelder M, Schott W, Nimsky C. Intraoperative magnetic resonance imaging during transsphenoidal surgery. J Neurosurg 2001;95(3):381–90.

[22] Schwartz TH, Marks D, Pak J, Hill J, Mandelbaum DE, Holodny AI, et al. Standardization of amygdalohippocampectomy with intraoperative magnetic resonance imaging: preliminary experience. Epilepsia 2002;43(4):430–6.

[23] Kaibara T, Myles ST, Lee MA, Sutherland GR. Optimizing epilepsy surgery with intraoperative MR imaging. Epilepsia 2002;43(4):425–9.

[24] Buchfelder M, Fahlbusch R, Ganslandt O, Stefan H, Nimsky C. Use of intraoperative magnetic resonance imaging in tailored temporal lobe surgeries for epilepsy. Epilepsia 2002;43(8):864–73.

[25] Buchfelder M, Ganslandt O, Fahlbusch R, Nimsky C. Intraoperative magnetic resonance imaging in epilepsy surgery. J Magn Reson Imaging 2000; 12:547–55.

[26] Nabavi A, Black PM, Gering DT, Westin CF, Mehta V, Pergolizzi RS Jr, et al. Serial intraoperative magnetic resonance imaging of brain shift. Neurosurgery 2001;48(4):787–98.

[27] Nimsky C, Ganslandt O, Cerny S, Hastreiter P, Greiner G, Fahlbusch R. Quantification of, visualization of, and compensation for brain shift using intraoperative magnetic resonance imaging. Neurosurgery 2000;47(5):1070–80.

[28] Nimsky C, Ganslandt O, Hastreiter P, Fahlbusch R. Intraoperative compensation for brain shift. Surg Neurol 2001;56(6):357–64.

[29] Wirtz CR, Bonsanto MM, Knauth M, Tronnier VM, Albert FK, Staubert A, et al. Intraoperative magnetic resonance imaging to update interactive navigation in neurosurgery: method and preliminary experience. Comput Aided Surg 1997; 2:172–9.

[30] Sutherland GR, Kaibara T, Louw D, Hoult DI, Tomanek B, Saunders J. A mobile high-field magnetic resonance system for neurosurgery. J Neurosurg 1999;91(5):804–13.

[31] Hall WA, Liu H, Martin AJ, Pozza CH, Maxwell RE, Truwit CL. Safety, efficacy, and functionality of high-field strength interventional magnetic resonance imaging for neurosurgery. Neurosurgery 2000;46(3):632–42.

[32] Hall WA, Martin AJ, Liu H, Nussbaum ES, Maxwell RE, Truwit CL. Brain biopsy using high-field strength interventional magnetic resonance imaging. Neurosurgery 1999;44(4):807–14.

[33] Kaibara T, Saunders JK, Sutherland GR. Advances in mobile intraoperative magnetic resonance imaging. Neurosurgery 2000;47(1):131–8.

[34] Nimsky C, Ganslandt O, Keller VB, Fahlbusch R. Preliminary experience in glioma surgery with intraoperative high-field MRI. Acta Neurochir Suppl (Wien) 2003;88:21–9.

[35] Nimsky C, Ganslandt O, Kober H, Buchfelder M, Fahlbusch R. Intraoperative magnetic resonance imaging combined with neuronavigation: a new concept. Neurosurgery 2001;48(5):1082–91.

[36] Schmitz B, Nimsky C, Wendel G, Wienerl J, Ganslandt O, Jacobi K, et al. Anesthesia during high-field intraoperative magnetic resonance imaging—experience with 80 consecutive cases. J Neurosurg Anesthesiol 2003;15(3):255–62.

[37] Nimsky C, Ganslandt O, Fischer H, Oppelt A, Vetter T, Distler P, et al. Kombination aus Kopffixation und Kopfspule für neurochirurgische Operationen. Siemens Technik Report 2000;3(6):64–5.

[38] Raabe A, Krishnan R, Wolff R, Hermann E, Zimmermann M, Seifert V. Laser surface scanning for patient registration in intracranial image-guided surgery. Neurosurgery 2002;50(4):797–803.

[39] Ganslandt O, Stadlbauer A, Nimsky C, Buslei R, Blümcke I, Moser E, et al. Integration of MR spectroscopy into neuronavigation for stereotactic definition of tumor infiltration zone. In: Lemke H, Vannier M, Inamura K, Farman A, Doi K, Reiber J, editors. CARS 2003, vol. ICS 1256. Amsterdam: Elsevier; 2003. p. 1339.

[40] Nimsky C, Ganslandt O, Buchfelder M, Fahlbusch R. Glioma surgery evaluated by intraoperative low-field magnetic resonance imaging. Acta Neurochir Suppl (Wien) 2003;85:55–63.

[41] Dina TS, Feaster SH, Laws ER, Davis DO. MR of the pituitary gland postsurgery: serial MR studies following transsphenoidal resection. AJNR Am J Neuroradiol 1993;14:763–9.

[42] Nimsky C, Ganslandt O, Hofmann B, Fahlbusch R. Limited benefit of intraoperative low-field magnetic resonance imaging in craniopharyngioma surgery. Neurosurgery 2003;53(1):72–81.

[43] Gupta T, Sarin R. Poor-prognosis high-grade gliomas: evolving an evidence-based standard of care. Lancet Oncol 2002;3(9):557–64.

[44] Laws E. Surgical management of intracranial gliomas—does radical resection improve outcome? Acta Neurochir Suppl (Wien) 2003;85(85):47–53.

[45] Nicolato A, Gerosa MA, Fina P, Iuzzolino P, Giorgiutti F, Bricolo A. Prognostic factors in low-grade supratentorial astrocytomas: a uni-multivari-

ate statistical analysis in 76 surgically treated adult patients. Surg Neurol 1995;44(3):208–23.

[46] Nimsky C, Ganslandt O, Keller VB, Romstöck J, Fahlbusch R. Intraoperative high-field magnetic resonance imaging: implementation and experience with the first 200 patients. Radiology, in press.

[47] Albert FK, Forsting M, Sartor K, Adams HP, Kunze S. Early postoperative magnetic resonance imaging after resection of malignant glioma: objective evaluation of residual tumor and its influence on regrowth and prognosis. Neurosurgery 1994; 34(1):45–61.

[48] Chandler KL, Prados MD, Malec M, Wilson CB. Long-term survival in patients with glioblastoma multiforme. Neurosurgery 1993;32(5):716–20.

[49] Lacroix M, Abi-Said D, Fourney DR, Gokaslan ZL, Shi W, DeMonte F, et al. A multivariate analysis of 416 patients with glioblastoma multiforme: prognosis, extent of resection, and survival. J Neurosurg 2001;95(2):190–8.

[50] Obwegeser A, Ortler M, Seiwald M, Ulmer H, Kostron H. Therapy of glioblastoma multiforme: a cumulative experience of 10 years. Acta Neurochir (Wien) 1995;137(1–2):29–33.

[51] Tzika AA, Cheng LL, Goumnerova L, Madsen JR, Zurakowski D, Astrakas LG, et al. Biochemical characterization of pediatric brain tumors by using in vivo and ex vivo magnetic resonance spectroscopy. J Neurosurg 2002;96(6):1023–31.

[52] Rock J, Hearshen D, Scarpace L, Croteau D, Gutierrez J, Fisher J, et al. Correlations between magnetic resonance spectroscopy and image-guided histopathology, with special attention to radiation necrosis. Neurosurgery 2002;51(4):912–20.

[53] Law M, Cha S, Knopp E, Johnson G, Arnett J, Litt A. High-grade gliomas and solitary metastases: differentiation by using perfusion and proton spectroscopic MR imaging. Radiology 2002;222(3): 715–21.

[54] Hall WA, Martin A, Liu H, Truwit CL. Improving diagnostic yield in brain biopsy: coupling spectroscopic targeting with real-time needle placement. J Magn Reson Imaging 2001;13(1):12–5.

[55] Dowling C, Bollen AW, Noworolski SM, McDermott MW, Barbaro NM, Day MR, et al. Preoperative proton MR spectroscopic imaging of brain tumors: correlation with histopathologic analysis of resection specimens. AJNR Am J Neuroradiol 2001;22(4):604–12.

[56] Beppu T, Inoue T, Shibata Y, Kurose A, Arai H, Ogasawara K, et al. Measurement of fractional nisotropy using diffusion tensor MRI in supratentorial astrocytic tumors. J Neurooncol 2003;63: 19–116.

[57] Kamada K, Houkin K, Takeuchi F, Ishii N, Ikeda J, Sawamura Y, et al. Visualization of the eloquent motor system by integration of MEG, functional, and anisotropic diffusion-weighted MRI in functional neuronavigation. Surg Neurol 2003;59(5):352–62.

[58] Tummala RP, Chu RM, Liu H, Truwit CL, Hall WA. Application of diffusion tensor imaging to magnetic-resonance-guided brain tumor resection. Pediatr Neurosurg 2003;39:39–43.

[59] Westin CF, Maier SE, Mamata H, Nabavi A, Jolesz F, Kikinis R. Processing and visualization for diffusion tensor MRI. Med Image Anal 2002;6: 93–108.

[60] Witwer BP, Moftakhar R, Hasan KM, Deshmukh P, Haughton V, Field A, et al. Diffusion-tensor imaging of white matter tracts in patients with cerebral neoplasm. J Neurosurg 2002;97(3): 568–75.

[61] Yamada K, Kizu O, Mori S, Ito H, Nakamura H, Yuen S, et al. Brain fiber tracking with clinically feasible diffusion-tensor MR imaging. Initial experience Radiology 2003;227(1):295–301.

[62] Hendler T, Pianka P, Sigal M, Kafri M, Ben-Bashat D, Constantini S, et al. Delineating gray and white matter involvement in brain lesions: three-dimensional alignment of functional magnetic resonance and diffusion-tensor imaging. J Neurosurg 2003;99(6):1018–27.

[63] Clark CA, Barrick TR, Murphy MM, Bell BA. White matter fiber tracking in patients with space-occupying lesions of the brain: a new technique for neurosurgical planning? Neuroimage 2003;20(3): 1601–8.

[64] Coenen VA, Krings T, Mayfrank L, Polin RS, Reinges MH, Thron A, et al. Three-dimensional visualization of the pyramidal tract in a neuronavigation system during brain tumor surgery: first experiences and technical note. Neurosurgery 2001; 49(1):86–93.

[65] Hastreiter P, Engel K, Soza G, Bauer M, Wolf M, Ganslandt O, et al. Remote analysis for brain shift compensation. In: Niessen W, Viergever M, editors. Medical image computing and computer assisted intervention (MICCAI). Berlin: Springer; 2001. p. 1248–9.

[66] Wolf M, Vogel T, Weierich P, Niemann H, Nimsky C. Automatic transfer of preoperative fMRI markers into intraoperative MR-images for updating functional neuronavigation. Institute of Electronics, Information and Communication Engineers Transactions Information and Systems 2001; E84-D(12):1698–704.

[67] Miga MI, Paulsen KD, Hoopes PJ, Kennedy FE, Hartov A, Roberts DW. In vivo modeling of interstitial pressure in the brain under surgical load using finite elements. J Biomech Eng 2000;122(4): 354–63.

[68] Ferrant M, Warfield SK, Nabavi A, Jolesz F, Kikinis R. Registration of 3D intraoperative MR images of the brain using a finite element biomechanical model. In: Delp SL, DiGioia AM, Jaramaz B, editors. Medical image computing and computer-assisted intervention (MICCAI). Berlin: Springer; 2000. p. 19–28.

[69] Gasser TG, Sandalcioglu EI, Wiedemayer H, Hans V, Gizewski E, Forsting M, et al. A novel passive functional MRI paradigm for preoperative identification of the somatosensory cortex. Neurosurg Rev 2004;27(2):106–12.

[70] Guye M, Parker GJ, Symms M, Boulby P, Wheeler-Kingshott CA, Salek-Haddadi A, et al. Combined functional MRI and tractography to demonstrate the connectivity of the human primary motor cortex in vivo. Neuroimage 2003;19(4):1349–60.

[71] Sutherland GR, Kaibara T, Wallace C, Tomanek B, Richter M. Intraoperative assessment of aneurysm clipping using magnetic resonance angiography and diffusion-weighted imaging. Technical case report Neurosurgery 2002;50(4):893–8.

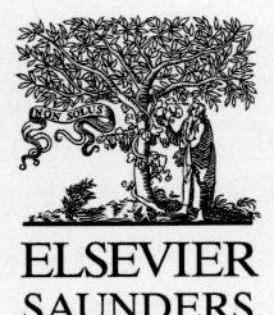

ELSEVIER
SAUNDERS

Neurosurg Clin N Am 16 (2005) 201–213

NEUROSURGERY
CLINICS
OF NORTH AMERICA

Future perspectives for intraoperative MRI

Ferenc A. Jolesz, MD

Division of MRI and Image Guided Therapy Program, Department of Radiology, Brigham and Women's Hospital, Harvard Medical School, 75 Francis Street, Boston, MA 02115, USA

Intraoperative MRI was introduced in 1993 [1]. Since then, it has been generally accepted as a valuable image guidance tool for neurosurgery, but it still applies relatively immature and diverse technologies; its clinical indications are not well defined, and its potential impact on everyday neurosurgical practice is not yet fully recognized. The reason for the early acceptance of intraoperative MRI is that it is not a so-called "disruptive technology," which necessitates the total transformation of a medical specialty. It has been easy to accept intraoperative guidance by MRI because it uses the same imaging modality for localization during surgery as it does for preoperative diagnosis. It also improves the now universally used intraoperative navigation by real-time, interactive, near–real-time imaging, with frequent volumetric updates. These can compensate for the unavoidable intraoperative deformations and brain shifts. The main reason for the relatively slow proliferation of this technology is not necessarily the high cost of MRI systems but the lack of clear definition of the requirements of the various types of intraoperative MRI systems. Neither the configuration nor the field strength of the MRI systems, nor their integration with the current conventional operating room environment and with multiple therapy devices, has been determined yet. It is also unclear whether intraoperative MRI is applicable only for tumor resection control or if it is relevant for any other neurosurgical procedure.

To realize the potential benefits of intraoperative MRI, one has to understand all the possible implications of this new approach. In a fundamental way, visualization beyond the exposed surface is an unrealized dream of surgeons who are looking at the "operational field" but de facto dealing with the "operational volume." Although the introduction of surgical microscopes changed the scale of dimensions, it did not reveal all three dimensions. It is obvious that the introduction of MRI in the operating room has expanded the limits of the surgeon's view of the operational field from two dimensional (2D) to three dimensional (3D). Intraoperative MRI also augmented the surgeon's eye via its portrayal of a more effective tissue definition than direct visual examination. Nevertheless, 3D volumetric imaging and MRI-based contrast mechanisms have already been used for MRI-guided tumor resection by conventional navigational systems. The main reason why intraoperative MRI was introduced to neurosurgery was to make up for deformation and to avoid incorrect localization and targeting. Therefore, the main advantage of intraoperative MRI is frequent image updates for neuronavigation.

Intraoperative serial imaging accounts for intraoperative shifts, or deformations, and demonstrates a progressively updated representation of the actual anatomy. The analysis of these data may tell us in the future how frequently we have to update the images during surgery and how much morphologic information it is necessary to correct for these deformations. With these data, we can answer one of the fundamental questions of image-guided neurosurgery, that is, whether elaborate and frequently repeated intraoperative imaging is necessary or if computer simulations supplemented by some intraoperative measurements can correct the unavoidable brain shifts.

Thus far, the greatest impact of intraoperative MRI is in glioma surgery [2,3]. The usefulness of MRI in localizing infiltrative tumor spread is obvious. Nevertheless, it is not clear that better

E-mail address: jolesz@bwh.harvard.edu

1042-3680/05/$ - see front matter
doi:10.1016/j.nec.2004.07.011

neurosurgery.theclinics.com

localization of the MRI-visible tumor margins can result in more effective tumor removal, and if it does, whether the outcome will be better. The main issue is to get MRI diagnostic sensitivity to define exact tumor margins, which may be an unachievable goal in the case of malignant brain tumors. Nonetheless, using multiparametric MRI not only helps to define tumor margins but can be used for functional tissue characterization. Functional MRI (fMRI), diffusion MRI, diffusion tensor imaging (DTI), magnetic resonance angiography (MRA), and magnetic resonance spectroscopy (MRS) can definitely help to achieve accurate and safe tumor resections and decrease the rate of complications of brain tumor surgery. There is a well-grounded rationale for using not only anatomic but functional parameters for surgical planning, but it has not yet been established that these time-consuming imaging tasks have to be done during surgery. Nonrigid registration of preoperative-to-intraoperative images may provide a solution. This solution has to be based on correct models of brain deformation; otherwise, it cannot be used for surgical guidance.

Some of the MRI-measurable physical or physiologic parameters (eg, temperature, diffusion, perfusion, flow) are especially useful for intraprocedural monitoring of interventions like thermal ablations or endovascular procedures. These quantitative parameters should be obtained using dynamic imaging sequences, or they cannot be used for the control of energy depositions or the detection of functional responses to vascular insults. This dynamic imaging requirement imposes serious requirements for MRI hardware and software. The closed-loop control also mandates the full integration of therapy devices with MRI, which is the reason why the future development of intraoperative MRI requires advances in imaging techniques and a series of further integration steps. The hardware and software components and the imaging features of MRI have to be integrated into the operating room environment. The various surgical instruments, tools, and therapy devices have to be strongly coupled with the software and hardware components of the imaging systems. In the future, intraoperative MRI has to be a fully integrated module of a complex image-based therapy delivery system.

Intraoperative imaging paradigms

Magnetic field strength and open configuration are conflicting physical features of intraoperative MRI systems. Because of this inherent contradiction, there is a need for a trade-off between image quality and access to the patient. The various imaging paradigms and magnet-table arrangements that have been introduced into clinical practice and tested have dealt with this contradiction in different ways and have provided various compromises and solutions.

The first intraoperative magnet is a result of a compromise between field strength and access. The concept of a vertically open-configuration intraoperative midfield magnet was developed by engineers from General Electric Medical Systems (Milwaukee, Wisconsin) and by the members of Brigham and Women's Hospital Image Guided Therapy Program. The system was deployed in Boston in 1991. That prototype system, nicknamed, "double doughnut," (as a product introduced as SIGNA SP; General Electric Medical Systems) consists of two cylindric magnets to create inversely overlapping external magnetic fields between them. An open imaging volume is formed between the two magnet bores [1]. The effective field strength of the system is at 0.5 T. This unique design allows relatively unrestricted and constant access to the patient's anatomy but provides only limited flexibility in patient positioning. In this arrangement, the table is across the magnets or positioned perpendicularly, providing some flexibility to access the head. The head can be accessed by two neurosurgeons, and the operative microscope can be integrated into the system.

The patient stays constantly within the imaging volume, and images are obtained repetitively or serially. Intraoperative guidance based on optical tracking and navigation for neurosurgical procedures (biopsies and open brain surgeries) is accomplished by near–real-time interactive MRI or with serial acquisition of volumetric image updates [4,5]. For other nonneurosurgical applications at various anatomic sites, the concept of frameless stereotaxy was applied as a suitable targeting method. The navigational aspects of this system were further augmented by the integration of a complex display and visualization platform, the 3D Slicer [6,7].

The 3D Slicer was originally developed to support image-guided neurosurgery performed in magnetic resonance therapy by providing real-time reformatting of a recently acquired volumetric image in response to interactive manipulation of a sterilized probe in the operative field. Since its initial development, the 3D Slicer (Surgical Planning Lab, Boston, Massachusetts and Artificial

Intelligence Lab, Cambridge, Massachusetts) has evolved into a general purpose platform for the analysis of collections of volumetric images as well as 3D models derived from such images. The 3D Slicer was designed to stay away from the 2D slice-by-slice view of imaging data by integrating 2D and 3D image data with geometric anatomic models and additional information, such as pointers and annotation. The 3D Slicer has been used to provide visual information in the operating room to guide neurosurgical procedures. Its basic infrastructure provides for modular extension, which has been used, for example, to provide an additional duplicate "slave" image of the user interface for display on a second screen in the operating room or to display the virtual image of tracked probes inside the open magnet.

The display and visualization platform also has a general capability for ensuring the accuracy of coordinate systems and organizing the transformations between various reference frames. It provides rigid and nonrigid registration methods for multimodality fusion between preoperative image data and intraoperative image data. This system will eventually include models of specific tracked instruments, such as the Ojemann stimulator, a bipolar cautery, and a suction device. The ultimate goal of this platform is to provide standardized methods for exchanging spatial coordinates among various therapy and imaging systems and to capture spatial-temporal events.

This design of the vertically open-configuration magnet and the related paradigm is still the most preferable solution for intraoperative imaging, especially for open surgeries. When the idea was conceived, technical factors limited the field strength and consequently constrained the gap between the two magnet components. As a result, image quality and resolution were suboptimal, and the surgeon's mobility was compromised in the narrow space. With advanced magnet-building technology, this exact configuration can be recreated at much higher field strength and with a substantially wider gap. In a less restricted environment, with more physician mobility and more flexible head positioning, this configuration still offers the best possible solution for MRI-guided neurosurgery. At a higher field strength (1 T and greater), spatial and temporal resolution can be improved to allow not only better anatomic detail but multiparametric functional imaging (eg, fMRI, DTI, MRA, MRS) during surgeries.

With improved hardware and software (eg, stronger gradients, dynamic-adaptive imaging sequences, parallel or multichannel methods), images could be obtained extremely rapidly, even continuously, without interrupting the flow of surgery. Even in this current intraoperative magnet, where the patient is always within the imaging volume, the intraprocedural imaging takes a considerable time and suspends the surgery. The surgeon's hand motion, occasional movement of surgical instruments, and radiofrequency (RF) noise from bipolar coagulation cause various artifacts that destroy the images. Using special imaging methods, incessant imaging that is relatively insensitive to motion, magnetic susceptibility, or brief electromagnetic noise can be implemented [8]. This potential technologic breakthrough can remove one of the major obstacles of intraoperative imaging—the neurosurgeon's unintentional but inherent resistance to suspend surgery or change the normal flow of the ongoing operation.

The ultimate solution for unlimited patient access is a so-called "flat" or "tabletop" magnet with an external remote magnetic field [9]. The advantage of this completely open configuration is full access to the head and maximal flexibility in head positioning. The major disadvantages are the inherently limited field strength, the relatively small homogeneous imaging volume, and the relatively large size of the magnet under the operating room table, which may prevent the surgeon from reaching the surgical field with his or her hands and by the microscope.

After the introduction of the first intraoperative MRI system, which was designed explicitly for image-guided neurosurgery, several other groups began to use existing commercially available magnet configurations for neurosurgical guidance. Low- and midfield strength, horizontal open-configuration magnets [3,10–12], and closed-configuration higher field magnets [12,13] were placed in operating rooms or in interventional suites, which were modified for the needs of neurosurgery. The magnets that were originally designed only for diagnostic imaging were adapted to image guidance. Most of the efforts concerned the MRI table, which had to be revised or redesigned to make it well suited for brain surgery and MRI.

Using these primarily diagnostic MRI systems, the imaging paradigms are more or less constrained by the actual magnet configuration. In all versions, the surgical procedure has to be done outside the magnet. Because the head is not within the imaging volume, the table has to move or swing in and out from the magnet. To avoid major modification of the operating room equipment and to get around the need for table motion, two commercial magnets were introduced. In both solutions, the magnet moves toward the head. The high-field (1.5-T) version is ceiling mounted, and during imaging sessions, it is pulled around to the operating room table [14]. The small low-field (0.12-T) magnet is mounted on the regular operating room table. It is partially open like the "double doughnut," with a gap that allows the magnet to slide around the head when imaging is needed [15,16].

As far as field strength is concerned, these two magnet designs represent the two diverging directions in intraoperative MRI. It is obvious that the higher the field, the better is the image quality, but the lower field solution is less costly and more adaptable to the operating room environment. The high-field magnet offers various imaging sequences (eg, MRA, MRS, diffusion) and functional imaging methods (eg, fMRI, perfusion), and the image is acquired much faster. At the lower field strength, there are fewer problems with safety and device compatibility. Midfield magnets offer some compromise, but finding the middle ground may not be acceptable for either side. Most surgeons' preference for the higher magnetic field is driven by the current advances in diagnostic neuroimaging, where the modern trend is pointing toward 3 T. Besides higher spatial and temporal resolution, the higher field offers the advantages of high-quality and low signal-to-noise MRA, fMRI, and DTI, which are now natural components of surgical planning (Fig. 1) [17,18]. Most neurosurgeons would like to have these features available during surgery. Advocates of low-field intraoperative MRI believe that the relatively low-quality images are still sufficient to define tumor margins and detect the shifts and deformations during surgery. Those who believe in the power of computer technology and in the advances of automated or semiautomated image processing may accept the midfield compromise. Nonrigid registration of preoperative high-field images to lower quality intraoperative ones may permit the use of MRI data that are available only at high fields. When biopsies or surgeries are performed under low or midfield intraoperative guidance, the preoperative high-field images can be registered to the low-field intraoperative data [19]. This augmentation of intraoperative imaging with information obtained before surgery shows promise. Multimodality guidance using not only multiple MRI-derived data but positron emission

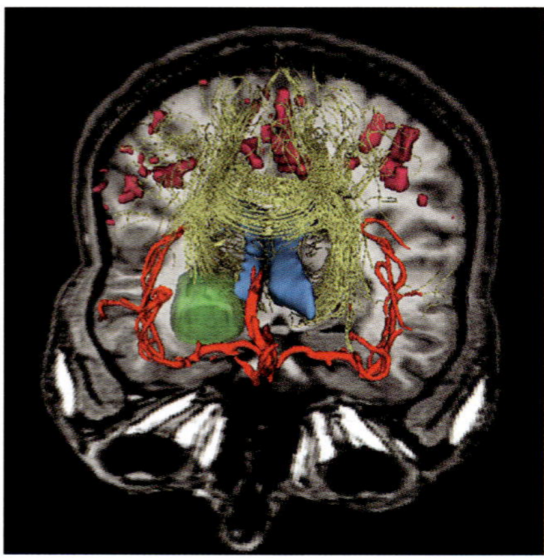

Fig. 1. Multimodality image fusion for surgical planning in a case of right temporal low-grade glioneural tumor. Three-dimensional (3D) tractography (yellow) derived from diffusion tensor imaging–MRI is rigidly registered with preoperative 3D spoiled GRASS and functional MRI (fist-clenching task). The 3D model of cortical activation is displayed in pink and the tumor is displayed in green.

tomography (PET), CT, and magnetoencephalography (MEG) should be an intrinsic part of surgical navigation. The preoperative data that are warped to the deformed intraoperative anatomy will reduce the rate of complications by providing an intraoperative model for real-time surgical planning at the operating room table that is essential for intraoperative decision making.

Field strength is not the only criterion when choosing magnet type. The flexibility in patient positioning and the surgeon's mobility are also critical; this is the main reason why neurosurgeons are adamant about using full-feature operating room tables. Good positioning of the head is critical for most open-brain surgery, and the use of surgical microscopes is also essential. These factors all influence the choice of imaging paradigms and the future design and ergonomics of image-guided operating rooms.

Potential benefits in intraoperative MRI

Surgical guidance augments and supports the surgeon in performing procedures by reinforcing the knowledge of the patient's anatomy and by providing explicit visualization of intraprocedural changes in the anatomy. This results in improved surgical decision making. Surgeons make decisions in the operating room based on the information that is available to them at that site at that time. Often, they do not have the luxury of time to reflect on these decisions. By providing surgeons with the most up-to-date morphologic data, combined with all the available image-based information, their decisions will inevitably lead to better patient care. Real-time accurate information will provide the surgeon with the means and confidence to remove diseased tissue while minimizing the margins of healthy tissue excised. This not only improves tumor resection control but facilitates management of complications.

Controlling the blood flow is the most technically challenging and time-consuming aspect of many operations, which often involves tedious dissection to ensure a vessel, nerve, or other critical structure is not inadvertently severed. The introduction of higher field MRI systems (up to 3 T) will make vascular imaging suitable for guiding vascular surgeries and endovascular interventions. It has already been shown that intraoperative diffusion imaging can detect early ischemic damage during surgery and can be used to monitor vascular procedures [20]. Diffusion MRI can be complemented with perfusion MRI, and surgeries and embolization of vascular malformations can be made safer by keeping an eye on the brain while the blood vessel is manipulated. In aneurysm surgeries, 3D visualization of the lesion can help by showing the position of clips and the relation to the neck of the aneurysm and related blood vessels from angles other than those the microscope provides.

If surgeons knew the exact location of all the vital structures within the operational volume, it would significantly increase the speed of dissection. Reducing operating time will decrease operating room costs and postoperative complications, thus improving patient outcomes. The union of 3D planning with real-time intraoperative guidance will optimize surgical techniques and reduce morbidity and treatment times. Some of the most important examples of these potential improvements are the intraoperative use of fMRI and DTI to prevent damage to critical cortical functions and pathways of essential connectivity, the use of PET or MRI perfusion data to distinguish necrotic from viable tumor tissue, and the use of diffusion MRI to recognize vascularly compromised tissues. Even more substantial advances are foreseeable in the future if tumor-seeking contrast agents or tumor-tagging biomarkers are introduced into neurosurgery.

To take better advantage of intraoperative MRI, several important steps should be taken. Among the steps necessary to realize the full potential of this technology, the most important are integration of intraoperative MRI scans with preoperative images obtained by other imaging modalities (multimodality fusion) and integration of the MRI methods with therapy devices/robots to transform open neurosurgical procedures into image-guided surgeries by changing surgical techniques and approaches. Without these advances, no major effect on disease outcome can be expected (Figs. 2 and 3).

One of the greatest benefits of intraoperative MRI is that the progress of brain deformations can be followed by serial intraoperative imaging [21,22]. Using this continuously updated information, preoperative images can be warped to the true anatomic position using nonrigid registration methods. Most of the specialized sequences (eg, fMRI, DTI, MRA) that are routinely used for surgical planning and intraoperative decision making can be obtained at high fields before surgery. Similarly, non-MRI images (eg, CT, PET, single photon emission computed tomography, MEG) can be adapted to intraoperative

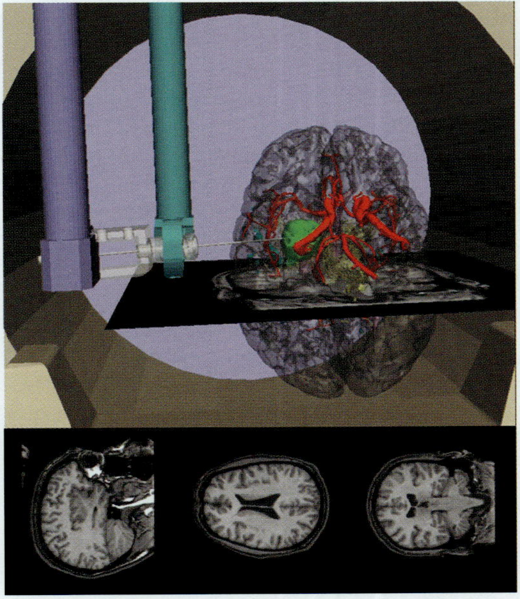

Fig. 2. Illustration of the interface between the 3D Slicer and the surgical robotic assistant. The robotic arm holding the biopsy needle is driven to the target (green) with the assistance of the 3D Slicer. The spatial position of the robotic arm and biopsy needle is tracked in real time and displayed in the 3D Slicer, along with image data.

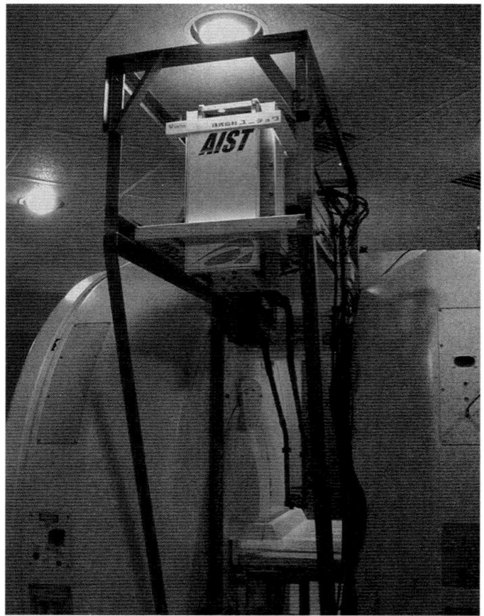

Fig. 3. The robot attached to the open MRI scanner.

brain images. This multimodality fusion is eventually incorporated by all commercial navigational systems but their use is limited because of the inability to map the images they provide correctly to the actual brain anatomy. These complex imaging data sets should be available during surgery and warped to the actual anatomy. In the future, intraoperative MRI systems will be able to display them concurrently with the real-time acquired MRI scans. With low-field intraoperative systems, this method can also be used to improve image quality. High-resolution images obtained before surgery and acquired at high fields can be warped into low-quality and low-field MRI scans. This "single modality image augmented fusion" can provide highly accurate image guidance. Structures that are invisible at lower field strengths because of lack of resolution and a low signal-to-noise ratio can be brought to light and can improve the surgeon's visualization and targeting. The combination of functional and anatomic images can improve the decision-making process, reduce complications, and result in improved outcomes.

Preoperative optimization of surgical approaches and trajectories is part of surgical planning. The preoperative plans usually consider all the available imaging data and combine them into a multimodality model. A simulation of surgery that includes multiple access routes and trajectories can supplement this model. This multimodality model and the related predetermined simulation strategy can be registered to the patient (usually with rigid registration); during surgery, additional "on the fly," modifications can be made by applying nonrigid registration to the changing anatomy. For preoperative data analysis, there is sufficient time for extensive and, presumably, more accurate, examination. In contrast, intraoperative data must be analyzed at a faster rate to reach a decision during the procedure. The surgical plan is interactively adapted to the intraoperative situation, and the real-time surgical planning assists surgical decision making. The predetermined plan of tumor removal can be compared with the actual resection to evaluate how the image guidance helped the surgeon to execute the original surgical strategy. This complex intraoperative interactive planning process is currently still cumbersome, however. In the future, more advanced image processing, visualization, and display techniques will be used in combination with software tools that emulate cutting, suction, coagulation, and other surgical manipulations.

The other important technical development that might follow the more widespread use of intraoperative MRI is related to the more complete integration of therapy devices into the interventional/intraoperative MRI environment. Fully integrated image-guided therapy delivery systems will be able to use localizing, targeting, and monitoring methods and will also be able to use quantitative image-based measurements to control various therapeutic procedures, such as robotic surgeries and image-guided thermal ablations. The use of image-derived quantitative parameters for the closed-loop feedback control of devices is a significant future development that may substantially change current neurosurgical practice. There have been early attempts to combine robots with intraoperative MRI [23] and to use intraoperative MRI to control thermal ablation devices (Fig. 3) [24–26].

One of the more ordinary consequences of intraoperative image guidance would be the transformation of traditional brain surgery into image-guided surgery. With more accurate and complete volumetric data, neurosurgeons should be able to operate more securely, with a faster and more economic approach. Thus far, there has been no reason for a more assertive and less cautious approach when intraoperative MRI is used. There is no indication of increased easiness, and no data suggest any decrease in the time of surgeries. This is despite the improved navigation and better understanding of functional anatomy and spatial relations. The improved distinction between normal and pathologic tissue and enhanced appreciation of the related anatomy have not yet led to novel approaches or overall re-evaluation of current surgical strategies. It is anticipated, however, that the changes in surgical visualization and navigation will eventually change the current practice of neurosurgery. As a direct consequence of improved image guidance, new surgical techniques, strategies, and approaches will be introduced into neurosurgical practice.

So far, there are few changes in neurosurgical techniques that can be attributed to image guidance. One of the potential changes involves positioning, however. Head position is an important aspect of brain surgeries. Head position and craniotomy location define the surgical approach to the target lesion and influence several aspects of surgery, such as localization, targeting, access, and visualization. In intraoperative MRI target definition, localization is augmented by MRI tissue contrast and visualization is complemented by MRI. As a direct consequence, tumor explorations can be changed and head position and craniotomy locations can be modified or customized. Similarly, surface visualization provided by surgical microscopes and volumetric MRI could be supplemented by endoscopes, and their role could be redefined in the context of intraoperative MRI. Instruments like flexible endoscopes, which traditionally had to be controlled by direct eyesight, can be located and positioned by MRI and can be tracked and inserted beyond the surface, where visual assessment of their position is not possible. Beyond surface visualization is especially important when thermal ablation probes (laser optical fibers, RF antennas, or cryoprobes) are introduced into the brain. In thermal ablation interventions, the human eye cannot provide guidance and the correct positioning of the probes as well as the monitoring of energy depositions is controlled by MRI. Consequently, if image-guided positioning is applied, the instruments can be manipulated by robots or other mechanical devices. MRI-guided robotic devices have been developed and tested in open-magnet configurations [23]; in the future, similar devices can be used in closed-configuration high-field systems.

Currently, most intraoperative MRI guidance is for the removal of malignant (low- and high-grade) brain tumors. In these image-guided procedures, MRI tissue characterization ability is exploited. MRI is used to delineate tumor margins and to detect residual tumor. It is obvious that MRI's high sensitivity may help to achieve more complete resection of tumors. Nevertheless, even MRI is limited in accurately delineating the entire spread of an infiltrative glioma, and most of the resection represents only debulking. Thus far, there is no definitive evidence that MRI-controlled extensive glioma resection results in any change in clinical outcome. The MRI guidance definitely improves the technical execution of surgery by providing 3D visualization, better understanding of spatial relations, and better delineation of critical functional anatomy. This advantage should eventually help not only malignant but benign tumor resections. Full comprehension of the operational volume versus the operational field, the appreciation of depth and distances, and the visualization of structures under the surface should eventually change the way surgeons approach intracranial pathologic findings.

Unresolved issues in intraoperative MRI

Images can be obtained during surgery in a serial fashion to provide image updates about the changing brain anatomy. Imaging, however, is time-consuming, and time is essential in surgery. Imaging not only interrupts the flow of surgeries but adds substantial extra nonsurgical time to the overall duration of the procedure. On the one hand, there is the surgeon's intuition to minimize the time for imaging, and on the other hand, there is the surgeon's need for accurate guidance. These two competing issues result in a compromise that defines the actual number of imaging sessions. Today, this important decision depends on the surgeon's instinct or preference and is not based on any scientific optimization method. It is unclear how much information is needed to correct intraoperative shifts and deformations and how often data acquisitions should take place to drive such an adjustment reliably. If intraoperative deformations and shifts follow a predictable course, computer-based simulation and modeling would help to reduce the need for image updates. The exact sampling interval required to update intraoperative images correctly depends on the particular deformation pattern, which presently cannot be foreseen before surgery. Without a relatively short sampling interval, the dynamic course and spatial extent of brain shift cannot be fully appreciated. Ideally, frequent or even continuous volumetric imaging is the only method that can guarantee accurate and real-time image guidance. Although MRI provides more information about brain morphology, other imaging modalities, such as stereo video systems, laser surface scanning devices, ultrasound, and CT, can also be used during surgery to reveal the changing anatomy. These methods may show changes of surface or internal anatomy during surgery, but the information they provide is not sufficient to provide full intraoperative guidance. Nonetheless, these methods can be used to reduce the need for frequent MRI updates. They can signal a significant degree of shift that indicates new volumetric updates. They can also be used for computer simulations that can model brain deformations. At present, neither the knowledge of the biomechanical properties of the brain nor the capabilities of computer simulation is sufficient to predict the various deformation patterns seen during surgery; therefore, the use of this adaptive model is limited.

In the future, we can use a series of imaging methods and processing algorithms to capture intraoperative changes during neurosurgery. Real-time automated segmentation methods will provide updated 3D models of the brain [21,27–29]. The combination of rigid and nonrigid registration methods, active surface-matching techniques, and the application of biomechanically more accurate models of brain deformation will eventually help to decrease the sampling rate needed for the full appreciation of changing brain anatomy during surgery. If a sufficiently accurate biomechanical model exists, the volumetric deformation field can be computed and used for intraoperative modeling.

The unpredictable nature of brain deformation is caused by extrinsic factors like retractors or by intrinsic factors like edema or hemorrhage. As a result of these unsystematic events, serial imaging cannot be substituted for simulation. Intraoperative MRI is a prerequisite of reliable and accurate intraoperative navigation.

MRI-guided thermal ablations

Previous clinical studies of thermal ablation in the brain have involved the use of focused ultrasound surgery (FUS) through an open skull, microwave, laser-induced ablation, and so-called "cryosurgery." Most studies have shown that thermal ablation of various brain lesions is feasible and safe. Relatively large lesions were treated with minimal morbidity. Unlike thermal ablation (eg, laser surgery, RF surgery, cryosurgery), FUS works without the introduction of a thermal probe, and if it is done through the intact skull, it is noninvasive. The converging ultrasound beams pass through the brain to the target, without damaging the intervening tissue and provides a small enough spot size (as small as 1 mm) for precision. The noninvasive nature of ultrasound surgery has special appeal in the brain, where the ability to treat or destroy deep tissue volumes without disturbing the overlying tissues is critical.

It was recognized several decades ago that converging focused ultrasound beams can be applied as a surgical technique to treat neoplastic tissue, particularly deep in the brain. FUS applies localized high temperatures to induce cell damage as result of protein denaturation and subsequent coagulation necrosis. The clinical application of this well-researched method was delayed because of the lack of a noninvasive imaging system to provide targeting and temperature monitoring in real time (see Fig. 4). MRI's excellent anatomic resolution, high sensitivity for tumor localization, and unique ability to image temperature changes all make FUS possible. Today, the full integration of MRI and FUS enables real-time, image-controlled, noninvasive, soft tissue coagulation in the breast and pelvis, and the clinical feasibility of MRI-guided FUS has been proven [30,31].

In neurosurgery, the clinical applicability of FUS is somewhat limited in the presence of bone and air or in gas-containing cavities in the skull. The bone has a high absorption and acoustic impedance compared with soft tissues. At bone–soft tissue interfaces, approximately one third of the incoming energy is reflected back, which may allow unacceptably high temperatures to develop within the bone. The loss of acoustic energy can be offset by focusing, but the focus can shift from the targeted location because of variations in skull thickness and refraction. The solution is to adjust the focus by applying corrections to the phase of the ultrasound source. Skull thickness can be estimated from CT of the head, and phased-array transducer elements can be independently controlled to adjust the phase and refocus the distorted beam [24,32,33]. The currently developed brain treatment system (Insightec, Dallas, Texas) overcomes acoustic aberrations of the ultrasonic beam using automated planning software based on a set of CT scan images.

MRI-guided FUS has major advantages over surgery and radiation therapy for the treatment of benign brain tumors. High-field MRI provides

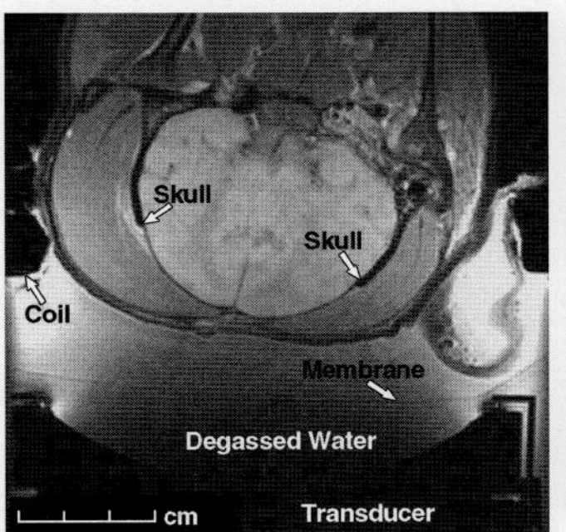

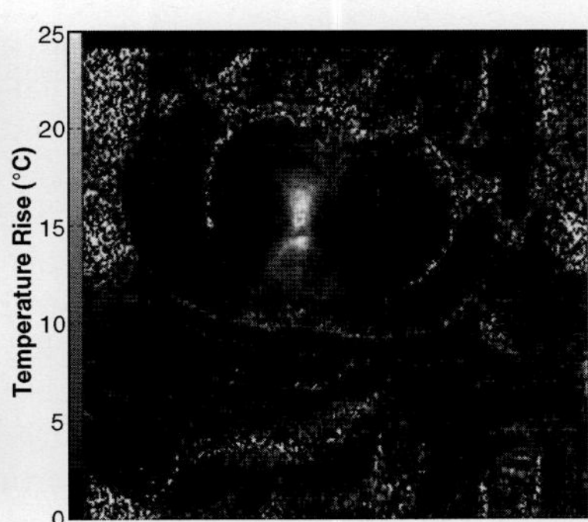

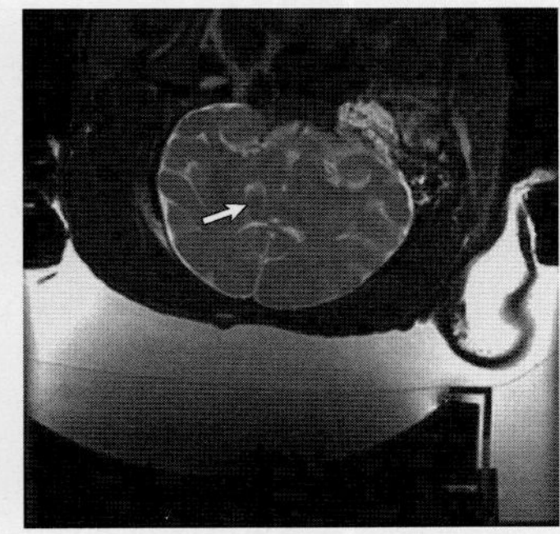

Fig. 4. (*Left*) Proton-density image of the brain of a rhesus monkey with a craniotomy. The monkey was placed on its back, and a bag of degassed water was used for acoustic coupling. (*Center*) Map of the temperature rise (generated from phase-difference gradient echo images) induced during a 10-second 63-W ultrasound exposure in the internal capsule just lateral to the thalamus. The peak temperature at the focus was greater than 90° C. The gap in the heating shown is caused by the ventricle, where there was no ultrasound absorption. A spherically curved transducer (radius of curvature/diameter = 10/8 cm, frequency = 1.5 MHz) produced the ultrasound field. (*Right*) T2-weighted image showing the resulting thermal lesion.

enough anatomic detail for correct targeting and real-time closed-loop control of temperature, and the deposited thermal dose ensures safe and effective treatment for benign tumors. The most serious shortcoming of thermal ablative treatment of malignant tumors is the lack of precise target definition by MRI. The surgical concept of a well-defined tumor mass is incorrect; instead, we deal with spatially disseminated tumor cells that may spread beyond the reach of the thermal treatment. This is a serious handicap for conventional and minimally invasive approaches. If a cure is not anticipated, however, a less invasive procedure is more justified for palliation.

MRI-guided FUS can be a major advance for functional neurosurgery. High-resolution MRI-defined anatomic regions can be targeted with high accuracy, and lesions of various sizes can be created. In combination with fMRI and DTI, functional changes can be monitored and changes in connectivity can be detected. There is some experimental evidence that lower power FUS may reversibly change nerve conductivity and/or neuronal function and can be used for functional testing before making permanent lesions.

In addition to tissue coagulation, the sharply demarcated thermal lesions have a zone around them that shows blood-brain barrier (BBB) leakage to larger molecules. This method could be used to open the BBB for chemotherapy or targeted drug delivery, but it is unpredictable and difficult to control. If BBB opening is mediated by heat, it is associated with potentially irreversible tissue destruction. Another more promising mechanism of ultrasound tissue interaction, cavitation, can also induce focal BBB opening. It is reproducible and reversible, and there is no neuronal damage within or around the sonicated area [34,35].

Cavitation refers to the collapse of rapidly developed gas bubbles at the focal point as a result of oscillations of pressure of the ultrasound field. Cavitation energy can be generated by preformed gas bubbles (ie, ultrasound contrast agents) injected into the blood stream just before the sonication. The collapse of a bubble is associated with a large concentration of energy, which creates high pressure, propagating a shock wave. This leads to direct mechanical tissue effects that change the cell membrane and vascular wall permeability. If the bubbles are intravascular, any adverse effects to the adjacent brain tissue is minimal, and the power levels used are orders of magnitude lower than that required for generating tissue ablation or the cavitation threshold. At the lowest power levels used, the sonications did not cause neuronal damage to the brain, and the BBB opening is completely reversible within 24 hours [35].

The opening of the BBB allows larger molecules to enter the brain [36]. This can have a significant clinical impact on the feasibility of local, noninvasive, targeted drug delivery or gene therapy. Specifically, FUS could provide targeted access for chemotherapy and gene therapy and allow the use of recombinant proteins, monoclonal antibodies, or antisense oligonucleotides as pharmaceutic agents for the brain. It could even provide a vascular route for implanting cells in the brain. The anatomically targeted and controlled opening of the BBB at a desired location would permit novel noninvasive methods of treating central nervous system diseases, such as brain tumors, seizures, and movement disorders. Using large molecular size peptides, neuroactive proteins, and various antibodies, new innovative therapeutic interventions should be available for dealing with organic brain diseases and mental disorders. In addition to the coagulative- and cavitation-based effects, high-energy acoustic beams can be used to occlude or block blood vessels [37,38]. Ultrasound techniques are therefore being developed to stop the bleeding resulting from trauma or catheterization (hemostasis) and for selectively blocking blood vessels. Blood vessel occlusion may be useful for the nonsurgical and nonendovascular treatment of arteriovenous malformations and for tumor treatment by interrupting blood flow to a tumor.

Image-based therapy delivery systems

Image guided thermal ablation requires the integration of therapeutic devices with imaging systems. This integration is a prerequisite of image-guided therapy, because location and feedback control of the energy disposition call for a fully integrated system. We are entering a new area of combined diagnostic and therapeutic applications involving advanced technology. There are still unresolved problems, the most important of which is the lack of sufficient data to establish the clinical efficacy of the minimally invasive techniques under trial. The few MRI-guided thermal ablations already performed contribute to the evaluation of the feasibility of these techniques.

Therapy systems must be linked with imaging systems to form complete therapy delivery systems. The successful deployment of these systems depends on a multidisciplinary team composed of surgeons, interventionalists, imaging experts, and computer scientists. Such an environment is radically different from the conventional operating room. Most notably, the surgeon's view of the surface of the operational field is complemented by images showing what is beyond the visible surface. This feature of MRI, in turn, leads to dramatic changes in surgical approaches and methods driven by a close integration of image-based information with surgical procedures. This new integrated setting, recently coined "The Operating Room of the Future," is not yet optimized and is the subject of intense research. The overall goal of image-guided therapy delivery systems is to integrate all the accessible information (preoperative and intraoperative imaging data) into a single complete operational therapy delivery system.

Images contain information used for diagnosis and therapeutic interventions—applications that are inextricably linked because of the close interplay between the process of diagnosis and therapy. Nevertheless, there are fundamental differences between the requirements for a diagnostic workup and an imaging study directed toward a therapeutic procedure. For correct diagnosis, specificity has greater significance than sensitivity. For therapy, sensitivity should be a fundamental feature. Images of the highest quality are requisite to accurate localization, targeting, and defining of instrument trajectories. All available imaging modalities, especially x-ray fluoroscopy, have been exploited in this regard. More recently CT, ultrasound, and MRI have been introduced into the operating room for intraoperative image guidance. At the same time, with the advance of computerized image processing and visualization tools, image guidance systems have been incorporated into various surgical and radiation oncology applications. These systems make use of images acquired before surgery to create anatomic models. The models, in turn, provide localization, targeting, and visualization of the 3D anatomy. Preoperative models, however, should be modified as the procedure progresses and the anatomy changes. The only feasible means of detecting physiologic motion, displacements, or deformations is via intraoperative or intraprocedural imaging. Monitoring of dynamic changes induced not by motion but by a variety of other functional or physical parameters may be altered or modified during interventional or surgical procedures. Although the primary goal of monitoring is to follow and update anatomic changes in position, other types of dynamic information (ie, flow, perfusion, cortical function) can also be extremely useful in optimizing this process. Although these therapy delivery systems can be tailored to different clinical applications, successful implementation depends almost entirely on interdisciplinary collaboration, an infusion of the most current surgical and radiologic methods, and cutting-edge biomedical engineering principles aimed at combining imaging and therapy devices. Few would argue that MRI-guided therapy is not the quintessential example of a truly interdisciplinary noninvasive approach to the diagnosis and treatment of disease.

Summary

MRI-guided neurosurgery not only represents a technical challenge but a transformation from conventional hand-eye coordination to interactive navigational operations. In the future, multimodality-based images will be merged into a single model, in which anatomy and pathologic changes are at once distinguished and integrated into the same intuitive framework. The long-term goals of improving surgical procedures and attendant outcomes, reducing costs, and achieving broad use can be achieved with a three-pronged approach:

1. Improving the presentation of preoperative and real-time intraoperative image information
2. Integrating imaging and treatment-related technology into therapy delivery systems
3. Testing the clinical utility of image guidance in surgery

The recent focus in technology development is on improving our ability to understand and apply medical images and imaging systems. Areas of active research include image processing, model-based image analysis, model deformation, real-time registration, real-time 3D (so-called "four-dimensional") imaging, and the integration and presentation of image and sensing information in the operating room. Key elements of the technical matrix also include visualization and display platforms and related software for information and display, model-based image understanding, the use of computing clusters to speed computation (ie, algorithms with partitioned computation to optimize performance), and advanced devices and systems for 3D device tracking (navigation).

Current clinical applications are successfully incorporating real-time and/or continuously updated image-based information for direct intraoperative visualization. In addition to using traditional imaging systems during surgery, we foresee optimized use of molecular marker technology, direct measures of tissue characterization (ie, optical measurements and/or imaging), and integration of the next generation of surgical and therapy devices (including image-guided robotic systems). Although we expect the primary clinical thrusts of MRI-guided therapy to remain in neurosurgery, with the possible addition of other areas like orthopedic, head, neck, and spine surgery, we also anticipate increased use of image-guided focal thermal ablative methods (eg, laser, RF, cryoablation, high-intensity focused ultrasound). By validating the effectiveness of MRI-guided therapy in specific clinical procedures while refining the technology that serves as its underpinning at the same time, we expect many neurosurgeons will eventually embrace MRI as their intraoperative imaging choice.

Clearly, intraoperative MRI offers several palpable advantages. Most important among these are improved medical outcomes, shorter hospitalization, and better and faster procedures with fewer complications. Certain economic and practical barriers also impede the large-scale use of intraoperative MRI. Although there has been a concerted technical effort to increase the benefit/cost ratio by gathering more accurate information, designing more localized and less invasive treatment devices, and developing better methods to orient and position therapy end-effectors, further research is needed. Indeed, the drive to improve and upgrade technology is ongoing. Specifically, in the context of the real-time representation of the patient's anatomy, we have improved the quality and utility of the information presented to the surgeon, which, in turn, contributes to more successful surgical outcomes. We can also expect improvements in intraoperative imaging systems as well as increased use of nonimaging sensors and robotics to facilitate more widespread use of intraoperative MRI.

Acknowledgments

Dr. Jolesz wishes to acknowledge Peter McLaren Black, MD, Ron Kikinis, MD, Kullervo Hynynen, PhD, Ion-Florin Talos, MD, and Simon DiMaio, PhD for their contribution to this article.

References

[1] Schenck JF, Jolesz FA, Roemer PB, Cline HE, Lorensen WE, Kikinis R, et al. Superconducting open-configuration MR imaging system for image-guided therapy. Radiology 1995;195(3):805–14.

[2] Black PM, Alexander E III, Martin C, Moriarty T, Nabavi A, Wong TZ, et al. Craniotomy for tumor treatment in an intraoperative magnetic resonance imaging unit. Neurosurgery 1999;45(3):423–33.

[3] Fahlbusch R, Ganslandt O, Nimsky C. Intraoperative imaging with open magnetic resonance imaging and neuronavigation. Childs Nerv Syst 2000; 16(10–11):829–31.

[4] Moriarty TM, Quinosnes-Hinojosa A, Larson PS, Alexander E III, Langham Gleason P, Schwartz RB, et al. Frameless stereotactic neurosurgery using intraoperative magnetic resonance imaging: stereotactic brain biopsy. Neurosurgery 2000;47(5):1138–46.

[5] Jolesz FA, Nabavi A, Kikinis R. Integration of interventional MRI with computer-assisted surgery. J Magn Reson Imaging 2001;13(1):69–77.

[6] Nabavi A, Gering DT, Kacher DF, Talos IF, Wells WM, Kikinis R, et al. Surgical navigation in the open MRI. Acta Neurochir Suppl (Wien) 2003; 85:121–5.

[7] Gering DT, Nabavi A, Kikinis R, Hata N, O'Donnell LJ, Grimson WE, et al. An integrated visualization system for surgical planning and guidance using image fusion and an open MR. J Magn Reson Imaging 2001;13(6):967–75.

[8] Kacher DF, Maier SE, Mamata H, Mamata Y, Nabavi A, Jolesz FA. Motion robust imaging for continuous intraoperative MRI. J Magn Reson Imaging 2001;13(1):158–61.

[9] Pulyer Y, Hrovat MI. An open magnet utilizing ferro-refraction current magnification. J Magn Reson 2002;154(2):298–302.

[10] Lewin JS, Metzger A, Selman WR. Intraoperative magnetic resonance image guidance in neurosurgery. J Magn Reson Imaging 2000;12(4):512–24.

[11] Bohinski RJ, Warnick RE, Gaskill-Shipley MF, Zuccarello M, van Loveren HR, Kormos DW, et al. Intraoperative magnetic resonance imaging to determine the extent of resection of pituitary macroadenomas during transsphenoidal microsurgery. Neurosurgery 2001;49(5):1133–1143; discussion 1143–4.

[12] Liu H, Hall WA, Martin AJ, Maxwell RE, Truwit CL. MR-guided and MR-monitored neurosurgical procedures at 1.5 T. J Comput Assist Tomogr 2000;24(6):909–18.

[13] Nimsky C, Ganslandt O, von Keller B, Fahlbusch R. Preliminary experience in glioma surgery with intraoperative high-field MRI. Acta Neurochir Suppl (Wien) 2003;88:21–9.

[14] Sutherland GR, Kaibara T, Louw D, Hoult DI, Tomanek B, Saunders J. A mobile high-field magnetic resonance system for neurosurgery. J Neurosurg 1999;91(5):804–13.

[15] Schulder M, Sernas TJ, Carmel PW. Cranial surgery and navigation with a compact intraoperative MRI system. Acta Neurochir Suppl (Wien) 2003;85:79–86.

[16] Hadani M Sr, Feldman Z, Berkenstadt H, Ram Z. Novel, compact, intraoperative magnetic resonance imaging-guided system for conventional neurosurgical operating rooms. Neurosurgery 2001;48(4): 799–808.

[17] Nimski C, Ganslandt O, Kober H, Moeller M, Ulmer S, Tomandl B, et al. Integration of functional magnetic resonance imaging supported by magnetoencephalography in functional neuronavigation. Neurosurgery 1999;44(6):1249–56.

[18] Mamata H, Mamata Y, Jolesz FA, Maier SE. Line scan diffusion high-resolution tensor images in normal and pathologic brain. In: International Society for Magnetic Resonance in Medicine Proceedings. Denver; 2000. p. 787.

[19] Bharatha A, Hirose M, Hata N, Warfield SK, Ferrant M, Zou KH, et al. Evaluation of three-dimensional finite element-based deformable registration of pre- and intraoperative prostate imaging. Med Phys 2001;28(12):2551–60.

[20] Mamata Y, Mamata H, Nabavi A, Kacher DF, Pergolizzi RS Jr, Schwartz RB, et al. Intraoperative diffusion imaging on a 0.5 Tesla interventional scanner. J Magn Reson Imaging 2001;13(1):115–9.

[21] Nabavi A, Black PM, Gering DT, Westin CF, Mehta V, Pergolizzi RS, et al. Serial intraoperative magnetic resonance imaging of brain shift. Neurosurgery 2001;48(4):787–98.

[22] Nimsky C, Ganslandt O, Cerny S, Hastreiter P, Greiner G, Fahlbusch G. Quantification of, visualization of, and compensation for brain shift using intraoperative magnetic resonance imaging. Neurosurgery 2000;47(5):1070–80.

[23] Chinzei K, Miller K. Towards MRI guided surgical manipulator. Med Sci Monit 2001;7(1): 153–63.

[24] Jolesz FA, Hynynen K. Magnetic resonance image-guided focused ultrasound surgery. Cancer J 2002; 8(Suppl 1):S100–12.

[25] Kettenbach J, Silverman SG, Hata N, Kuroda K, Saiviroonporn P, Zientara GP, et al. Monitoring and visualization techniques for MR-guided laser ablations in an open MR system. J Magn Reson Imaging 1998;8(4):933–43.

[26] Zientara GP, Saiviroonporn P, Morrison PR, Fried MP, Hushek SG, Kikinis R, et al. MRI monitoring of laser ablation using optical flow. J Magn Reson Imaging 1998;8(6):1306–18.

[27] Warfield S, Talos F, Tei A, Bharatha A, Nabavi A, Ferrant M, et al. Real-time registration of volumetric brain MRI by biomechanical simulation of deformation during image guided neurosurgery. Comput Visual Sci 2002;5:3–11.

[28] Kaus MR, Warfield SK, Nabavi A, Black PM, Jolesz FA, Kikinis R. Automated segmentation of MR images of brain tumors. Radiology 2001; 218(2):586–91.

[29] Tsai A, Yezzi A Jr, Wells W, Tempany C, Tucker D, Fan A, et al. A shape-based approach to the segmentation of medical imagery using level sets. IEEE Trans Med Imaging 2003;22(2):137–54.

[30] Hynynen K, Pomeroy O, Smith DN, Huber PE, McDannold NJ, Kettenbach J, et al. MR imaging-guided focused ultrasound surgery of fibroadenomas in the breast: a feasibility study. Radiology 2001;219(1):176–85.

[31] Tempany CM, Stewart EA, McDannold N, Quade BJ, Jolesz FA, Hynynen K. MR imaging-guided focused ultrasound surgery of uterine leiomyomas: a feasibility study. Radiology 2003; 226(3):897–905.

[32] Hynynen K, Sun J. Trans-skull ultrasound therapy: The feasibility of using image derived skull thickness information to correct the phase distortion. IEEE Trans Ultrason Ferroelectr Freq Contr 1998;46(3): 752–5.

[33] Clement GT, Hynynen K. Correlation of ultrasound phase with physical skull properties. Ultrasound Med Biol 2002;28(5):617–24.

[34] Hynynen K, McDannold N, Vykhodtseva N, Jolesz FA. Noninvasive MR imaging-guided focal opening of the blood-brain barrier in rabbits. Radiology 2001;220(3):640–6.

[35] Hynynen K, McDannold N, Vykhodtseva N, Jolesz FA. Non-invasive opening of BBB by focused ultrasound. Acta Neurochir Suppl (Wien) 2003;86:555–8.

[36] Greenleaf WJ, Bolander ME, Sarkar G, Goldring MB, Greenleaf JF. Artificial cavitation nuclei significantly enhance acoustically induced cell transfection. Ultrasound Med Biol 1998;24(4): 587–95.

[37] Hynynen K, Colluci V, Chung A, Jolesz FA. Noninvasive artery occlusion using MRI guided focused ultrasound. Ultrasound Med Biol 1996;22(8): 1071–7.

[38] Delon-Martin C, Vogt C, Chigner E, Guers C, Chapelon JY, Cathignol D. Venous thrombosis generation by means of high-intensity focused ultrasound. Ultrasound Med Biol 1995;21(1):113–9.

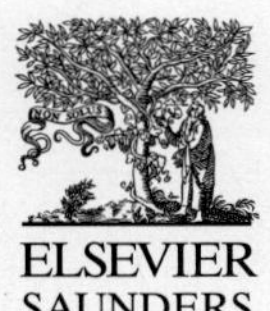

ELSEVIER
SAUNDERS

Neurosurg Clin N Am 16 (2005) 215–221

NEUROSURGERY
CLINICS
OF NORTH AMERICA

Index

Note: Page numbers of article titles are in **bold face** type.

1042-3680/05/$ - see front matter
doi:10.1016/S1042-3680(04)00133-0

G

H

I

J

L

M

N

W

Changing Your Address?

Make sure your subscription changes too! When you notify us of your new address, you can help make our job easier by including an exact copy of your Clinics label number with your old address (see illustration below.) This number identifies you to our computer system and will speed the processing of your address change. Please be sure this label number accompanies your old address and your corrected address—you can send an old Clinics label with your number on it or just copy it exactly and send it to the address listed below.

We appreciate your help in our attempt to give you continuous coverage. Thank you.

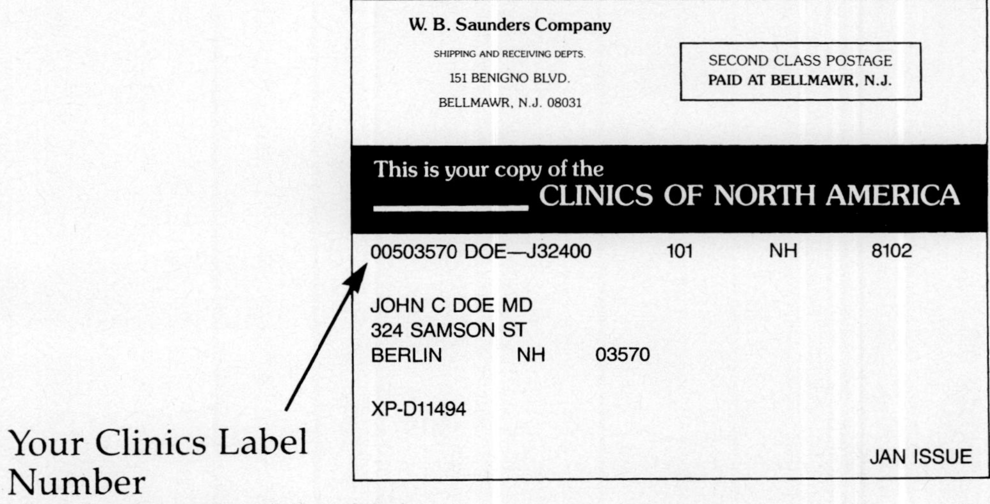

Your Clinics Label Number

Copy it exactly or send your label along with your address to:
W.B. Saunders Company, Customer Service
Orlando, FL 32887-4800
Call Toll Free 1-800-654-2452

Please allow four to six weeks for delivery of new subscriptions and for processing address changes.